T0342569

Bad Souls

ELIZABETH ANNE DAVIS

Bad Souls

MADNESS AND RESPONSIBILITY

IN MODERN GREECE

Duke University Press   Durham and London   2012

CONTENTS

Note on Orthography and Pronunciation

For Greek terms that appear in this book, I have chosen not to offer transliterations in the Latin alphabet, but rather to present my English translations alongside the original terms in monotonic Greek alphabet. My incorporation of Greek language into this text in place of transliterations is intended to facilitate the comprehension and evaluation of modern Greek readers. For those who do not read modern Greek and who are interested in orthography and the pronunciation of Greek terms, I offer the following guide. Please note, this guide is intended only as a general reference and does not reflect regional, contextual, or idiosyncratic variants.

Note: The phrase *αυτός έφα* (Latin: *ipse dixit*), which appears as a heading on p. 58, means "he (himself) said it." Referring originally to the authoritative speech of Pythagoras that went unquestioned by his disciples, this phrase designates the evidentiary status of a claim for which the only proof is that it has been said.

LETTERS

A α	a, uh	flat, about
B β	v	very
Γ γ	g, y	gear, year
Δ δ	dh, th	then, smoothe
E ε	eh, ai	end, sundae

Z ζ	z	zoo
H η	ee	ease
Θ θ	th	think
I ι	ee	ease
K κ	k	keep
Λ λ	l	lot
M μ	m	mumble
N ν	n	none
Ξ ξ	x, gs	extra, exit
O o	oh, ah	slow, dog
Π π	p	piano
P ρ	r	run
Σ σ (-ς)	s	sound
T τ	t	tell
Y υ	ee	ease
Φ φ	ph, f	phonograph, fog
X χ	ch, h	challah, human
Ψ ψ	ps	lapse
Ω ω	oh, ah	slow, dog

CLUSTERS

γγ, γκ	ng	fungus
μπ	b	ambit
ντ	d	ending
αι	ae	sundae
ου	oo	loose
ει, οι	ee	ease
αυ	av, af	avenue, after
ευ	ev, ef	ever, effort

Acknowledgments

I owe an unredeemable debt of gratitude to my interlocutors in Thrace, only some of whom appear in this text. I want first to thank those I have called Anastasia, Fatmé, Kleandis, and Smaro, who told me their stories "from beginning to end" and trusted me to write them; Selvinaj, who did not make it; and many others in treatment who helped me grasp something of their experience. I thank as well the clinicians at the hospitals, health centers, and institutes in Thrace who let me in and shared their time, their work, and their thoughts with me. Out of respect for their privacy, I cannot thank these people by their real names, but I hope they may recognize something of themselves in this book, and understand my deep appreciation for their contributions to it.

This book began as a doctoral dissertation, and I want to express my profound gratitude to my advisors at Berkeley who, in their distinctive ways, shaped and supported my project from its inception: to Lawrence Cohen, Wendy Brown, Paul Rabinow, Maria Kotzamanidou, and especially to Stefania Pandolfo, whose sensibility, wisdom, and friendship have been inestimable gifts to me. Tremendous thanks go as well to those friends, colleagues, and mentors who have discussed this work with me over the years, read parts of the evolving text, and contributed insight, advice, and encouragement: Anne Allison, João Biehl, Jim Boon, Vangelis Calotychos, Vincent Crapanzano, Olga Demetriou, Kathy Ewing, Cristiana Giordano, Brian Goldstone, Carol Greenhouse, Michael Herzfeld, Andy Lakoff, Rena Lederman, Anne-Maria Makhulu, Jonathan Metzl, Megan Moodie, Diane Nelson, Anand Pandian, Neni Panourgiá, Beth Povinelli, Anu Rao, Natasha Schüll, Pete Skafish, Rebecca Stein, Livia

Velpry, and Ara Wilson. I thank the anonymous reviewers at Duke University Press, who provided thoughtful and essential guidance; Tsering Wangyal Shawa, for beautifully mapping Greek Thrace and its larger world; and Ken Wissoker, without whose generosity, encouragement, and patience this book could not have materialized. Finally, I thank my colleagues in the Department of Anthropology and the Program in Hellenic Studies at Princeton University, who so swiftly and graciously made this place a lively and happy home as I was bringing the project to a close.

Parts of this text have been presented at various venues, including the University Seminar in Modern Greek Studies at Columbia University, the Liberalism's Others Working Group of the Center for the Critical Analysis of Social Difference at Columbia University, the Faculty Work-in-Progress Seminar of the Program in Women's Studies at Duke University, the Gender and Disability lecture series of the Program in Culture, Health, and Medicine at the University of Michigan, and the inaugural Symposium of the Modern Greek Studies Program at the University of Illinois, Urbana-Champaign; as well as the Departments of Anthropology at CUNY Graduate Center, Columbia University, Yale University, Duke University, and Princeton University. I am grateful to the participants in these events for their helpful questions and comments, as well as to the organizers for making them possible.

I have been fortunate to receive generous support for this project over the years. Different phases of my research in Greece from 1999–2004 were funded by the National Science Foundation, the Foreign Language and Area Studies Program (U.S. Department of Education), the German Marshall Fund of the United States, the Social Science Research Council, the Hewlett Foundation, and the Robert H. Lowie endowment administered by the Department of Anthropology at UC Berkeley. Writing was sustained by a Charlotte W. Newcombe Doctoral Dissertation Fellowship from the Woodrow Wilson Foundation, a Simpson Memorial Research Fellowship from the Institute of International Studies at UC Berkeley, and a Mellon Postdoctoral Fellowship in the Society of Fellows at Columbia University.

Bad Souls

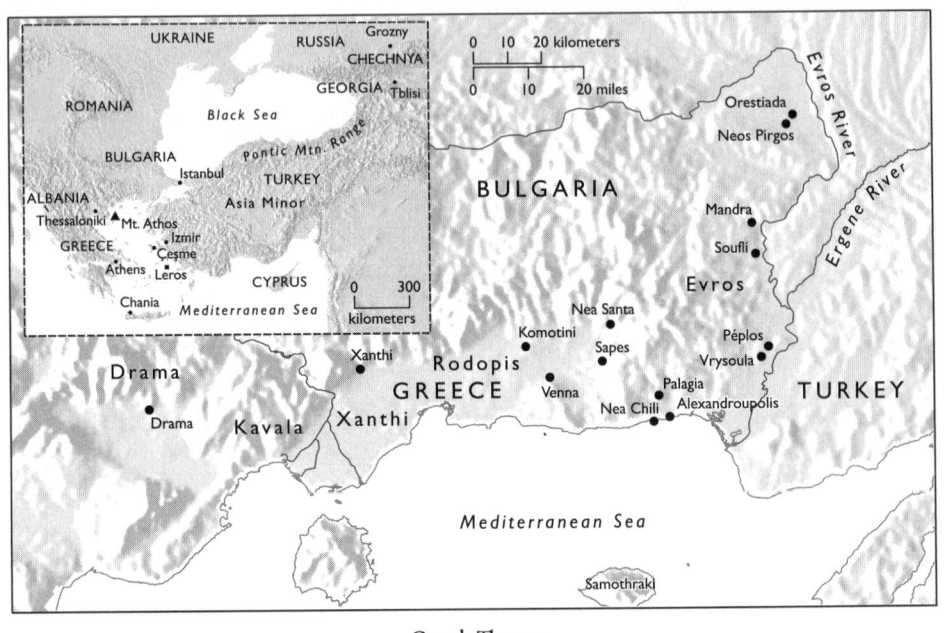

Greek Thrace

INTRODUCTION

"Psychology" is merely the thin skin on the surface of the ethical
world in which modern man seeks his truth—and loses it.
—MICHEL FOUCAULT,
Mental Illness and Psychology (1954)

*You wouldn't have guessed. She didn't seem urgent. I took her history. She was . . . I
don't know. Sad. She didn't feel well. She was kind of listless. So I ordered a sedative,
and I let her rest. That's what she wanted. This was Saturday afternoon.*

(Alexandra lights a cigarette. She often chain-smokes at these staff
meetings, and often turns in a performance. She is known for her wit.
But it's stranded in this story, requested by the other therapists, who have
only heard rumors. She warns them each time she reaches for sarcasm:
she has to laugh so she doesn't cry.)

*Martina said she was from out of town. Her doctor had an Athens number. But
her surname was local, very distinctive. The head nurse thought she knew the family.
So we looked into the archives and found an old file for her. It turned out she had bipolar; she was treated at the old hospital ten years ago. She was living with her older
brother then. He was devoted to her—he took care of her after her parents kicked her
out of the house. Martina didn't tell me this, but I assume she was the source of his
marital problems. Because he left his wife. He took Martina with him to Athens, and
she was getting treatment there. His wife stayed with his parents in their village, a
half hour from here. But they reconciled recently—that's why Martina was back in
town. When the brother took his wife on a vacation, he left Martina with their parents in the village. But she didn't get along with them. She got upset, and she wanted
to stay at the clinic until her brother got back from his trip.*

*Right after I admitted her, I had to run to the neonate unit to deal with our old
patient, Stamatia. That was bizarre. She'd picked up an infant and wouldn't give him*

up. She kept screaming that they'd stolen her babies. She lay down in a bed, holding the little thing in her arms. The nurses were so pissed off when I got there.

That's where I was paged. So I ran back to the clinic. The nurse told me Martina was acting desperate. She was still in her room. She was crying, wailing. I couldn't understand her, she wasn't really speaking at first. But she wound down. She was upset about her brother. I told her I was giving her an antidepressant that would make her feel better. She was calm when I left.

It must have been twenty minutes later, maybe thirty. I was in the other wing, in the office. The nurse said that Martina was lost. Couldn't find her. Her roommate said she'd left the room to take a little walk. But we couldn't find her anywhere in the clinic.

So we started a search. We got all the nurses looking. We called the hospital administration. We called the other units. I couldn't believe it—they were so cooperative. You know, we lose patients a lot, they go wandering, they cause trouble. So the other units, they don't like us very much. They refuse to do anything with our patients; they just call us to come pick them up. But this time everyone was really helpful—as if they knew. Finally I had to call Dr. Lamberakis. He was on call, he came in. He lives right downtown, he got to the clinic in ten minutes.

And it was hours. It was night by then. All the units in the hospital were on watch for Martina. And then I got a call from hematology, they wouldn't say why, they just told me to go to this spot. You know that courtyard between our wing and the main building, where the labs are, and there's a stairwell in the back. That courtyard is pretty well hidden, it's hard to find. A couple of security guards had covered her with a plastic sheet by the time I got there. I won't describe the spectacle.

She used the back stairwell to get up to hematology, which is on the top floor. And I guess she found the door open to the nurses' lounge, and just jumped right out the window. That's six stories she fell. Maybe more, because the ground slopes downhill from the main building there.

So they dealt with the body, I had nothing to do with it. I had to go back to the clinic to start "the procedure." That's what the police called it. The first thing I did was light a cigarette. They asked about her admission, about her family, what she said to me, what medications she was on, how did she get away. They didn't get the concept of "open ward." Thank god the other units responded the way they did, or else we would have been blamed for not doing a thorough search of the hospital. They questioned Dr. Lamberakis, too. They searched her room, collected her things to give to her family. They got her file. Lamberakis kept checking in on me, asking if I was OK. Every time he had to leave to take care of something, he'd tell me: "I'm going now, I'll be at such and such a place, call me if you need me, I'll be right back." He was pretty shaken. People kept saying it was the first suicide on hospital grounds in twenty years. You know, they kill themselves outside, once they're discharged, but never at the clinic. It's too hard to do it inside—there's no privacy.

And of course I had to stay until morning, because I was still on duty. There were some other incidents. Sotiris had a violent fit, we had to restrain him. And I found out that Chrisoula had been trading favors for cigarettes with other patients, so I had to intervene.

And we have two other bipolar patients who are very unstable. There's been a lot of commotion over the suicide. So now we have these chains up in the clinic. Dr. Michailidis decided. He said we have to keep the patients inside to protect them, until we can find a better solution. They hate being locked in, they feel imprisoned, they're nerve-wracked. The staff can't come and go freely, either. The climate is really tense. Honestly, I've never seen it so bad, we're in really bad shape right now.

❄ ❄ ❄

The oily old chains are secured with a padlock around the handlebars of the double doors in the main wing. There is no other way to effect a barrier; lockdown had not been anticipated in the open design of the new clinic. The blockade divides the patients' rooms, nursing station, and consultation offices from the doctors' offices, public restrooms, and the passageway leading to the main hospital. Chains have also been laid on the emergency exit doors at the far end of the patients' wing, and on the internal doors to the kitchen, which connects one wing to the other. A nurse is supposed to mind the front desk by the main doors at all times, to let staff and visitors in and out; but often the post is left empty, and people gather continually by the doors, muttering, waiting for a key. One patient adopts the job of monitoring the doors and calling for an aide if someone needs to pass through. Nurses grumble about the aggravation and the foolishness of the blockade. Doctors complain that the clinic is not an "institution"—even institutions don't use chains anymore!—and locking patients in is a sure way to undermine their therapy. Is this a return to the dark days of their profession? The clinic director dismisses criticism and is disparaged behind his back. The chains become an obsessive topic in group therapy sessions. Patients express anxiety, resentment, shame at being contained like lunatics. They remark on the hypocrisy of the directorial rationale—the two-sided nature of their security, the refusal to name and to take responsibility: It's just easier for them to keep us locked up! Then it doesn't matter how treatment's going. The chains persist, day after day. They become a chronic condition.[1]

As the scope of liberal democracy expands globally, and its concomitant rights and duties are conferred to increasingly varied kinds of subjects—not just individual persons of age, but also children, protected groups, animals, corporations—mental illness remains a resistant, troubling experience, unaccountable to law in many ways. Since the international movement for patients' rights began in the 1960s, debates over the capacities and incapacities of the mentally ill have engendered confused and conflicting claims of responsibility for these "vulnerable persons" on the part of governments, doctors, advocates, and patients themselves.

Bad Souls is an ethnographic study of responsibility among psychiatric patients and those who give them care in Thrace, the northeastern borderland of Greece. I examine responsibility there in the context of national psychiatric reform—a process designed, mandated, and funded largely by the European Union as a humanitarian condition of Greek accession in the early 1980s. Reform policy aimed to shift psychiatric treatment from custodial hospitals to outpatient settings, challenging patients to help care for themselves. This "democratic experiment" has contributed to a profound questioning of Greece's marginal share in the goods and advances associated with modernity in the West—particularly human rights and progressive medical science. Amid this questioning, decades into reform, I observed grave uncertainty in the practice of Greek psychiatry, arising from the speculative nature of diagnosis and pharmacotherapy and from the perpetual problem of communicative ambiguity in clinical encounters. While this uncertainty is not unique to Greek psychiatry, the moralism of responsibility has come to govern the determination of truth in the clinics of Thrace in quite distinctive ways, with particular and pressing stakes.

This book is organized around three topoi of responsibility that emerged in my research on Greek psychiatry. Part 1 examines suspicions of deception shared by patients and therapists, which insinuated a peculiar intimacy into therapeutic relationships even as they worked to disqualify some patients from recovery. Part 2 traces the emergence of local "cultural pathologies" that diagnostically marked minority patients, and embodied their variegated dependence on therapists and state care. Part 3 considers the humanitarian confrontation with patients presenting the "inhuman" face of severe pathology, thereby challenging the presumptions of personal freedom written into the legislation of reform. Exploring these sites of diagnosis, persuasion, healing, and failure, I show how the normative cultivation of responsibility implicated therapists in patients' ethical relationships with their illness—relationships fostered by daily practices of self-medication, self-examination, and self-control devised to help them avoid relapse and hospitalization, and thus to enhance their health and dignity. These ethical relations between self and self, and self and other, activated new therapeutic dynamics of autonomy and dependency, while madness itself—as an ontological form and a retreat from society—was withdrawing from the space of the clinic.

I conducted the research for this book between 2001 and 2004 in Thrace, a largely rural region between the Turkish and Bulgarian borders of northeastern Greece.[2] Its sparse population includes a number of "cultural minorities" that remained, at that time, largely segregated from Greek society: Muslim communities of Gypsies, Turks, and Pomaks,[3] as well as a growing group of Pontii (Πόντιοι)—immigrants of Greek ancestry and Greek Orthodox affiliation from former Soviet states.[4] Since the 1990s, as these communities expanded and their connections to Turkey and Russia grew increasingly politicized—ramified by a surge in illegal human traffic into Europe from the north and the east—cultural difference came into view as a problem in local clinics, buttressed by new research projects and training curricula in transcultural psychiatry.[5] In the psychiatric settings where I worked, these minority groups were perceived to make disproportionate and often illegitimate demands on local health and social services. Yet patients from these groups were bound to others whose identities and legitimacy were less critically marked.

After more than a century of secluding the mentally ill in remote custodial hospitals, state authorities in Thrace have attempted to reintegrate psychiatric patients into society during the past twenty-five years of reform. These patients struggled against a folk genetics of madness that rendered them a social liability to their families and against the threat posed to their recovery by a stigmatized identity "in the community."[6] At the same time, in this part of Greece, as opposed to many other places in the global periphery where medical knowledge and institutions have been transposed from elsewhere, there was a marked absence in local clinical settings of cultural beliefs and practices that might make illness and healing intelligible outside the biomedical paradigm of psychiatry. On the contrary, culture often appeared to patients and therapists alike as a *cause* of mental pathologies and treatment failures. These conditions—in which an authoritative medical apparatus appropriates and objectifies the cultural import of illness, and communities fail to provide an alternative experience of care—radically constricted possibilities for psychiatric patients in Thrace to inhabit their world meaningfully just when, historically, such possibilities appeared to be opening up. This book documents the singularity of their experience, their isolation from a collective world of meaning, and their exile to a liberal landscape where they had either to take responsibility for themselves or to craft pathological modes of dependency.

Most of the research for this project took place in two principal psychiatric settings. One was the public inpatient clinic and associated outpatient clinic at the General Regional University Hospital of Alexandroupolis, a small facility attached to the medical school at the University of Thrace. In 1978, its inpatient clinic was the first psychiatry ward to be established in a general hospital in Greece, with a mandate to treat patients for brief periods and to sustain their well-being outside the hospital with systematic outpatient supervision—a new model for psychiatric services that would eventually replace large custodial institutions throughout the country.

The other setting was the Association for Social Psychiatry and Mental Health in Alexandroupolis ("the Association"). This was the local branch of a semiprivate national organization founded in the early 1980s that— with grants from hospitals, private donors, the Greek Ministry of Health, and the European Union—provided free psychiatric and psychological care to patients living "in the community."

Both agencies, in addition to treating residents of Alexandroupolis, operated mobile units throughout the Evros and Rodopis prefectures of Thrace, providing care to patients in their homes and at rural health centers, from as far north as Orestiada to the island of Samothraki, off the southern coast. Both agencies also functioned as training centers, where much of the day-to-day therapeutic labor was undertaken by recent graduates of medical school pursuing either a psychiatry specialist's license (at the hospital clinic) or a master's degree in social psychiatry (at the Association).

While they shared some patients and some personnel, the hospital clinic and the Association performed, on the whole, quite different kinds of work. The hospital clinic provided full-time treatment to patients in acute crisis for periods of no more than a month, as well as intermittent follow-up supervision.[7] The Association, on the other hand, tended to patients' quality of life and long-term stability outside the hospital through regular therapy, social and occupational activities, and, in some cases, supervised housing. Though both agencies relied on psychoactive medication as a foundation for treatment, they diverged in their philosophies of therapeutic practice. The Association adopted a more psychoanalytic orientation: therapists interpreted their patients' symptoms as expressions of conflicts arising from their psychosocial development, while attending in treatment sessions to the unconscious dynamics of their therapeutic relationships. The hospital clinic, on the other hand, offered a range of therapies in addition to pharmaceutical treatment, including supportive and family counseling, group therapy, and cognitive-behavioral therapy, but few hospital clinicians had any training in psychodynamic theory and practice. They remained largely biopharmaceutical in orientation, regularly conducting studies on the efficacy and side effects of the medications they prescribed, and occasionally hosting clinical trials of new ones.

The patients treated at these two sites learned techniques of communication and self-reflection that shaped their desires and capacities for responsibility. In this book, I aim to document those techniques without reproducing, in my own analysis, the interpretive frames of psychoanalysis and biopsychiatry that helped authorize them at the Association and the hospital clinic. For patients who fell into both orbits of care, the discrepancies in diagnostic interpretation and therapeutic approach yielded many disagreements over the proper course of treatment. Nevertheless, both agencies avowedly shared a basic responsibility to keep patients alive, healthy, and functional "in the community." This explicit mission, animated by an ethos of cooperation (συνεργασία) between therapists and patients, defined the domain of contention over responsibility in the psychiatric sites of Thrace.

This contention recurred among therapists in the meetings, classes, discussions, and case presentations I observed throughout my time in Thrace. Most often, though, it arose between therapists and patients in treatment sessions. Consider one confounding dialogue that took place at the public outpatient clinic in the General Hospital of Komotini, the capital city of the Rodopis prefecture, about fifty kilometers from Alexandroupolis and another twenty from the Turkish border. The clinic was run by Dr. Karras, appointed the previous year when the hospital in Komotini first created a post for a psychiatrist. He worked without assistance, in a mode of urgency, charged with up to twenty scheduled patients each day in addition to many who dropped by without appointments. I joined him at the outpatient clinic during the final weeks of my field research.

On one of those days, along with a dozen other patients, we saw Michalis, an edgy, pallid man in his early twenties who lived with his older brother in a Pontian township nearby, where they had settled after leaving Ukraine seven years before. Earlier that week, Michalis told us, he had received a phone call from the police, ordering him to report for a week-long maintenance exercise at the army camp in Alexandroupolis. *I want to go,* he said to the doctor, *but my brother said I should ask you first.* Later, Karras explained to me that Michalis had been discharged from army service when he suffered his first psychotic break at the age of nineteen, fitting a familiar pattern in Greece for the emergence of schizophrenia in young men. The military did not keep track of his medical history, so Michalis remained on the active list despite his disqualification. It was left to his psychiatrists to produce official waivers each time he was called up for maintenance training. And so Karras explained to him again, that morning, that the army exercise was out of the question: *It'll be too hard for you, Michalis, and dangerous for your health.* He completed the waiver form, certifying a diagnosis of schizophrenia.

This bureaucratic transaction completed, Karras asked in his routine way about Michalis's health and progress. *I'm the same,* Michalis replied. *But I miss drinking ouzo, now that I'm forbidden.* Karras promised to tell his brother that one glass of ouzo a day was permitted: *You don't have to give up drinking completely, but you have to be careful. Too much ouzo will keep your medications from working. And it causes bad behavior.* Michalis seemed to absorb this information—and then added abruptly, quizzically, as if sounding Karras out: *I've been thinking about going down to Athens to see my people. I want to find out from them how this happened to me, how I got sick.*

Karras unraveled the obscure significance of this statement. It emerged from this questioning that "his people" in Athens were the ones Michalis had used to hear talking to him "inside his head." Seizing on this sign of emergent delusion, of imminent relapse, Karras began a gentle interrogation: *What do you expect to happen on this trip, Michalis? Do you think these people, unknown [ἄγνωστοι] to you, would take you in if you showed up? Probably they'd just throw you out!* He laughed.

Michalis stared, not registering the joke, which must have been addressed to me in any case. From what vantage could he have understood Karras's pretense to credit the existence of these people, and his attribution to them of respect for social norms as against Michalis's own unseemly, unreasonable expectations? Observing the rift he had created, Karras shifted into a diagnostic mode more familiar to Michalis:

—You know it's not possible to hear the voices of people who are so far away. Don't you think they might be part of your illness? Did you hear their voices before you got sick?

—No, I didn't hear them before. Probably they're part of my illness. But the problem is, now that they're gone, I don't know who knows. . . . If I can't talk to them, then to whom can I address myself to find out what happened, who's responsible?[8]

—But Michalis, these people are just like those other voices you used to hear. Remember when you thought Irene Papas was talking to you?[9]

—(Michalis laughs.) I used to think all kinds of funny things. I used to talk to a Russian secret agent working undercover in America.

—(Karras smiles with him.) You spoke in Russian, it was like a secret language. But you don't hear those people anymore, right? It's just that you remember what it was like to hear them.

—That's true, I don't hear them anymore.

—And isn't it better that way?

—Well, no, it's not better. I miss them.

—What do you miss about them?

—They kept me company. They cared about me, they looked after me.

—But you were really scared of them, Michalis. They made you so nervous. You used to tremble when they talked to you, right in front of me. Do you remember that?

—I remember . . . but I'm different now. I know they're just part of my illness, and I'm not scared of them anymore. I would know how to handle them now.

Karras nodded quietly and opted out of the exchange. He asked how Michalis was doing with his medications, and Michalis confirmed that he was taking them as instructed. With an air of resolution, Karras directed him to the front desk where he could get an official stamp for his waiver form.

The hospital in Komotini contained no psychiatric ward; it presented to patients no space of protection, nor any threat of confinement, and the therapeutic encounter transpired hastily, in the provisional quarters of an outpatient office. Here, psychiatrist and patient negotiated their responsibilities in different, perhaps incommensurable, registers. Michalis addressed Karras as a benevolent advisor, requiring his scrutiny and approval. He took the doctor's advice on moderate conduct as "forbidding" even a taste of ouzo, which he had decided he was willing to forego. He acquiesced to plans—for his employment, diet, and medication regimen, as for army training and travel to Athens—determined by deliberations between his doctor and his healthy brother. The medications he took faithfully had evacuated the voices from his head, and he had achieved a retrospective and metapositional vantage, mediated by his encounters with Karras, on what he conceded was his "illness"—a vantage that Karras used, for the most part effectively, to fortify his own authority as an expert caregiver.

And yet, in the account he demanded from "his people," Michalis pronounced the limits of that authority. Karras's insistence on Michalis's responsibility for his health was refracted in his own discourse, but responsibility emerged there in a different form. He pressed the doctor to validate his need to know who was responsible for his illness, but did not address to the doctor his demand for an account. It was "his people," instead, who bore the authority to know, and the prospect of redress. Michalis's liberation from auditory hallucinations had come at the cost of his access to these people. His impossible desire to visit them, sustained by the knowledge that they were *probably not real*, expressed an enigma posed by the responsibility he had achieved as an outpatient. He could handle them now that he was in treatment, but he missed the care they had given him even as they nourished the illness he sought to heal. Karras, with all his advice and certificates and medications, could not provide that care to him. Nor was Michalis able to care in that way for himself.

Karras was in no position to countenance this dimension of responsibility for Michalis's illness. He kept to diagnosis, focusing on the hallucinatory advent of the voices rather than the moral demand Michalis addressed to them. Karras compared these voices to others that Michalis used to hear—voices that resembled "his people" only in their hallucinatory form, not in terms of what he might seek from them. Karras tried to persuade him to understand these voices only as aspects of his illness, offering as evidence that they disappeared when he began treatment with antipsychotic medication. His diagnosis disqualified Michalis from performing his civic duty of army service, and thus from responsible citizenship, at the same time as it protected his stability as an outpatient. This ambiguous exclusion, for Michalis, was doubled by his precarious sociopolitical status as a Pontios, an immigrant with a claim to Greek ancestry but a marginal affiliation with Greek society; his ties to "his people" were evidently much stronger. From Karras's position, there was nothing to say about the moral question that Michalis preserved as he lost these internal interlocutors, or about his own debarment as a source of redress. Responsibility had taken an unanswerable turn.

IN RELATION TO OTHERS

As many scholars of modern Greece have shown, the development of Hellenism in the nineteenth century—a strategy of Greek modernization, Europeanization, and emancipation from Ottoman imperialism—conferred on modern Greek letters a unique and proprietary claim to the archaic and classical roots of Western civilization.[10] This claim was leveraged by the special universalism that Greek culture, history, and language have long borne in scholarship and the arts outside Greece. This standing is evident still in contemporary social theory, expressed in its perpetual recursion to the classical heritage—that indispensable corpus of philosophy and literature, and that repertoire of mythic personae, from Apollo and Dionysus to Oedipus and Antigone, who stand as allegorical figures of *anthropos*:[11] the human, object and subject of anthropology, that so powerfully shapes our analysis of political organization, social conflict, kinship, sexuality, language, and history.[12]

Bad Souls, too, recurs, if only erratically, to the classical past—to the ancient ancestry of the shadowy yet vital figure of *psyche* (ψυχή): soul, mind, spirit.[13] Classicists observe a tension in the semantic range of this term, tracing a decisive historical shift from Homeric to Platonic usage. In the Homeric sources, psyche often names a double, replica, alter ego, wraith, or shade: a reflection of the self that survives the death of the body but whose form after death is no more substantial nor rational than a dream or shadow.[14] The psyche that appears in Plato, on the other hand, seems already integrated and immanent to personhood: a "seat of 'thought, desire and will,'" a robust self defined by moral agency.[15] As a nonclassicist, and a foreign guest in modern Greek studies, I do not make any proprietary claims about the classical origins of the modern Greek concept of the psyche. Nor do I offer evidence for its historical continuity or direct genealogical transmission from classical sources.[16] But I do register the peculiar gravity of the ancient psyche that weighs on clinical meanings of *psyche* in Thrace today.[17]

Modern psychiatric knowledge has, until recently, been predicated on a developmental model of the human psyche, an interior domain of mostly unconscious activity that generates symptoms as symbols of motive.[18] Increasingly, this model of psyche, in Greece and elsewhere,[19] is being displaced from clinical medicine to the domain of the humanities by a liberal model of coherent and transparent mental life, which invests psychiatric patients with conscious intentionality and dignifies them with human rights. In these divergent models, I see that ancient tension within psyche as, on the one hand, a double, the reflection of a self fragmented by alien and unruly desires and weaknesses; and on the other, the agency of an integrated self that can wittingly and freely decide on a project of self-improvement.

In my examination of the modern Greek psyche as a seat of ethical subjectivity, I draw from one of the most influential recursions to the classical corpus in recent social theory: Michel Foucault's multivolume genealogy of ethics.[20] Foucault's return to Aristotle, Artemidorous, Epictetus, Marcus Aurelius, and other ancient philosophers of the soul has popularized the analysis of an expanding constellation of nondecisionist yet transformative practices of "care of the self" geared to ethical "mode[s] of being."[21] A number of recent ethnographies have mobilized this Foucault—taken as the heir of Aristotelian, as against Kantian, ethics—to distinguish an ethical field of habits and techniques from the purely rational, deliberative task of aligning intentions with duties.[22] In Bad Souls, I pick up a thread from this emergent anthropology of ethics to examine psychiatric reform in Thrace: namely, the thematization of ethics as relational practices.

In the course of its modern history, psychiatry has yielded a profusion of theories and techniques bearing on the moral treatment of mad persons, and on the therapeutic ethics of such treatment. But the humanitarian framework of community-based treatment, with its demand for patient responsibility tied to life outside the hospital, constitutes a decisive new ethical development.[23] I therefore treat "responsibility" not only as a programmatic element of psychiatric reform, but also as an expansive ethical notion in contemporary Greece, engaging identifications with an enigmatically Western modernity and its moral goods of progress and freedom. Among the ethical philosophies here contributing visions of responsibility and its limits are political liberalism, the foundation of psychiatric reform policy and of its emphasis on the autonomy and dignity of the rights-bearing patient; social welfare policy, with its imperative of tolerance toward the mentally ill, and its dream of the state as the guardian of human well-being; and the humanism of psychodynamic and pharmaceutical treatment, which advance different conceptions of personal responsibility as the basic criterion of mental health.

These visions of responsibility together provide a rich vocabulary for articulating the moral and ethical features of clinical encounters in contemporary Greece. They do not, however, meet the demand for responsibility that defines the dynamic between parties to those encounters. Contemporary psychiatry, in Greece as elsewhere, lacks sound etiological concepts and reliable therapies for mental illness. This dearth of clinical knowledge is intimately tied to the question of responsibility. With the obsolescence of psychoanalysis, and the enduring inadequacy of biopsychiatry, what I often observed being worked out in clinical encounters in Thrace was blame for the persistence of mental pathology. Was it due to the dishonest patient, who evaded help on the basis of obscure and illegitimate motives (a question I address in part 1)? Or to cultures that fostered pathological behavior, exposing individuals to traumatic poverty and violence while foiling any means of redress (part 2)? Or to an inhumane system of care provision, which confounded the freedoms essential to patients' therapeutic progress, even as it renounced the asylum model of care (part 3)?

It is in the context of this urgent questioning, at the convergence of intractable pathology with humanitarian psychiatry, that the ethics of responsibility for mental illness may transform into a moralism about whom to blame. If, as Émile Durkheim proposed, morality describes the laws, rules, or norms that bind individuals in a solidary collective,[24] then it is crucial to observe a distinction between ethics, as a relationship the self has with its own morality, and moralism, as a concern for the morality of others.[25] This distinction mirrors the fundamental asymmetry in therapeutic relationships, in which the morality of the patient alone is foregrounded as a concern for both parties: a problem of ethics for the patient, but an undertaking of moralism for the therapist.

The distinction between ethics and moralism helps pin down and particularize the enigma posed by Michalis in the previous section of this text—*to whom can I address myself?* This question expresses the implication of therapeutic relationships in the enduring paradox of personal responsibility broached by psychiatric reform. To the extent that patients are enrolled in psychiatric care by an agency other than their own robust and autonomous will—by a therapist, a family member, a clinical institution, a community—the responsibility they cultivate requires another ground than the liberal premise of personal freedom undergirding the project of reform. The constitutive task of their ethical subjectivity is to assume responsibility for a duty, or a destiny, or a desire that is determined elsewhere than in the self and otherwise than by the self, but that is discovered and directed through self-examination and self-transformation.[26] Yet as Foucault and theorists in his line are careful to observe, the self that performs such ethical work on itself does so "in its relation to others," and this is no less the case for psychiatric patients in Thrace today than it was for the ancient disciples of Epictetus.[27]

In this book, then, I focus on the relations with others that configure the reform of psychiatric patients in Greece. I document the dispersal of responsibility across multiple subjects in community-based care—primarily patients and therapists, but also case workers, friends, family members, community members—that has given rise to distinctive forms of collaboration. Like their fellow citizens, patients are expected to function as responsible members of a community; but unlike them, many patients are ascriptively or subjectively disabled from the capacities and desires that define responsible citizenship.[28] This disjunctive demand for patient responsibility inaugurates a collaborative mode of ethics by which therapists in a sense complete the subjectivity of their patients as they enlist them in treatment. In this process, therapists make moral decisions for patients that they seem unable to make for themselves, supplying the responsibility they lack. Patients, for their part, attempt to free themselves from illness by submitting themselves to treatment. In these relationships, designed to expand the responsibility of patients in proportion to their freedom, therapists occupy a shaky ground between guidance and coercion.[29]

These collaborative relationships, emerging as a therapeutic norm with psychiatric reform in Greece, differ markedly from the therapeutic relation of psychoanalysis, animated by the unconscious dynamics of transference and countertransference. In part, the difference can be attributed to the limited influence of psychoanalysis on psychiatry in Thrace, an issue I address in part 1. But the new model of therapeutic collaboration can also be understood in terms of a more overtly liberal vision of the patient as a coherent and fully conscious subject, one endowed with legal rights and the capacity to enter and uphold agreements about treatment. In this vision, the patient's role in the therapeutic relationship is conditioned by his or her growing awareness of a responsibility to self-care, and an increasing competence at achieving it. The clinician's role entails a professional duty to safeguard the therapeutic relationship, as well as a moral commitment to human rights and the ongoing reform of psychiatric practice and policy.

In my experience in Thrace, these therapeutic relationships often yielded something like enhanced ethical subjectivity on both sides. As therapists supplied responsibility to their disabled patients, they, too, became responsible subjects of the moral discourse of reform. Yet the radical asymmetry of the power dynamic in these relationships produced asymmetrical effects beyond the reciprocal responsibility in terms of which therapists and patients collaborated with one another or, instead, failed one another. While therapists often banalized failures of responsibility as routine professional frustration or indifference, these same failures put the well-being of patients at stake, and sometimes their lives.

These asymmetrical effects of psychiatric reform might appear as breakdowns in "responsibilization"—that "key vector" of neoliberal governance to which so much attention has lately been paid, especially in the social science of the psyche.[30] In part 3 of this book, I address the special problems that severe mental illness poses to that style of analysis. Here, I only propose that, to the extent that neoliberal governmentality calls on the individual to cultivate its own autonomy and responsibility as a citizen and consumer, it cannot accommodate the therapeutic relationship as a site of ethical subject formation. The history of psychiatric reform in Greece is more than a story of governmentality—of how self-governance comes to be the dominant mode of population governance in the modern state.[31] It is more, too, than a story about consumption and risk management in healthcare, as therapeutic points of contact proliferate, outpatient services saturate local communities, and patients increasingly seek medication and counseling to enhance their self-care.[32] It is, above all, a story about collaboration between patients and therapists, and the impasses of their collaboration.

In this book then, I explore the reworking of therapeutic relationships in Thrace through persuasion and negotiation, as against methods of confinement and constraint associated with the inhumane institutional care of the past. Throughout, I observe moments when these therapeutic relationships worked: when they called forth a partnership, and yielded some measure of responsibility and health. When they did not work, however, these relationships often prompted moralism. Many patients, for their part, assimilated this moralism into their emerging ethical disposition toward their illness: as the judgment to which they must account their behavior, and as the guilt arising from their failure to behave responsibly. Other patients—or the same ones, at other moments—greeted it with a countermoralism of their own. In this text, I document the discursive and nondiscursive forms of their countermoralism. I explore the communicative strategies by which patients, turning the discourse of responsibility back onto the clinic, recalled therapists to their own duties and debts, both as caregivers and as organs of the welfare state. I also consider certain clinical symptoms of mental illness as moral claims that could not function discursively in that way. Some patients—particularly those from minority communities in Thrace— were disappointed in their pursuit of clinical resources: medications and disability subsidies, as well as personal attention and care. I suggest that, in this context, some patients articulated demands for clinical resources through affective, corporeal, and behavioral symptoms of mental illness.[33] These symptoms reflected and deflected the moralism of responsibility by which their discursive strategies were often defeated, challenging a psychiatric science notoriously unable to standardize mental disorders within a secure diagnostic apparatus.[34]

That patients registered moral claims and refusals by way of symptoms does not mean that this strategy was deliberate or even conscious; as I document throughout this text, strategic communication occupies a range of intentionalities and instrumentalities. Likewise, the discourse of responsibility has many dialects, operating in disparate contexts; it calls forth different modes of communication in the clinic from those it commands in the welfare office or at the police station. Symptoms describe a communicative mode peculiar to the clinical context. Whether the symptomatic communication of patients in that context attains or amounts to *ethics* is an open question that I elaborate throughout this book.[35] This question is not limited to strategies and counterstrategies of moralism, but extends to theory more generally. I understand the patients I present in this book to be theorists of the psyche, and theorists of relations. Treatment offered some of them some tools for reflection; their experiences of alterity shaped their use of those tools to think in other ways. In these pages, I attempt to trace the vagrant course of that ongoing theorization.

Bad Souls is organized in three main parts following from a prelude. The prelude offers a narrative of Greek psychiatric reform, and a comparative analysis of its design for devolving responsibility for the mentally ill. Incited and supervised by the European Union, the Greek project of reform was founded on the human rights of the mentally ill—most important among them the rights to consent to treatment, to live in the community "as far as possible," and to receive the "best available" mental health-care. As the Greek state proved to European auditors its responsibility in promoting the welfare of its most vulnerable citizens—protecting them both from relapse and from stigma in the communities to which they were liberated—therapists and patients in turn were obliged to prove their responsibility as members of a progressive political community.

The three main parts of the text that follows address broad thematics—truth, culture, freedom—that stand both as instruments and as sites of responsibility in Greek psychiatry. In part 1, I focus on communication between patients and therapists, showing how they negotiated the ethical task of assuming responsibility for mental illness. The clinical encounters I write about here took shape around experiences of mental illness that appeared to resist treatment. Therapists often pointed to deception by their patients as the main factor in these treatment failures. They struggled to determine their patients' psychological aptitudes for truth, and thus for responsible self-care, according to clinical profiles of pathological dishonesty. I analyze the diagnostic and practical logics they deployed to discern lies in their patients' speech, and to interpret those lies as symptomatic (or not) of particular mental illnesses. Yet these logics proved quite limited in their capacity to contain the meaning of patients' speech—and patients often developed doubts of their own about the honesty of their therapists. I suggest in part 1 that mutual suspicions of deception in these encounters actually helped fortify and sustain therapeutic relationships, even as they inhibited successful psychiatric care.

In part 2, I take the problematic of suspicion as a bridge to cultural difference in Thrace, which I elaborate through a sustained dialogue between psychiatry and anthropology. In this region known for its fraught border with Turkey and its "dangerous minorities," presumed cultural differences presented by minority patients in clinical settings often appeared as etiologies of pathology to therapists trained in the new diagnostics of transcultural psychiatry. In this diagnostic field, the array of classic "hysterical" symptoms had undergone an informal division—between, on the one hand, somatic complaints presented by rural patients, often attributed to a "traditional" culture shared by rural Greeks and Turks; and on the other, the behavioral symptoms of personality disorders, especially among Gypsies. Behaviors such as lying, stealing, addiction, and violence were considered most diagnostic of this group's pathogenic culture, one saturated with everyday traumas and deprivations. Yet this same constellation of "antisocial" symptoms appeared as readily to therapists as culturally normative behavior under conditions of extreme poverty and marginality.

This political-economic account of mental pathology, which implicated therapists as agents of state care, was at odds with the relativism framing their transcultural diagnostics. In light of this contradiction, I query the evident concern on the part of therapists to preserve a clinical mandate in their cross-cultural encounters. I suggest a range of complex identifications between Greek therapists and minority patients that troubled the cultural parameters of both categories. I also consider the ways in which patients eluded or embraced the identities imputed to them by cultural diagnostics. I explore the possibility that, through their affective, corporeal, and behavioral symptoms, minority patients made moral claims on their therapists and the state that could not be expressed in political propositions—claims that often very effectively indebted their therapists to them.

In part 3, I address the ethical implications of psychiatric reform for patients and therapists in Thrace. I show that the "democratization" of psychiatry here has radically altered expectations of treatment for therapists and patients alike. The liberalization of patient care under psychiatric reform—the ostensible liberation of patients from mental illness by psychoactive medications, and the cultivation of their personal responsibility with supplementary techniques such as therapeutic contracts and group therapy—has opened to them the enjoyment, within limits marked by "danger," of the right to certain legal and political freedoms. But these therapeutic techniques required an ontological freedom that eluded many patients, addressing them in vain as autonomous subjects who could choose to become responsible. I contend that this breach between their legal personae and their ethical faculties helps account for the intractability of severe pathology under psychiatric reform.

During the past twenty-five years of psychiatric reform in Greece, patients have moved from custodial hospitals to "the community"; the treatment of mental illness has progressed from debilitating "heavy" medications to carefully calibrated and customized cocktails; and the clinical profile of severe mental pathology has shifted from chronic schizophrenia to acute neurosis. Contemporary Greek psychiatry is marked by the withdrawal of archetypal "wild" madness from clinical encounters, as by the disappearance of the asylum itself—not only as an institution of confinement, but also as a potential refuge for the severely ill.

In my view, this complex historical shift has produced a new array of moral and ethical challenges that cannot be addressed by the humanitarian politics of liberation. From this retrospective vantage, reform appears rather as a liberal effort to humanize madness, thwarting a genuine confrontation with unreason and the unknown. This confrontation demands a more radical questioning of our subjective relationship to truth—an ethical task that necessarily opens the prospect of not knowing.[36] The present fragility of psychiatric knowledge, in Greece and elsewhere, indicates that reason is destabilized by the unintelligibility and intractability of mental illness. As unreformable patients living "in the community" make plain, madness has not been successfully routinized or banalized in the science of psychiatry. This science pushes at the frontiers of pharmacology, neuroimmunology, and genomics without assimilating severe pathology, rationalizing the unreliability of clinical care in the present by deferring to future knowledge. The political work of psychiatric reform—to expand the rights and duties of patients along with the scope of state care—proceeds in terms of this ethical failure to abide the unknown.

It is one of my aims in this book to show that the moralism of responsibility places normative limits on this failure that are particular to the aftermath of psychiatric reform. If responsibility describes the normativity of mental health, here, then a persistent negativity—what Ellen Corin describes as "unbinding"—can be discerned in the irresponsibility with which patients confound community-based care.[37] This negativity qualifies the freedoms that can be practiced ethically by these patients liberated from the asylum.

In this book, I attempt to present together, in their mutual interference and effacement, the normative and the negative faces of madness.[38] The text dwells in the profound and multiform disjuncture between the experience of mad persons and the medical-juridical vision of "the human" that holds sway in contemporary Greek psychiatry. It shifts between the broad scale of Greek culture and history and the intimate scale of ethical relations in the present, showing how madness in Thrace dismantles the oversymbolized figure of *anthropos*. What stands in its place is a different figure, named for me by a patient as he struggled to explain his failure to emerge as a responsible person from a twenty-year struggle with depression and schizophrenia: *Maybe I'm a bad soul [κακόψυχος]*. A shade of psyche, this "bad soul" — denoting, in common usage, a craven person disabled by moral cowardice and irresponsibility — is the psycho-medical and ethical concept of subjectivity that drives this book.[39] It is a concept of madness, of an ill nature, of a sickness born in and with the self: an unaccountable form of existence, a source of want, an object of blame, a binding of dependency — a fate from which freedom is something more than health.

Prelude:

The Spirit of Synchronization

NATURAL ENVIRONMENT

I met Yiannoula in late October, the first time I accompanied the hospital clinic's mobile unit on its route through the countryside northwest of Soufli, an old silk industry town just a few minutes from the Turkish border. Toward noon we stopped at the outskirts of a tiny village, a cluster of cottages rising up the hillside from a small dirt road. Thanos, the team's psychiatric resident, told me that the patient who lived here was psychotic and possibly mentally retarded; she suffered, as well, the devastating long-term side effects of neuroleptic medication. *But she's behaviorally adjusted to her illness*, he said. *She's able to take care of herself, and she asks for help when she needs it.* Yiannoula was sitting on her stoop with a loaf of bread when we arrived and rose awkwardly to greet us. She was in her fifties but looked decades older: wizened, toothless, with thinning white hair. But she had a cheery, girlish air as she gamely invited us inside.

In the vocabulary of psychiatric reform, Yiannoula's house was a "natural environment"—a place of her own "in the community," instead of a custodial institution. Her place had two rooms, one on either side of a small foyer. A kitchenette with a gas burner and sink was wedged into the back of her bedroom. This room contained her only window, as well as the coal stove that choked the house with smoke and engraved its surfaces with soot. No electricity, no bathroom. Her sparse furniture stood low to the ground; the bedroom ceiling sagged over the stove, let-

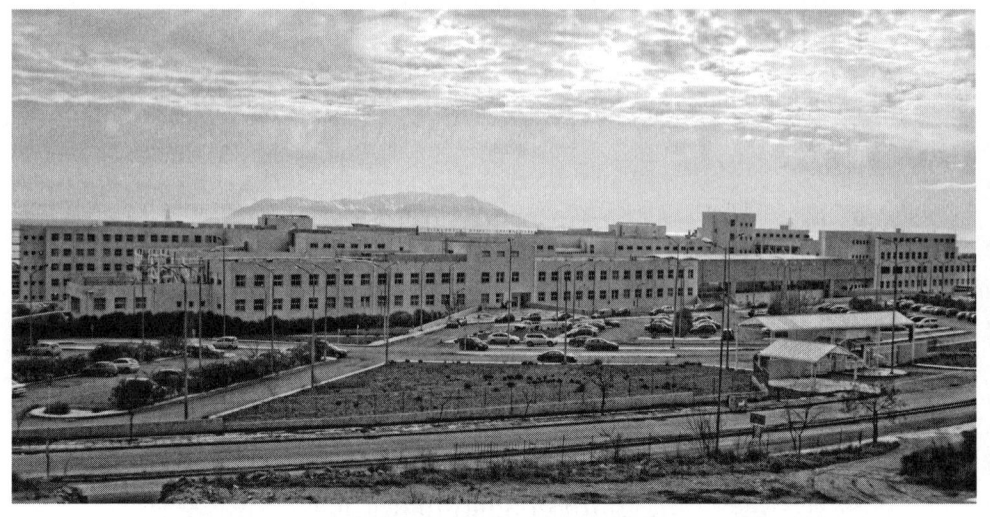

The new General Regional University Hospital of Alexandroupolis (back view), 2010.
Courtesy of Dimitris Korfiotis

ting chunks of tinny insulation onto the floor from the exposed rafters. Roula, the team's social worker, checked my reaction. *In the villages you see a lot of houses like this,* she said. *They're a horror inside, but they look just fine from the outside. Do you have houses like this in America?* Thanos told me the place had been infested with mice when they last visited, so they had asked the community—in this case, the village mayor's office—to send someone to clean and repair it. Basic upkeep was a community responsibility.

Yiannoula's income amounted to the 150 to 200 Euros she received each month from welfare and disability subsidies. She was unable to travel to the health center at Soufli for checkups, so the mobile team would visit her at home once a month to give her an injection of Aloperidin (US Haldol) and refill her prescriptions. She took sedatives and anticholinergics in addition to her antipsychotic medication. Too many pills for her to keep straight. A pile of near-empty pillboxes accumulating in her foyer indicated that she had not been taking them correctly. Stratis, a psychiatric nurse, straightened them out, extracting the lone pill or two from each box, consolidating like with like, and leaving Yiannoula only enough to last until their next visit. She could not read, so he went over the directions with her, pointing out the blue and white and yellow pills, counting out the dosages, repeating a rhyme that would help her remember. As we exited the house, she clung to him, pleading with him to come back the following week.

We left Yiannoula to visit her daughter, Aliki, who lived five minutes away on the other side of the village. She shared a small house with her husband and their two children, along with her brother, Sakis, who occupied a rickety shed by the driveway. Yiannoula's son and daughter were, like her, diagnosed indeterminately with "psychotic syndrome." They usually saw the mobile team at the health center in Soufli to receive medication and supportive counseling, but they had not shown up for their appointments in weeks. Yiannoula had not seen them, either—her contact with her children was rare and haphazard, despite their proximity.

Dogs and cats scattered from the yard as we pulled up the driveway. Aliki appeared to be running into the house, while Sakis skulked behind a pile of garbage near his shed. Hiding. Roula went inside after Aliki, and emerged with her trailing sheepishly. Like her mother, Aliki was toothless, heavy, dirty. Her bare arms were bruised and scratched, pocked with small bite marks. She stood silent and stared at the ground, as if waiting to be scolded. Roula told us that the house was a shambles inside; Aliki had not been cleaning. When Stratis asked her how she had been feeling lately, she said she was sleeping a lot. *And I'm hearing voices again. I was afraid when I heard your van, that's why I ran away.*

Stratis fetched Sakis from the shed. He was older than his sister, unkempt and jittery but jolly. We clustered in the yard to negotiate. The team tried to persuade Aliki to come to the clinic for a few days in order to get some rest. *We can adjust your medications so you won't feel so afraid,* Thanos told her. *If you come now, it'll be easy for us to help you. But if you wait, you'll just get worse. And when you finally come to the clinic, you'll have to stay much longer. Nobody wants that.* But Aliki would not budge. Sakis piped up from time to time, offering and then pleading: *I'll come! I'll come instead of her!* But Roula said he would have to wait: *Today is Aliki's turn—you can come next time.*

The team did not prevail that morning. Aliki continued to evade their glances and suggestions. We left with the understanding that if she did not turn up at the clinic in a day or two, they would see her at the Soufli health center the following week.

The mobile unit made another trip to Yiannoula's village a month later. Her home was in drastically worse shape by then. Trash and dozens of empty milk bottles were strewn across the yard. The bedroom ceiling had fallen in over the stove. Mice scuttled around the baseboards. The team was appalled. Thanos asked Roula to investigate Yiannoula's options for alternative housing. She did not qualify for any of the state-funded sheltered residences in the area, both because of her age—most of the group homes were reserved for younger patients—and because she had never resided in a psychiatric hospital and was therefore ineligible for the deinstitutionalization housing programs run by the Association. Roula, apparently exasperated, said, *It's absurd for restrictions like these to be placed on mental health resources. Why should someone like Yiannoula be excluded?* She told me Yiannoula had lived by herself in this tiny house for many years. *It used to be worse—it didn't have any windows or a stove. But slowly, bit by bit, the community made small improvements.* Later that day, Roula reported the fire hazard in Yiannoula's bedroom to the mayor's office. But the community would not respond until the end of winter, when a fire destroyed the roof and Yiannoula was obliged to take up residence at the hospital clinic in Alexandroupolis.

Yiannoula's daughter Aliki had not kept her appointments at Soufli since the last home visit, so we went to see her again that afternoon. She came straight out of the house, barefoot despite the cold and the mud from that morning's rain. She had gained weight, and her bare arms were again scarred, this time with burns, which she blamed on a cooking accident. Roula suggested that she was getting clumsy due to her poor health.

This time, the negotiations were swift. The team was adamant that Aliki be admitted to the clinic immediately. She resisted at first: *I get dizzy on the bus, I hate it. And I can't afford a taxi.* Stratis offered her cab fare to force her hand, and then she admitted that she just did not want to come to the clinic, though she agreed she was not well. *I fight with my husband a lot, especially when he's drinking. The children are unhappy, they cry all the time.* Her brother Sakis was worse, too; he was raving quietly to himself when Stratis approached him. He still seemed eager to go to the clinic, and this time he was given permission, so long as Aliki came with him.

Both patients were given injections as a stop-gap measure until persuasion could overcome Aliki's resistance to the clinic. Her husband arrived as we were preparing to leave. He had been in town, drinking ouzo at a coffee house, as he readily told us. He was better turned out than his wife and brother-in-law, and although he seemed sedated and absent-minded, Roula was able to engage him in a conversation about the conditions at home. He claimed that his own health was fine—he was not hearing voices—and he denied fighting with Aliki. He agreed immediately to borrow a car and bring her and Sakis to the clinic the following day. He showed interest in Roula's offer to complete paperwork at the clinic that would allow them to combine all of their individual welfare and disability subsidies into a single amount for the entire household. This would not only accelerate the payments but earn them an extra subsidy for the children as well.

Two days later, Aliki and Sakis had been admitted to the hospital clinic. I found them in group therapy, sitting silently side by side. They would stay for a week before returning home.

❊ ❊ ❊

By the beginning of February, Yiannoula had been admitted to the clinic as well. Roula had not been able to get good information from the community, but it seemed that a fire had damaged Yiannoula's house—ignited either by her own stove, or by some teenaged boys from the village who had played pranks on her in the past. Yiannoula was what the staff called a "social admission": her mental condition did not warrant inpatient treatment, but her living conditions were untenable and dangerous, especially in winter. So she would stay at the clinic until the community repaired her house or devised an alternative arrangement.

When her case was presented at the weekly staff meeting, doctors who did not know Yiannoula expressed surprise at her circumstances. It was unusual for a patient at her age, with her diagnosis, to live on her own for so long. Stratis, who knew her well, said, *She's not really on her own—she has the mice to keep her company!* (A nurse sitting next to me, watching me take notes, laughed and told me I should be sure to write this down, "mice and all.")

This was the first in a series of more or less affectionate jokes that followed Yiannoula around the clinic. People said that when she had left home to come to the clinic, she set out some vegetables for the mice in her bedroom so they would not starve in her absence. One morning, she defecated in a side yard of the clinic by the parking lot, in plain sight of the main office where we were gathered for a staff meeting. A nurse told us that Yiannoula had complained about the toilets in the clinic: *She only knows how to go outdoors!* The psychologist suggested they build an outhouse for her in the side yard of the clinic. They spoke of her fondly as a simple soul—childlike, docile, helpless—without fear that her dignity might be compromised by residence at the clinic; and she stayed for several months more, away from her village and her family.

Deinstitutionalization was the primary task of psychiatric reform in Greece from the early 1980s onward—as in other European states where the reform process was already well underway by the 1960s. Chronically ill residents of state psychiatric hospitals would be discharged to the community, where treatment and rehabilitation would be provided in outpatient settings. These same community-based services would also aid in prevention, helping new psychiatric patients avoid hospitalization altogether.[1] This radical transformation of psychiatric care demanded not only massive financial investment in training and infrastructure but also participation and sensitivity on the part of the communities that would host discharged and other outpatients. Programs for raising public awareness about mental illness were thus frequently written into reform legislation.

These changes in psychiatric policy and practice describe a generic and highly mobile apparatus of reform that has accompanied movements of political liberalization worldwide since the 1950s. Yet a distinctive story of reform in Greece is told by the academic psychiatrists who run its public institutions. This narrative originates in a brief historical moment when Greek politics and medicine occupied the same progressive path toward health and freedom. It is a tale of alienation and political awakening among citizen-doctors during the dictatorship (1967–74) who, afterward, activated their ambition of transforming the state and the way it fulfilled its responsibilities to its most vulnerable citizens.[2] Psychiatric reform appears in this narrative as both a paradigm and an allegory of modernization.

The particularity of Greek reform is a key question animating the popular textbook on community-based psychiatry published by Panayiotis Sakellaropoulos, a renowned leader of psychiatric reform in Greece and the founder and president of the Association. For Sakellaropoulos, psychiatric reform in France, the site of his own professional training, forms the comparative context for reform in Greece: the scale by which its progress can be measured with a critical eye, registering the movement of psychiatry through its evolutionary history.[3] The introduction to the textbook, presented in Greek and French, even in its title— "Introduction to Applications of a Contemporary Psychiatry"—broaches the question of what is new in Greek psychiatric reform that cannot be attributed simply to the *application* of the generic apparatus itself, transposed in quick succession from England, France, and the United States to Belgium, Germany, Spain, Portugal, and finally Greece, after "a delay of several decades," leaving only Italy to invent and implement its own "remarkable" program of reform:[4]

> The application of the fundamental principles [of reform] can lead to different types of functioning, according to the personality of the leaders, their training, experience, the point of view of other caregivers, the country or region where its tasks are undertaken, and of course, the available budget. The services always have an evolutionary and dynamic character: they are born, they develop, and they decline. Thus, in Western Europe, psychiatric reform has not ceased to evolve and renew itself. In Greece, the application of its fundamental principles has improved, in certain regions, the quality of psychiatric care. . . . The connection of the past to the present, as well as certain historical reminders, permits us to rediscover the reasons and the processes that have led to the current forms of psychiatric care.[5]

In a brief history of critical events — those leading up to and provoking the florescence of reform in Greece, in a series parallel to that of the French experience but dislodged in evolutionary time — Sakellaropoulos presents the struggle of an "avant-garde movement" against the conservatism of the state. Efforts led by Sakellaropoulos himself in the 1960s included a pediatric psychiatry clinic in Athens, designed on an "anti-asylum" model. But, he writes, the state intervened in the functioning of this clinic, blocking the development and funding of appropriate administrative structures. Next, an experimental unit was created at a major Athens hospital to provide "gestalt therapy" and "humane" medical care to psychiatric patients, as against insulin and electroshock treatments. The dictatorship put an end to this experiment. Yet according to Sakellaropoulos, a transformation in "mentality" among psychiatric personnel had already transpired by then that could not be reversed.

Many newcomers to the psychiatric profession in the 1970s, after the junta, arrived with an investment in the human rights of patients and a commitment to the practice of critical psychiatry originated by their radical counterparts in Great Britain and Italy. Some told me they had chosen the psychiatric specialty precisely because this "backward" branch of medicine had the worst reputation for abuses of power. A new "interest in the freedom and rights of the individual," itself partly engendered by the dictatorship, impelled these new specialists toward a radical reform of state care.[6] In the late 1970s, this freshly politicized community of doctors put together a number of policy proposals and pilot projects for new psychiatric services targeted to the underserved rural populations of Macedonia and Thrace. These efforts yielded the country's first day hospitals and community mental health centers.[7] They also produced a mass of demographic and clinical data that drove and shaped the establishment of the National Health System in 1983.[8]

Among these early studies was a report on the current state of psychiatric care in Greece, published in 1980 by Costas Stefanis and Michalis Madianos, professors of psychiatry at Athens University and clinicians at the university psychiatry clinic of Aeginition Hospital, Athens—members of the most elite institutions of the highly centralized Greek psychiatric academy.[9] Their report in fact presented that centralization as the greatest obstacle to psychiatric reform. The authors compared psychiatric services in Greece with those in seven other nations of the European Economic Community (EEC) according to specific aspects of care provision that, they concluded, marked the difficulty of Greece's "synchronization" with European policies:[10] "The conservatism of [our] system, with its institutional anachronism and organizational defects, comes into conflict with aspects of the global program of structural modifications, especially in our country's attempt in the social sector to coordinate with the countries of the European Community, where the decentralization of the system of psychiatric care constitutes a keystone of social policy."[11]

Decentralization emerged as the linchpin of synchronization—itself the essential mechanism of reform that became, over the subsequent decade, its primary objective. Lodged thus from the outset in a position out of synch with other Europeans, Greek reformers addressed infrastructural adjustments and technical innovations as temporal rather than therapeutic devices. For example, Stefanis and Madianos argued against a plan, proposed by a state agency at a national conference on health in 1979, to increase the number of beds in existing psychiatric hospitals. They contended that this action, though it would immediately help alleviate inhumane conditions of overcrowding at these hospitals, would only consolidate the centralized organization of care. They proposed instead to accelerate the process of decentralization by allocating the new beds to inpatient units in general hospitals and small, regional psychiatric hospitals.[12] Though these regional hospitals never materialized, the inpatient units in general hospitals did, along with all the other suggestions in the 1980 report. These included the founding of a national advisory board on mental health, national legislation establishing new services for the mentally ill, mechanisms for differentiating psychiatric admissions in existing hospitals according to diagnosis, the separation of psychiatry from neurology as a distinct clinical specialty with a corresponding residency program,[13] the creation of postgraduate programs in social psychiatry that included clinical training at community mental health centers, the improvement of administrative relations between psychiatry wards and other medical departments in hospitals, and the development of undergraduate programs in psychology at all Greek universities.

Stefanis and Madianos concluded their report in 1980 with a demand that "our country . . . replace the traditional model of organization of psychiatry services . . . with modern services open to the public."[14] Nevertheless, they warned that this process of modernization, global as it surely was, would also be idiosyncratic and gradual in Greece. It behooved clinicians to proceed with careful attention to Greek particularities:

> The fact is that we find ourselves in a period of social transformation. New understandings of the etiology and nature of mental disorders, and especially a new awareness of the social rights of disadvantaged persons and our social responsibility toward them, are determining the implementation of many of these new measures in the domain of Mental Health. It is also true that, in most cases, a cost-benefit analysis of these measures happens only in retrospect, in the context of a spirit of synchronization disposed to justify each effort that distances itself from traditional conceptions of how to cope with mental illness. Thus changes are often made without any prior analysis of the existing realities in each country or region, by passively transposing organizational schemas that operate in other societies and cultural circumstances, with the effect not only of *not* improving the approach to mental illness, but also of undermining the basic principles that ideologically support the new systems of provision for psychiatric services.
>
> We believe, in order to avoid such unintended "side effects," that the goal of synchronizing the existing system must include recognizing the need to study the benefits of new measures in relation to the existing cultural, socioeconomic and administrative conditions in our country.[15]

This ambivalent critique of synchronization—itself an image of Greece's tie to Europe as a leash by which the nation was dragged toward its presaged future—preserved an attachment to the universalist apparatus of psychiatric reform: a legislative framework, and an infrastructure mandated by that legislation for new clinical services, support services, and personnel training. The transformation of Greek psychiatry was patterned in this way by Greek membership in the EEC, ratified in January 1981. The previous several years, during which psychiatrists had conducted the early research on reform, constituted a period of evaluation and preparation for accession. The EEC and its successor, the EU, served as guide, patron, and auditor to Greece throughout this process.[16] Reform thus acquired the peculiar temporality of synchronization from the very beginning; failures would, from that point onward, acquire the import of the state's failure to keep up.

In its more generic, international narrative, psychiatric reform appears as a universalizable technology of the state: a set of policies, institutions, and practices whose place in the history of law and governance can be found in the global expansion of human rights and policies of social welfare in the twentieth century. But at the turn of the century, the ambitions and successes of psychiatric reform might appear obsolete to social scientists tracking the evolving relationship between psychiatry and the state since the 1980s. The nearly worldwide eclipse of psychoanalysis by statistical and pharmaceutical psychiatry in this period,[17] and of state health and social services by managed healthcare and private self-help movements, have been associated in the scholarly literature with the rise of technologically enhanced rational individualism diffusing through international consumer markets for psychiatric medications and expertise. For many, these developments signify a new biopolitical logic wrought by the devolution of state responsibility both to private managerial bodies and to individual subjects of care.[18]

Perhaps the best-known work in this literature is Robert Castel's *The Management of Risk* (1981), a grand historical synthesis in the tradition of Foucault's *Madness and Civilization* (1961). Here, Castel observes a "mutation" in contemporary psychiatry attending the rise of a "post-disciplinary order." What is deformed in this mutation, he argues, is the policy of sectorization devised in postwar France, driven by the radical politics of antipsychiatry that aimed to liberate patients from coercive

institutional power. According to this policy, the old *dispositif* (apparatus) of the asylum would be replaced with the new *dispositif* of the sector,
though it shared with the asylum its principled rubric of public assistance. With the sector, psychiatric care would be diffused in "intermedi-
ary structures" throughout the social field. Each municipal system in
each prefecture of the country would be divided into small, discrete geographic units deploying treatment teams to address all psychiatric needs
within that community.[19]

Fears that the policy of the sector, as a ruse of power, might facilitate
the expansion of social control by the state were not borne out. Castel reports that the sectorial *dispositif* never fully materialized in France,
since the state made only limited investments in the requisite infrastructure, and the old hospital system retained control over the training and
hiring of clinicians. During the 1970s, the weak and partial sectorization
of psychiatry was dismantled by three events: first, the rise (or return)
of scientific positivism and medical objectivism, in a backlash against
psychoanalysis; second, the invention of new techniques and technologies for identifying and managing high-risk populations; and third, the
emergence of a culture of everyday psychologism outside the clinic.[20]

Castel furnishes a number of phrasings—some more absolutist than
others—for the "mutation" that finally "passed across the threshold"
of this situation, historically antecedent to the present.[21] It is, he says,
a shift from the sector to the profile, from the scene of treatment to
the scene of management. It is the obsolescence of the therapeutic encounter, the relation, the contract, and the continuity of care; and the
emergence of risk profiles compiled in the autonomous space of compu-
tation. It is the dissolution or disappearance of the subject—of the "concrete individual" with a social identity and a personal history—into a
combinatory of "interchangeable" and "heterogeneous" factors describing populations with new "destinies" irreducible to the old "geography
of the social."[22] On his account, it is no longer in clinical encounters
between doctors and patients that "diagnostic synthesis" is achieved,
but rather in the crafting of policy by managers and administrators.[23]
Diagnosis itself is unleashed from treatment, coming to function as the
pure and extractable product of expertise rendered by commissioned
technicians rather than devoted caregivers. No longer determining pathology, diagnosis instead assigns individuals a distance from the norm
corresponding to an identitarian path within a new social field of competencies—thereby legitimating, with scientific (or "pseudoscientific")

knowledge (or "pseudoknowledge") the administrative instrumentaliza-
tion of social conditions.[24]

While clinical encounters continue to take place on this novel psychiatric terrain, Castel argues both that they are progressively less important to administrative policy and that they are "no longer able to keep
pace" with developments in the field of psychiatry itself, constituted
in the "triangle" linking experts to the private sector and the state. In
this triangle, experts put their knowledge on the market, performing
an "auxiliary" function rather than a therapeutic vocation.[25] The private
sector—which includes charitable organizations as well as "marginal"
ones, such as "encounter groups" animated by the politics of a now
aging "counter-culture"—puts this expertise to work, meeting the increasingly numerous and discrete needs and desires of local populations.
These functionally "diffuse" and structurally "capillary" organizations
operate, in theory, more efficiently than public services, both because
they reach greater numbers of patient-clients and because they achieve
greater accountability through internal audits.[26] The neoliberal state,
succeeding a welfare state that bore responsibility for the entire network of care, takes a regulatory role in this distribution of expertise and
treatment. No longer aiming to "create, execute, and finance directly,"
but instead to "centralize and plan the data, rationalize the implementation of services, fix strict norms of functioning, and control the results,"
the state leaves the field of psychiatry to run itself like a business.[27]

After its publication in 1981, *The Management of Risk* set off a wave of
critical inquiries into neoliberal psychiatry in the sociopolitical con-
federacy of what Castel calls "'advanced industrial' (or, as one prefers, 'post-industrial' or 'post-modern') societies."[28] But while novel
elements, clinical and economic, have certainly shaped the theory and
practice of psychiatry since the 1970s, I suggest that this now dominant neoliberal narrative offers a misleading account of contemporary
psychiatry in Greece, as in many states where the public sector remains
the primary scene of medical care. Three decades after the publication
of Castel's book, and more than fifty years after the introduction of
the sector in France, psychiatric reform in Greece is still taking shape
around that *dispositif*, behind the frontier of technological and political
"mutation."

This ostensible lag is not, however, a matter only of the comparative development of national political economies according to a global
scale. In the field of psychiatry itself, the clinical encounter—the scene

of treatment—bears the same relationship to risk management that Greece bears to France. Greek psychiatry, whether in the public or private sector, remains invested in the clinical treatment of pathology diagnosed in "concrete individuals." While the urban centers of Athens and Thessaloniki present a different array of services, there is no mass market in Thrace for "psy" technologies,[29] as Nikolas Rose calls the expanding range of private organizations and practices that "empower" individuals to discover, reform, and liberate themselves according to the normative values of responsibility and autonomy and to the special sociality of neoliberal governmentality that is managed but no longer "disciplined" by a diffuse state apparatus.[30] If this type of activity is what uniquely constitutes "the new," then it is happening elsewhere. So when psychiatrists in Thrace remarked, as I often heard, that Greek psychiatry was "backward" or "behind" (πίσω), they were indicating a double deficit: one in the standard of psychiatric care, and another in the state of society.

The following section dwells on this twofold problematic of "the new" and its attendant rhetoric of backwardness, as the technical and ideological framework of psychiatric reform in Greece. This problematic—in its domestic and extrinsic versions in Greece—plays into a presumptive and circular tendency in contemporary social theory to restrict the analytic purchase of novelty to a certain knowledge/power grid organizing the societies judged most advanced according to these same measures. While Castel observes a mutation in psychiatry that dispels the subject along with the therapeutic encounter, psychiatry in Thrace is tied to the clinical scene of the sector, where the pathology of individual patients persists as an urgent and emergent problem for the state. The radical transformations in care represented by the *dispositif* of the sector, here, have hardly yet begun. If Greek psychiatry is indeed facing the advent of neoliberalism, the sector may be doomed—but it is not obsolete.

THE MOST BASIC NOTIONS OF HUMAN DIGNITY

With the restoration of democratic government in Greece after the fall of the junta in 1974, the conservative New Democracy party (ND) was elected to power. Already the Greek state, resurfacing from dictatorship, was poised to take responsibility for implementing psychiatric reform; already the process was conceived within a certain legislative framework borrowed from Western Europe. The ND government passed two measures regarding mental healthcare in the mid-1970s: one stipulated re-habilitation services for the mentally ill, and the other conferred legal status on voluntary admissions to psychiatric hospitals, authorizing state coverage of treatment sought by patients on their own initiative. The ND administration was dislodged in 1981 by the more activist PASOK party (Panhellenic Socialist Movement) under the leadership of Andreas Papandreou. In 1983, his government passed Statute 1397, creating the National Health System.[31] Article 21 of the statute mandated a five-year plan for decentralizing mental healthcare, which would diffuse through new community mental health centers as well as psychiatry wards and outpatient clinics in general hospitals.

The new National Health System was to consolidate and extend the primary healthcare network instituted in 1956 with a law that ordered a compulsory year of community medical service, called a "rural [year]" (το αγροτικό), for all graduates of Greek medical schools.[32] These rural doctors—each responsible for one large village or several small ones, and often equipped with nothing more than a consultation room, a first-aid kit, and a stock of common antibiotics and analgesics—were "first-contact" workers whose role in the new National Health System would be to refer patients appropriately to more centralized, specialized facilities. The disparity between this primary healthcare network of young, inexperienced general physicians and the future National Health System was vast, in terms not only of infrastructure but also of personnel.

On its accession to the EEC in 1981, Greece submitted several memoranda to the commission regarding "problems arising from [its] membership," especially in regard to "structural inadequacies." The commission appointed a research and review team of "independent experts" on health—representatives from Greece, other EEC nations, and the World Health Organization (WHO)—which found in December 1982 that the Greek psychiatric system had "serious problem[s]":

> In Greece, as elsewhere, emphasis in the past has been placed on the treatment of patients in psychiatric hospitals, while care in the community framework has remained relatively undeveloped. This tendency to privilege hospital care has contributed to the hyperconcentration of buildings, in their decrepit and poorly maintained condition, with insufficient services, characterized by therapeutic inactivity, an atmosphere infused with passivity and despair among patients, as well as low morale and intolerable working conditions for the staff—in short,

a general situation that renders the pursuit of treatment especially difficult. These conditions reinforce the stigmatization of mental illness and the inhumane, costly, and unacceptable features of hospitalization.[33]

These memoranda and findings resulted in the passage, in March 1984, of the EEC measure 815/84 "on exceptional financial support in favour of Greece in the social field." The final report of the EEC on measure 815/84, published eleven years later, offers a terse history of the program, beginning with the state of psychiatric care in Greece before its inception. It quotes the preamble to the Greek National Health System bill of 1983, in which the Greek Ministry of Health reported: "It is broadly accepted that psychiatric care [in Greece] is totally inadequate. The manner of dealing with psychiatric patients often comes close to denying the most basic notions of human dignity. Radical reform is needed to change this intolerable situation."[34]

At that time, psychiatric care in Greece was restricted to ten state psychiatric hospitals, of which the five largest were located in Athens, Pireaus, Thessaloniki, Chania (Crete), and the island of Leros.[35] The EEC proposal echoed dozens already generated within the psychiatric academy in Greece. It mandated a redirection of building and funding from these large residential hospitals to community-based services. Stipulations included the relocation of chronic patients from hospitals to sheltered residences in the community, social and vocational rehabilitation programs in outpatient settings, and an investment in preventive care in local mental health centers, short-stay inpatient wards, and other "alternative mental healthcare services and facilities." The program also earmarked funding for retraining fellowships to be granted to psychiatrists and support staff.

The EEC granted a portion of 120 million ECU to Greece to implement this psychiatric reform project over a period of five years, from January 1984 to December 1988—the same period projected by the Greek Ministry of Health for the development of the new National Health System.[36] Initially, the EEC grant was supposed to cover 55 percent of public expenditures on reform projects.[37] Fundable activities included acquiring medical equipment, training personnel, building or extending infrastructure for outpatient care, and developing pilot projects for alternative services. According to commission documents, "expenditure on the mere improvement of mental asylums was expressly excluded from the scope of [the] Regulation."[38]

The five-year plan, it turned out, proved overly ambitious. In September 1987, Greece requested a three-year extension of the reform program, due to significant delays in implementation and a consequent "low rate of absorption" of funds.[39] The extension was approved without any modification to the funding package, but the commission appended a requirement for the Greek government to establish an evaluation committee of experts, including commission representatives, that would report on Greece's progress three times a year to the commission.[40] The report of 1988, in which the extension was approved and recommendations were made for the evaluation committee, noted: "It would be advisable for such assistance to assume a more systematic form following the pattern set recently by certain provisions applying to other Community interventions. A relevant amendment to the Regulation would enable the Community and the Hellenic Republic to improve the management of the programme by setting up strict criteria for the rational utilization of available resources."[41]

Delays in reform were attributed in this way to the managerial disorganization and instrumental irrationality of Greek medical experts and administrators who, despite this reprimand, continued to miss important targets and deadlines. By December 1989, a year and a half later, only 14.2 of only 32.5 million ECU—about 44 percent of 27 percent of the total award from the EEC—had been disbursed for completed psychiatric reform projects.[42] At that time, the evaluation committee appointed in July 1988 had not submitted a single report. Representatives of the commission's Court of Auditors therefore conducted spot checks of 135 projects to which funding had been committed, and found that many of these projects had not even begun.[43] The commission moved to "postpone indefinitely" the approval of new psychiatric projects in December 1989. Funding for new projects was suspended, and funding commitments for seventy-six projects approved between 1984 and 1988 were canceled because that work had still not begun.[44]

In its report of 1990, the Court of Auditors found in the Greek contribution to psychiatric reform "a high level of improvisation and the absence of any precise preparation of the investments to be financed," a problem the auditors regretted that Greece had not redressed by enlisting the expertise of commission members. Most of the Greek labor expended on reform, they reported, had focused on formulating national policy on mental healthcare and a plan for the distribution of resources; very few specific projects or beneficiaries had yet been named.[45] Moreover, the auditors noted with alarm that the projects executed had mostly improved and consolidated the existing psychiatric hospital infrastructure, in effect producing the opposite result from that intended by the program, which was to reduce the role of long-term residential hospitals in the provision of psychiatric care.[46]

In a bid to recapture EEC financing and support, Greek delegates presented in March 1991 a revised proposal for psychiatric reform to be undertaken from 1991 to 1994. This proposal detailed specific projects for establishing alternative mental health services according to the new legislative framework for the National Health System that would pass in 1992. Statute 2071/92 stipulated, among other provisions, the construction of community mental health centers, a legal specification of modes of hospitalization, and a new framework for patients' rights.[47] Once the erstwhile evaluation committee had been reconstituted, and the special program called "Leros I" set in motion,[48] the commission approved the new Greek proposal in December 1991. Apart from one six-month extension, approved in December 1994, the reform project proceeded to its completion in 1995 without substantial delay or complaint.[49]

The EU issued its final report on measure 815/84 in 1996.[50] In the report, Greece's progress in psychiatric reform was assessed according to several indices. The first of these described the transformation of material infrastructure. The report listed Greek achievements in this direction: the creation of "25 Community Mental Health Centres, 28 Psychiatric Units in General Hospitals, 7 Acute and Short-Stay units, 9 Guidance and Day Treatment Centres, 23 Pre-Vocational/Vocational Training and Rehabilitation Centres and Workshops, and 42 Hostels providing alternative residential accommodation,"[51] in addition to forty-nine pilot projects exploring "new methods of care," and eight training programs for psychiatric staff and professionals.[52]

A second index of progress described the geographical distribution of new services. Here the report observed that 48 percent of new reform projects in Greece were undertaken outside Athens and Thessaloniki, the two largest urban areas in Greece, where more than half the nation's total population resided. A third index described the relocation of patients from residential psychiatric hospitals. Here the report noted a 37.2 percent reduction in the number of patients living in such hospitals between 1982 and 1995, and a 38.5 percent reduction in the number of beds in those hospitals—without a corresponding increase in private psychiatric clinics. The fourth index described the personnel-to-patient ratio in psychiatric care settings. Here the report showed a 132 percent increase in the number of psychiatrists in Greece between 1984 and 1995, 900 percent in psychologists, 280 percent in social workers, and 29 percent in psychiatric nurses. It also noted the 40 percent participation rate of psychiatric staff in new training programs offered for the first time in 1994–95. A final index, not included in the EU report, described the duration of admission in psychiatric hospitals or wards. Progress on this front had already been apparent to the Court of Auditors in 1990, when the average length of admission had decreased to 87 days from an average of 260 days in 1983.[53]

In its final report from 1995, the EU pledged that, after the lapse of measure 815/84, European support for Greek psychiatric reform would continue "in the context of the Community Support Framework 1994–99 for Greece, with financing from the Structural Funds." Technical assistance from the evaluation committee "expired" within the legislated time frame, but the European reform of the Greek state continued in a new fifteen-year plan called Psychargos, approved by the EU in 1998 and passed in bodies of Greek legislation in 1999 (Mental Health Act, Statute 2716/99) and 2001 (Reform of the National Health System). Psychargos outlined three phases of reform between 2001 and 2015, emphasizing the final completion of deinstitutionalization with the closure of all state psychiatric hospitals by 2015, the sectorization of mental healthcare services throughout the country, and the formation of patients' cooperatives to promote their social and economic integration and destigmatization.[54]

The European reform packages amounted to a targeted investment in public sector healthcare—the bedrock of a robust welfare state—and the corresponding bureaucratic structures for the efficient planning and implementation of social welfare programs. Stelios Stylianidis, a prominent social psychiatrist, psychoanalyst, and reformer, notes that the absence of such welfare programs had, throughout the post–Second World War period, marked the gap between Greece and other western European nations: " 'Social welfare' is a recent notion in Greece. The country's 'prosperity' has not, in the past, permitted the development of structures and systems of protection as complete as those in other industrialized nations. Greeks have therefore 'relied' more on personal initiative and familial support than, as elsewhere, on direct financial 'participation' in care [on the part of the state]."[55]

The imaginary of the welfare state invoked here—some twenty years after Castel had announced the "retreat of the welfare state" in France—is both a technique and an achievement of psychiatric reform. As Stylianidis sees it, this is a state able, for the first time in Greece's beleaguered and often autocratic modern history, to take responsibility for the well-being of its citizens: to step in where the culturally conservative institution of the family had been.

It did not weaken the appeal of this imaginary that the welfare state itself did not actually materialize in Greece before the private sector usurped its role of assistance to the mentally ill, as Sakellaropoulos points out.[56] He identifies the obstruction of innovation on the part of the state as the chief factor in the diversion of reform efforts to the private sector in the 1970s—an obstruction to which he protests, "It is impossible that the private sector should have more privileges and administrative flexibility than the State and public psychiatry."[57] When his multivolume textbook was published in 1995, Sakellaropoulos characterized as the chief administrative task of social psychiatry the recuperation of the state as an ally in reform.

Private psychiatric care, provided in consultation offices and small clinics, had historically been sought almost exclusively by middle-class patients in Greece—those with the means to undertake long-term psychotherapy for "neurotic" disorders or, for the more severely ill, to avoid the state mental hospitals that were the only sites of public psychiatric care before the development of the National Health System. Private treatment remains more expensive than public healthcare, and it is only partially reimbursable by insurance. Clinicians have incentives to refer patients in acute crises to more profitable private clinics.[58] Fee schemes for private care are largely unregulated, permitting the rapid growth of private insurance plans with an increasing profit margin for clinicians in private practice.[59]

By 1989, with the growth of public outpatient and community-based services, private psychiatric clinics were declining in number.[60] That year, only forty private clinics were in operation in Greece—down from forty-nine in 1977—of which twenty-eight were located in Athens.[61] During the late 1980s and mid-1990s, when public community-based services were proliferating, many private clinics turned to IKA ('Ίδρυμα Κοινωνικών Ασφαλίσεων, or Social Insurance Institute), the semipublic healthcare and insurance agency, to subcontract their services.[62] But in 1996, the year in which the EU completed its final evaluation of Greek psychiatric reform, about 44 percent of the ninety-five hundred psychiatric beds in Greece were still located in private clinics.[63] According to Stylianidis, the "equilibrium" reached between public and private psychiatric care, after fifteen years of reform, was likely to be disrupted in the near future. The private sector, he observed then, was "in the ascent," due to persistent structural weaknesses in the public sector and "a certain 'retreat' of the state."[64] And thus, once again, at the turn of the century, Greece found itself out of synch with European socioeconomic and political progress. The welfare state was threatened by the advancement of the private sector—but preemptively, before the state could take responsibility for the mentally ill and saturate the public sector with social welfare programs.

According to this analysis, the comparative vigor of the private sector in contemporary Greek psychiatry does not mark the advent of neoliberalism so much as the weakness of the welfare state. Welfare remains the reigning ambition of reformers in Greece, just as reform remains the reigning ambition of psychiatrists. It is only within the structure of a self-conscious time warp that community-based psychiatry could organize the devolution of responsibility for the mentally ill from the state to individual patients without departing from the biopolitics of welfare.

THE MISSION

For the psychiatric academy in Greece, the first and dominant mode of professional modernization during the process of reform was the production of local psychiatric knowledge, as against the mere translation of psychiatric texts and techniques from elsewhere. This did not, in the beginning, yield a body of biological or clinical knowledge that might constitute a local contribution to a global science. Instead, the professional authority of the Greek cadre of academic psychiatrists was largely invested in their expertise on Greek culture, society, and economy—the field of obstacles, such as stigma and illiteracy, that threatened to impede community-based care. A new humanitarian ethos in the profession denigrated traditional Greek psychiatry for colluding with these obstacles of "custom" to produce dependency on state hospitals for the custodial internment of the mentally ill.

This framing of local culture as an obstacle positioned Thrace as a national laboratory of psychiatric reform. The poorest region in mainland Greece, the most rural, the most eastern, and the most "backward,"

Thrace presented the greatest apparent need for reform. Early experiments therefore targeted the region, creating alternative services in the public and the private sectors, years before policy changes transpired at the national level.

The key figures in psychiatric reform compose a small circle in Thrace. Several of the current generation of senior academic psychiatrists at the University of Thrace attended medical school in Athens during the late 1970s, moving to Alexandroupolis in the early 1980s for their residencies in order to work with Sakellaropoulos, then the director of the university psychiatry clinic. His own mentor, Charalambos Ierodiakonou, who later headed the university psychiatry clinic at the General Hospital of Thessaloniki, was at that time chair of the department of psychiatry at the then new teaching hospital in Alexandroupolis.

It was Ierodiakonou who developed and oversaw the early reform of public psychiatry in the Evros prefecture of Thrace. As he explained in his WHO report of 1983, the main goals of this effort included outreach to the rural population, the prevention of crises and relapses, and continuity of care, all aided by the systematic organization of medical records.[65] His first innovation was to establish, in 1978, a psychiatry ward at the General Regional University Hospital of Alexandroupolis—a twenty-two-bed, short-stay, open inpatient unit with an associated outpatient clinic, the first of its kind in Greece.[66] By 1981, his team had attached to this ward a community mental health center in downtown Alexandroupolis, as well as mobile units throughout the eastern countryside of Thrace that provided care to patients in their homes and at rural health centers. Ierodiakonou began immediately to craft studies of these new services and the unique impediments to their implementation presented by the rural population of Thrace.[67]

This research formed the basis for national reform in two ways. From the point of view of policy, it served as the principal reference of concrete proposals for drafters of the National Health System and European legislation. From the point of view of execution, it offered a model for further reform efforts in Thrace, as well as in other provincial regions,[68] including those undertaken by Ierodiakonou's former students. For one, Sakellaropoulos founded in 1981 the Greek Association for Social Psychiatry and Mental Health ("the Association"), a private, nonprofit "scientific organization" whose charter was to provide free psychiatric and psychological care to the public. Its first project was the establishment of mobile units in Amfissa, in central Greece, but it soon opened a branch in Athens. In 1985, in cooperation with the hospital in Alexandroupolis, it opened a third branch in Alexandroupolis and established mobile units in Sapes and Komotini, small cities in Rodopis, the majority-Muslim prefecture of Thrace that had remained out of reach to Ierodiakonou's public services in Evros.

Over the course of the next ten years, in addition to treatment units, the Association oversaw in Thrace the creation of the first group home for deinstitutionalized chronic patients from Leros (1987), two vocational cooperatives (1988), institutes for child psychiatry in Alexandroupolis and Xanthi (1996), and a number of socialization groups, counseling groups, and vocational integration programs in cooperation with municipal welfare offices. In 2000, with funding from the Greek state, the Association undertook an ambitious project to build and staff a collection of sheltered residences to accommodate deinstitutionalized patients from the state psychiatric hospital in Thessaloniki, four hundred kilometers away. All of these reform projects were bound, explicitly and programmatically, to the "philosophy and the principles of social psychiatry,"[69] now the dominant model for the devolution of state care to individual therapists and patients in Thrace.

These transformations in infrastructure and law accomplished by psychiatric reform in Thrace entailed a transformation of practice as well. Early efforts at building a National Health System from the foundations of the extant primary healthcare network required, in theory, the training or retraining of first-contact workers—rural doctors and nurses, as well as nonpsychiatric specialists employed at hospitals and IKA health centers.[70] None of this personnel had received even rudimentary training in psychiatry or psychology, and reformers feared that they would protract rather than combat the medical neglect of the mentally ill, even as psychiatry was revolutionizing itself in the academy.

Undertrained psychiatrists themselves presented a further challenge to reform. Those senior clinicians who had attended medical school in Greece had been trained in outdated psychoneurology curricula that did not include psychotherapy or social psychiatry. Even the younger generation of psychiatrists had still, in the mid-1980s, acquired their clinical experience only in traditional state hospitals, because new community-based services had not developed sufficiently to support formal training residencies.[71] Reformers observed with concern the absence of specialized training in psychiatric nursing, a deficiency that, twenty years later, remained to be addressed at the national level.[72] Several pilot projects funded by the EEC in the 1980s offered residency fellowships in other EEC member states for Greek psychiatrists. Domestically, the specialty curriculum was adapted to the five-year program now standardized across Europe, including compulsory exposure to a range of psychotherapeutic techniques.

In a report on the state of Greek psychiatry in 2000, Stylianidis observed that Greece, having no "national school" of psychiatry, accommodates a wide range of contemporary approaches, from psychoanalysis and psychodynamic therapy, to cognitive-behavioral therapy, to biopharmaceutical treatment. The heterogeneity of these "theory-driven practices," he writes, reflects a variety of influences from outside Greece, introduced by way of senior clinicians trained abroad, most frequently in the United States, France, Germany, and Great Britain. However, while psychoanalysis has borne a certain progressivist and humanist prestige in Greece since the 1910s, it was never incorporated into institutional or academic settings as it was, for example, in France; and its influence has for the most part remained limited to small intellectual circles in Athens and Thessaloniki. According to Stylianidis, biopharmaceutical research represents the main direction of academic psychiatry in Greece today, signifying a broad "valorization" of the "scientific model," with its diagnostic criteria and procedures of quantitative assessment, codified in international manuals—primarily the *Diagnostic and Statistical Manual of Mental Disorders* (the DSM, published by the American Psychiatric Association) and, at a distant second, the *International Statistical Classification of Diseases and Related Health Problems—Mental and Behavioural Disorders* (the ICD, published by the WHO). On this foundation, the Greek psychiatric infrastructure has developed in accordance with the European model and its emphasis on sectorial community-based care.[73]

Psychiatric reformers in Greece, whose efforts have yielded this state of the field, promoted "humane" practices and conditions over the "inhumane" customs and institutions of the past. This divergence did not, as in the United States during the same period, take the form of an ideological battle between biopharmaceutical and psychodynamic approaches or worldviews. Social psychiatry, as it developed in Greece and especially in Thrace, was the vector by which the humanization of psychiatry accompanied its pharmaceuticalization.[74]

The Association promoted this biohumanitarian perspective in a series of "awareness-building" seminars offered to the public in 2002–3 in Alexandroupolis. According to the seminar proceedings, distributed to each participant as well as at local schools and health centers, the practice of social psychiatry is tied to sectorization and community-based care, provided in therapeutic and residential settings. Beyond treatment itself, which aims at forming a stable and continuous therapeutic framework, social psychiatry encompasses social and vocational rehabilitation and support, advanced training of psychiatric personnel, and sensitization of the community.[75] This core set of practices is meant to facilitate timely intervention into the course of mental illness, and especially the prevention of relapses. The philosophy of social psychiatry, to which these practices are explicitly bound, promotes the following "mission": to secure a high quality of care; to respect the personality and identity, the needs, the dignity, the personal choices, and the wishes of the patient; to provide a stable, safe, and peaceful setting for patients' treatment and everyday life; to restore patients' independence and cultivate their responsibility.[76]

The first seminar in the series—which I attended in the fall of 2002 along with a small group of teachers, priests, police officers, and concerned citizens—introduced the general problematic of psychiatric reform in Greece. We were told that, before reform, psychiatric patients were locked up in state hospitals, "as if in prison," in order to conceal them from society and to protect society from them. The psychoactive medications administered in these hospitals merely suppressed disruptive symptoms, without treating underlying illnesses. The "dehumanizing" effects of institutionalization thus mirrored the clinical symptoms of psychosis: lack of will, low self-esteem, weak ego, disintegration of identity, and loss of social function. Institutionalized patients often lived no more than a "vegetable existence." The humanization of therapeutic practice in the 1980s thus depended on the development of better medications. New antipsychotic and antidepressant drugs, with fewer and safer side effects, achieved a "revolution" in treatment. Patients tolerated their medications rather than resisting them, and as a result they suffered less frequent and milder relapses. As their long-term health took a better course, the time frame of their treatment decreased and, for some, pharmaceutical treatment appeared for the first time as a "short-term approach." This accomplishment opened the space for psychotherapy, which expanded within individual treatment regimes and beyond—into the social, familial, and occupational realms of patients' lives.

According to the Association staff who gave the seminar, social psychiatry in Greece came to address the nonmedical as well as the medical needs of patients—including their "need to love and be loved," to make connections with other people, and to live and think independently. These needs accompanied the liberation of patients from institutions and their restoration to a "natural environment," usually their family home. However, such environments presented special challenges, as relationships between patients and family members were often fraught with shame, ambivalence, and fear. When these "stressors" threatened the stability of patients living at home, social psychiatrists could offer group counseling in an effort to reform the family. Relatives could be educated about the nature and treatment of mental illness and the destructive power of stigma; they could work out their guilt and fear in a therapeutic context, and learn techniques for constructive communication. If, however, a family remained unable to provide a stable environment for a patient, a sheltered residence or group home could be arranged where the patient could be entrained in the "healthy rhythm" of a social life.

With a psychiatry ward nearby at the hospital in Alexandroupolis to address urgent cases, and in the near distance the state psychiatric hospital at Thessaloniki to furnish custodial care in the last resort, the Association invested most of its staffing and infrastructure in Thrace in this new and expanding therapeutic environment in the community. According to Lazaros, a psychologist at the Association, its two vocational rehabilitation programs proved this paradigm of care. Most patients working at the cooperatives were schizophrenics, and their participation entailed supportive therapy along with medication. *Schizophrenia is the most debilitating illness,* Lazaros told me. *It devastates every aspect of a person's life, from work to family to physical health, and these patients are unlikely ever to recover completely. So they always carry with them "the break" made by their illness: they can remember who they used to be before, and they have to bear this loss of self in addition to all their clinical symptoms.* He explained that vocational rehabilitation was designed to help patients combat the grief and frustration occasioned by this loss of self: by following a routine, becoming productive, and collaborating with others, they could recover some of the dignity of their former lives as they constructed a new life around their reduced capacities. The nominal wages patients earned at the cooperatives were meant to symbolize this recuperation of dignity and sociality—though many told me they counted on the money itself as a supplement to their disability income. A therapeutic space of rehabilitation, largely autonomous from the hospital, was the condition for this dignity and this sociality to emerge from the patients' exercise of responsibility.

During the same week in February that Yiannoula was admitted to the hospital clinic for "social reasons," the Association staff met to discuss the case of one of her three sons, a patient of theirs for more than a decade. I had met Pavlos months before, at the Association's farming cooperative. At that time, he described what had seemed to me a fantasy about his family. He told me that he had been raised by a priest in Athens, but that his real family, whom he had not seen since childhood, lived in a village in the hills beyond the farm where we were standing. *They're all sick*, he said, *and it's not good for my health to see them*. It was not until this staff meeting at the Association, months later, that I understood he had been telling me the truth, repeating the words his therapists had spoken to him many times—and that I finally saw converge the parallel tracks of his case at the Association and Yiannoula's at the hospital clinic.

According to Daphne, his psychiatrist, Pavlos had begun to relapse several weeks before. His "descent" was marked by the resurgence of an old delusion that he had a wound in his head. His second therapist, a psychologist, reported that certain elements of his delusional complex had become "frozen and pronounced." And lately, a new element of "religious megalomania" had emerged: *Pavlos is saying now that he's been chosen by God for a special purpose, that God speaks directly to him, and he has greater insight than most people—including his therapists!*

Pavlos was to be the subject of a case presentation that evening by Dr. Politis, a psychiatrist and psychoanalyst who headed the Association at that time. Before Pavlos arrived, Politis provided a medical and biographical history. He had known Pavlos since they began therapy together some ten years before. According to Politis, they had a "special relationship." *You should know*, he instructed the audience, *that Pavlos has a certain reverence for me, which will affect the way he relates to me during the interview.*

According to the history Politis presented, Pavlos was the last biological child born to Yiannoula. His brother and sister, Sakis and Aliki, now lived in the same village as their mother, near Soufli. Another brother, who was "healthy," had "escaped" the family, and now lived elsewhere in Greece. Yiannoula had abused Pavlos as a young child—*not because she's bad*, Politis insisted, *but because she was not equipped to handle her situation. Imagine being psychotic and raising four children without a husband or any financial means!* Once, she burned Pavlos's arm in the fireplace to get rid of an infection; another time, she tried to strangle him to stop his crying. At the age of eight, Pavlos was removed from her custody and adopted by a Catholic missionary and his wife, who lived in Athens and took in abused and abandoned children. Pavlos lived with their large family for many years, but he returned to Thrace at the age of fifteen to enroll in a vocational training program. It was then that he began treatment at the Association.

According to Politis, Pavlos was an unusual case: *It's not clear that he's truly psychotic. Due to the way he was raised, especially in his early childhood, he never had the chance to develop normally. And so he remains mired in the fairy-tale world of a child. His delusions have a mythological quality, rather than clinical characteristics. He gives the impression that he's mentally retarded, but this is not an organic problem. Again, it's the effect of his compromised social development.* When Daphne raised the problem of Pavlos's recent relapse, Politis gently corrected her diagnostic language: *Better to use terms like "myth" and "dream" than "delusion" and "megalomania." Pavlos is in a different category of illness from the rest of his family.*

During the interview itself, in response to Politis's questions, Pavlos offered a straightforward narrative of his life. (In the discussion afterward, his other therapists expressed surprise at the precision and fluidity of his speech; they were more accustomed to a scattered rush of fragments and tangents.) When Politis asked how he had been feeling lately, Pavlos mentioned trouble with what he called his "emotional wound" — a hole in his head. He attributed it to his rejection by a girl at a bus stop: *I used to see her all the time. I thought we were friends; I thought she liked me, but that day she showed me she didn't. That's when the pain started.* Politis gently challenged this story, and Pavlos eventually admitted, *I guess I was wounded earlier, by my mother.*

Later in the interview, Politis asked Pavlos for his thoughts on the Association. *What does it do for you to come here? Does it help you?* Pavlos immediately agreed: *Yes, it's great, it helps me. You all really care for me.*

— *But what about the bad, Pavlo?*
— *There's no bad!*
— *Well, from everything we experience we take both good and bad, right?*

Pavlos nodded agreement. Politis tried once more: *Are you agreeing with me just to please me? Don't be afraid to tell me the bad things — surely there must be something bad, and we need to know about it. It will help us to help you.*

Pavlos again agreed. *Well, there's lots on the good side. The people here take good care of me. I like having conversations with them. Dr. Daphne always helps me stay in "the here and now," and not get stuck on the past. But, on the bad side . . . I've lost a lot of strength and flexibility since I started coming to the Association. From my medications. I've gotten fat and slow, and I'm really tired. I'm only twenty-five years old, I should have more energy. That's why I want to start acupuncture and yoga, to get back the strength I used to have.*

In the discussion afterward, Politis flagged this comment as a moment of "clear logical thinking" on Pavlos's part: *He really understands what it means to be healthy.*

❋ ❋ ❋

In July, having long since recovered from his winter "descent," Pavlos visited his adoptive family in Athens, as he did every summer. They planned to drive him back to Thrace at the end of the month. He had asked them if, while they were in the area, they would take him to visit his "natural family" for the first time in fifteen years. His adoptive parents responded ambivalently, and called Daphne for advice. At a staff meeting, Daphne told us she considered such a visit completely out of the question: *It would really damage Pavlos to see the environment his mother and siblings are living in. Pavlos is by far the healthiest member of the family, and it would be a shock for him to see the people and the conditions that he came from.*

That Pavlos had escaped those people and those conditions as a child, without developing "true psychosis" or suffering organic damage, was crucial to his qualification as an adult subject for therapy. Though his regular therapists seemed to see Pavlos as a typical schizophrenic, Politis discovered for them his superior faculties, including some understanding of his health, which rendered him responsible, "to an extent," for his own care. And indeed Pavlos had already proven himself an eager and capable participant in the entire spectrum of outpatient services offered by the Association: in addition to undertaking regular pharmaceutical treatment and counseling, he lived in a group home, worked at the farming cooperative, and attended a socialization group.

The comparison, on the basis of competency, between Pavlos and his family—who, being more ill, received less therapeutic support—gained explicit articulation only in the directive to keep a distance between them. His therapists sought to protect Pavlos from the threat still posed to his mental health by his family: the threat of poverty and social isolation that Yiannoula and her other children faced; inhumane conditions that forced them all, at one time or another, to take refuge in the hospital clinic, disputing the benefit of life "in the community." But was it these conditions that his therapists imagined would come as a shock to Pavlos? Or was it, rather, the discrepancy between these conditions and his own that posed the threat? Would Pavlos, bearing an attachment to his family that his therapists did not share or support, find this discrepancy confusing, unjust, or shameful? Did they fear that their responsibility for this confusion, injustice, or shame would be exposed by his visit? Enclosed in the secret of Pavlos's family was a contradiction in the practice of community-based psychiatry: a restriction of its humanitarian universalism by the logic of scarce resources, which permitted a correlation to emerge between the competencies of patients and the conditions of their lives "in the community."

Yet more than resources were invested in the competence of patients like Pavlos. Clinical work at the Association carried, for some, the anticipation that patients might present the possibility of a meaningful therapeutic relationship. This anticipation, marking scarcity of a different kind, was engrained in their psychodynamic training, and modeled by Politis himself, who had emphasized his "special relationship" with Pavlos from the start.

But that relationship had its limits. Before his case presentation at the Association, months before, Politis had told the assembled audience that Pavlos used to love to play the recorder, which he called a "flute." His adoptive parents had given the flute to him when he came to live with them, and he took to it eagerly. *He played it for years, with their encouragement,* Politis told us. *He put on little performances for the whole family.* But Pavlos had left the flute with his family in Athens when he moved back to Thrace. He had often spoken about it with Politis. *He said he left it with his family because it was broken and needed repair. But it's significant that Pavlos has put off this repair for so long. It's like his emotional wound, you see. He's made a sacrifice of it, symbolically.*

During their interview, Politis broached the flute straight away. He asked Pavlos to tell us what he had told Politis about it in the past. Pavlos said that he could not really remember. Politis tried to remind him but hit a dead end with Pavlos, who seemed confused by his leading questions. Politis frowned and moved on. In the discussion afterward, one of the therapists in the audience observed that Politis had "really pushed" Pavlos at that moment, and showed disappointment in him. Politis agreed: *I was attempting to establish a genuine therapeutic relation with Pavlos; I thought the flute was a way to do this. But I failed, because Pavlos isn't capable of thinking* symbolically. He can't make the connection that the flute is more than just an object—that he lost it because he lost other things, and that he's holding on to that loss. Those of you who work with Pavlos should understand that you'll never be able to do true psychotherapy with him. He can't achieve insight into his own psychology. The best we can do is support him. But that's already a lot.

PART 1

False Face

ON DIAGNOSIS AND METHOD

The process of mutually sustaining a definition of the situation in face-to-face interaction is socially organized through rules of relevance and irrelevance. These rules for the management of engrossment appear to be an insubstantial element of social life, a matter of courtesy, manners, and etiquette. But it is to these flimsy rules, and not to the unshaking character of the external world, that we owe our unshaking sense of realities. To be at ease in a situation is to be properly subject to these rules, entranced by the meanings they generate and stabilize; to be ill at ease means that one is ungrasped by immediate reality and that one loosens the grasp that others have of it. To be awkward or unkempt, to talk or move wrongly, is to be a dangerous giant, a destroyer of worlds. As every psychotic and comic ought to know, any accurately improper move can poke through the thin sleeve of immediate reality.
—ERVING GOFFMAN, "Fun in Games"

On a late spring morning at the hospital in Alexandroupolis, I sat with Lina, a first-year psychiatric resident, and Dr. Angelidi, her supervisor, as they saw visitors to the outpatient clinic. A nurse called for the next patient, and two women entered the consultation room without a medical file that would indicate a history of treatment here. The older of the two, training her gaze at the floor rather than at the two doctors, did not speak as she awkwardly took a seat on the far side of their desk. Her

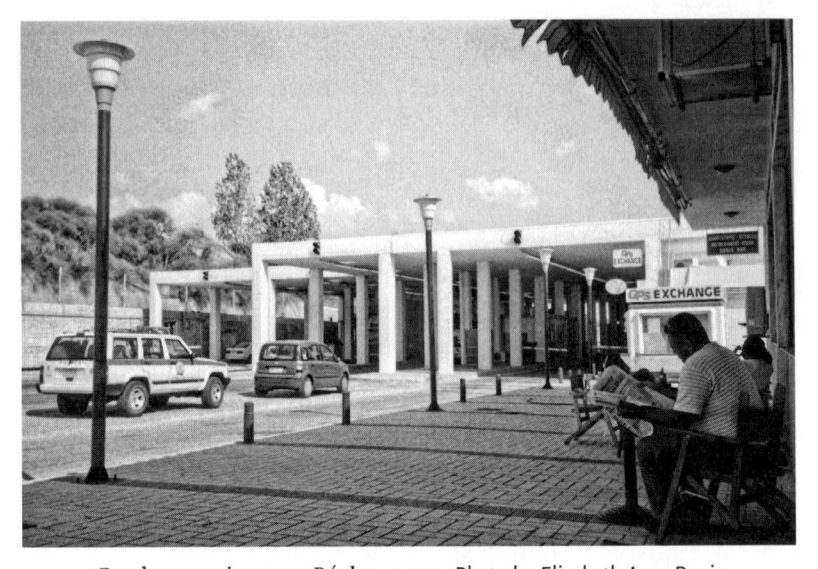

Border crossing near Péplos, 2004. *Photo by Elizabeth Anne Davis*

young companion, when invited to join her, spoke out loudly: *No, I'm not sick. Just write a paper* [χαρτί] *for this poor soul!* They were seeking a certification of diagnosis (γνωμάτευση).

Angelidi addressed the silent woman seated across from her: *Tell me why you've come, dear.* The young woman again spoke in her place, again loudly: *Listen, first I'll talk, then you can talk.* Lina shook her head and threw down her pen. They were off to a bad start.

> Angelidi: *Please sit down. I'm trying to talk to the patient.*
>
> Young woman (still standing): *She doesn't talk. I told you, I'm doing the talking.*
>
> Lina (to the young woman): *All right, then you can tell us what's wrong with the patient.*
>
> Young woman: *She's sick* [άρρωστη] *and she's stupid* [χαζή]. *You give her a plate of food to eat and she just throws it on the floor. She can't do anything for herself.*
>
> Angelidi: *But what's her diagnosis? What illness* [αρρώστια] *does she have?*
>
> Young woman: *I don't know. Look in her booklet and you'll see what medications she takes.*
>
> Angelidi: *But that doesn't tell me what illness she has!*
>
> Young woman: *Can't you tell from the medications?*

Angelidi (reading through the prescription booklet): *She sees a doctor at Komotini Hospital? Why didn't you take her there today?*

Young woman: *I don't know, I thought it was the same to come here.*

Angelidi: *No, it's not. The doctor in Komotini knows the patient already, and knows what illness she has. So that doctor can write her a paper with the diagnosis. I don't know her at all—I'd have to see her three more times before I could diagnose her for sure.*

Young woman (pausing): *Three more times we have to come back here?*

Angelidi: *It would be much easier for you to take her to her regular doctor in Komotini.*

Young woman: *Why can't you just write the paper for her? It wasn't easy for me to come here. This woman has no one, no family or friends to take care of her, she's poor, she has nothing. She's obviously very sick.*

Angelidi: *She may be sick, but I don't know how she's sick. That's what I have to write on the paper.*

After another round of refusals, the two women left without a paper certifying the patient's diagnosis. Dr. Angelidi explained to me when they had gone that the young woman may have been attempting a scam: the patient, who was indeed "obviously sick," no doubt already had a certification from her doctor in Komotini. *So maybe her friend was looking for another paper that she could put in a false name,* Angelidi said. *Then she could sell it, or use it herself, as a way to get disability income.* For all parties to this encounter, diagnosis meant knowledge of disability, and thus official means for a patient who couldn't "do anything for herself" to earn support from the state. Withholding diagnosis was a way for Angelidi to avert deception on this score, even if the patient was, to her mind, legitimately ill. But while the conflict between the clinicians and the patient's advocate here may have arisen partly from this unspoken mistrust, it was elaborated in terms of incompatible conceptions of diagnosis. For Angelidi, diagnosis named a process of getting to know the patient over time, in order to determine the specific illness entity that disabled her. The young woman, by contrast, took diagnosis as knowledge of a general condition of illness: knowledge that could easily be deduced from medications, or from one look at the sick patient. This knowledge required an expert appraisal, but the young woman took that appraisal as a mere formality and an immediate entitlement for the patient.

Diagnosis derives from the Greek word *diagignoskein* (to discern, distinguish), comprising *dia-* (through) and *gignoskein* (to come to know, perceive): the art or act of identifying a disease from its signs and symptoms.[1] In this section, I explore the manifold gnosis within diagnosis, and the arts of discernment on which that knowledge turned in the clinics of Thrace.

Games of Truth

In 1980, reflecting on the changing character of the social sciences "in recent years," Clifford Geertz named Erving Goffman the leader of a "swarm of scholars" contributing to "the game analogy" as an emerging genre of social theory. For Geertz, the versatile "gamelike conceptions of social life" that Goffman so voraciously deployed depended on a conception of social actors as strategists, committed to playing "enigmatical games whose structure is clear but whose point is not." It is this pointlessness that brought Geertz to discern, in Goffman's work, not only a nonhumanist approach but also a "radically unromantic vision of things, acrid and bleakly knowing . . . but no less powerful for that."[2]

Perhaps an unlikely comrade in other ways, Foucault meets Goffman on that terrain of games. He finds there a point that Geertz could not see in Goffman's depiction of social actors' "self-rewarding" submission to rules: namely, to maneuver around the effects of power on the field of truth. To an interviewer's question about access to "truth in the political sense," by which he meant a truth that, if aired, would break up the "blockages" of power, Foucault replied, "This is indeed a problem. After all, why truth? . . . I think we are touching on a fundamental question here, what I would call *the* question for the West. How did it come about that all of Western culture began to revolve around this obligation of truth which has taken a lot of different forms? . . . Things being as they are, nothing so far has shown that it is possible to define a strategy outside of this concern. It is within the field of obligation to truth that it is possible to move about in one way or another, sometimes against effects of domination which may be linked to structures of truth or institutions entrusted with truth."[3] Foucault's response indicates that truth in the "political sense" that interests his interviewer promises only a delusory liberation from power. He proffers the alternative notion of truth as a game, radically circumscribed by its implication in power. He defines *truth game* as "a set of rules by which truth is produced . . . a set of procedures that lead to a certain result, which, on the basis of its principles and rules of procedure, may be considered valid or invalid, winning or losing."[4] Since there is no effective strategy of thought outside the "field of obligation to truth," critique can be achieved "only . . . by playing a certain game of truth," but "differently," at a distance.[5]

Likewise, truth games for Foucault are not just "concealed power relations"; thus one can examine power relations in the truth game of psychiatry, for example, without "impugning [its] scientific validity or therapeutic effectiveness."[6] Rather than being falsified by its alliance with power, it is precisely in this alliance that truth becomes a strategic possibility. Foucault defines *strategy* as the rationality by which an end is sought; as the seeking of advantage in relation to an opponent's strategy; and as the means of obtaining victory, particularly when it is a matter of depriving an opponent of those means. These three definitions, he says, "come together in situations of confrontation—war or games."[7] Since they are played according to rationalities, principles, and rules, I will observe—and this is a point about psychiatry that I will demonstrate ethnographically throughout this book—that if truth games, like wars, may be declared won or lost only once they are over, they can also be conducted badly and interminably.

In this book, I treat clinical diagnosis as a truth game, not only at the level of institutionally legitimized power indicated in Foucault's definition, but also at the level of confrontation between parties to the diagnostic encounter—a confrontation between discrepant strategies of truth. This second level of the truth game is the object of Pierre Bourdieu's theory of practice: a theory, as he proposes in *The Logic of Practice*, of "what it is to be 'native.'"[8] This is to be the player of a game—to be engaged in the "*real play* of social practices" such as ritual, gift exchange, and work.[9] Bourdieu mobilizes game-playing as a metaphor for the kind of knowledge employed in these practices, in order to evoke the "practical sense" manifested in a player's "skill, dexterity, delicacy, or *savoir-faire*" in a game, or the "feel for the game" implied by "native membership in a field."[10] In "actual" games, like chess, he argues, the game is "clearly seen for what it is, an arbitrary social construct";[11] but in the social practices that he treats as metaphorical games, players remain unaware of the constructed nature of the stakes and presuppositions. Game-playing in this sense requires "self-deception" of a particular kind, which Bourdieu labels the *illusio* of the game—the player's interest, his or her investment in what is at stake, as opposed to the objective truth of the game's social function.[12] Nativity entails having already passed through the gradual process of initiation by which the disposition to play the game is learned and its objective truth repressed. It means having a body that "takes metaphor seriously" and "believes in what it plays at."[13]

Bourdieu's theory of practice as native game-playing is a sharp tool for analyzing the unconscious nature of strategy, without hypostatizing any particular unconscious—least of all, perhaps, the one modeled by psychoanalysis. This theory of practice makes sense of the fact that certain kinds of questions "never arise" when players are "caught up in the game."[14] Questions about the coherence of the game, broached by contradictions between its theoretical and practical elements, remain unasked by players because they play the game over time, rather than within the totalizing temporality of the synchronic model. As opposed to this theoretical logic of the model, Bourdieu describes the logic of practice as "fuzzy," "convenient," "easy to master and use," "poor and economical": in the temporality of action, its loose and imperfect nature does not impeach its coherence.[15] Theoretical questions about coherence are not, for Bourdieu, of the same order as those "excluded" as "unthinkable" by the logic of practice—those that expose the objective truth of the game, which is to say its social function, and the relations of domination hidden within it that naturalize and legitimize the strategies of the privileged.[16]

In the next section, I turn to the former questions—those that "never arise" in practice—to analyze clinical diagnosis. My procedure is to discern the moral judgments expressed in diagnostic practice, as articulated by experts, and to assemble these judgments into something like a logic of the diagnostic truth game. This logic is a "common sense" that I believe clinicians, as its more privileged players, might recognize if asked, but that they are not disposed to articulate, since what this logic is transparent to is not their practice but my critical inquiry.[17]

Yet this threshold of transparency is the point at which Bourdieu ceases to guide my approach to the practice of clinical diagnosis. For Bourdieu, practice itself and theoretical knowledge about practice occupy discrepant orders of logic. They may be reconciled only through the conceptual instrument of habitus—both the "embodied history" of practice and the "immanent law" that regulates and describes it functionally.[18] The moral judgments that I present in this text, on the other hand, are of the same logical order as the diagnostic practices in which they are embedded, as well as the order of my own analysis and the critical responses of patients. My position as an outside observer therefore does not confer an essentially special capacity to perceive the logic of this game. It is entirely possible for a player to see this logic at work in clinical practice, to assimilate it theoretically, and to speak with me about it. I imagine that such a conversation could take place without creating a logical impasse—and certainly without, as Bourdieu puts it, "totally breaking the spell" of practice.[19]

Likewise, I cannot describe psychiatric practice as a habitus of "learned ignorance."[20] This practice, like my own clinical work, is a matter of theoretical second-order reflection that participates in the development of theory about itself, and that is therefore permeable to reflection about it. What differentiates my intervention from the clinical practice of psychiatrists, then, is not a special claim to objective description, but rather its alliance to a different goal: not therapy, but critique.

It is in light of this transparency of practical logic to itself that I characterize the clinical encounter as a game—although not metaphorically, as Bourdieu would have it, since its constructedness is very much in play. This game does not exclude as "unthinkable" questions about its ultimate truth. In their everyday confrontation with patients, the clinicians I cite here were well aware of disputation over the truth of diagnosis, and thus over the legitimacy of their authority to practice it. Far from being uncritical automatons caught in *illusio*, these clinicians self-consciously operated in a space of play, where they occupied a variety of moral positions within and between partial regimes of truth. Like Quesalid, the unhappy shaman depicted by Claude Lévi-Strauss in "The Sorcerer and His Magic," they were ethically engaged in a conscious deliberation on the truth of their practice, often becoming convinced in the process of its efficacy, yet finally unable to determine their own good faith.[21] They were aware that the apparatus of clinical diagnosis naturalized their privilege and authority, which arose from grounds additional to their mere expertise; and that the truths it yielded were inconclusive, unstable, and strategic. In practice, as I observed it, this awareness was voiced—not as transcendental truth, but as context-specific doubt—in consultations and arguments among clinicians, in their negotiations with patients, and in my conversations with them. It is this lack of scientific and moral certainty in the clinical orientation to truth—this witting absence of secure grounding, often expressed in the mode of irony—that leads me to view diagnosis as an "actual" game.

The practical logic of clinical diagnosis thus comprehends its own strategy, even as it reproduces that strategy. My attention to commu-

nicative disruptions in diagnostic encounters is intended to shed light
on this double consciousness by which clinicians speak the discourse of
truth while, in its margins, speaking a discourse of doubt. This double
consciousness does, as Bourdieu predicts, yield an impasse—but this
impasse is not located where he finds it, between theoretical and practical logic. Rather, as the renowned activist psychiatrist Franco Basaglia
insisted, it resides in the "social fabric" and in the political economy that
promote a humanitarian ethics for psychiatry but withhold the resources
and confound the reorganization of governance that might allow this
ethics to materialize in practice.[22] As I showed in the prelude to this text,
Greek psychiatrists perceive this impasse as a moral as well as a governmental deficit, expressed in a rhetoric of backwardness—a rhetoric that
orients itself to the fantasy of truth symbolized by modern, Western, progressive medicine, and more specifically, by scientific advances in biopsychiatry.

αυτός έφα

The critique of psychiatry as a discourse of truth is a fertile and crowded
field, both within psychiatry itself and in associated disciplines in the
social sciences. One approach, arising with the early phases of international psychiatric reform, voiced a denunciation of institutional psychiatry from a position of explicit moralism. The foundational thought
of Basaglia in Italy, of R. D. Laing in Great Britain, and of Thomas Szasz
in the United States, among others, sought to reveal the construction of
psychiatric truth through coercive power, both to liberate patients from
their institutional domination and to develop new therapeutic avenues
to the truth of madness.[23] In its more strident moments, this critique of
psychiatry appears as precisely the sort of delusory emancipatory project
that Foucault dismantles with his analytic device of the truth game. Goffman, in his work on asylums, redirects this critique toward a different
objective: he evacuates the unmasking process of its therapeutic mandate, revealing the psychiatric institution as a field of power that mirrors
social relations outside the institution, particularly hierarchical "service
relations."[24] But since mental illness, from this point of view, can only
provide a framework for status-seeking strategies inside the institution,
Goffman declines to account for madness as a question of truth.

A more contemporary and less emancipatory critique of psychiatry has
emerged from the field of medical anthropology. Wedded to the ethno-

graphic task of describing and contextualizing healing practices while "bracketing" the truths that authorize them,[25] some medical anthropologists have provisionally ceded the ground of truth to those authorized in the field of psychiatric power.[26] The ethical distance they effect by bracketing truth carries a responsibility not to question its authorization, as a matter of descriptivist restraint in elaborating local criteria. Since healers of the psyche deal with vulnerable people who suffer, this practice of bracketing truth renders the anthropological inquiry a moral field, in which controversies in knowledge about madness are adjudicated in terms of the moral authority of the healers. Bracketing truth thus sharpens the moralizing vector of the anthropological critique, but without offering a resolution to the ethical predicaments posed by the production of knowledge about madness in a field of power. In suspending alliance to any truth game, this bracketing risks concealing the determination of truth by one particular game—the one in which most anthropologists are "native" players.

Clinical diagnosis is the key to the problematic status of truth in contemporary psychiatry. Its global truth game is increasingly monopolized by cutting-edge research conducted for multinational pharmaceutical corporations in psychopharmacology and, at its speculative outer limits, pharmacogenomics.[27] But this monopoly, arising through the imbrication of laboratory research with expanding international consumer markets,[28] reinforces the dependence of pharmaceutical research on clinical knowledge. The development of new medications and diagnostic techniques begins and ends with profiles of patient populations generated in the clinic, whether these are profiles of illness identified through standard diagnostic interviews, or purportedly more specific medication-response profiles that suspend ontological questions about illness-entities.[29] Diagnosis remains the leading procedure by which psychiatric knowledge attains to truth.

It is therefore crucial to observe the provisionality of clinical diagnosis on two levels. First, diagnosis is based primarily on patients' reports about their own experience and behavior, and therefore wholly mediated by speech in all its potential ambiguity and duplicity. In this sense, language has even more diagnostic significance in community-based psychiatry than in antecedent forms of institutional care, as therapists come to rely ever more heavily on what patients say about their lives outside direct clinical supervision.[30] Second, the link remains tenuous between the clinical profiles generated through diagnosis, on the one hand,

and the biochemistry, neurophysiology, and genetics of mental illness, on the other. Advances in diagnostic specificity in the clinic, or in laboratory knowledge of neurotransmission, do little to consolidate or concretize the link between them. The vulnerability of clinical knowledge thus substantially implicates biochemical, neurological, and genetic knowledge of mental illness.

This question of "the unknown," rooted in the unreliability of speech, looms large in psychiatry in all its developing scientific facets. It has been posed persistently to psychiatry, both within and outside the field, at least since the political critiques and therapeutic experiments of the 1960s, now broadly associated with the antipsychiatry movement.[31] While the backlash in psychiatry and adjacent fields has dismissed antipsychiatry as simplistic, moralistic, and antiscientific, psychiatry today remains vulnerable to criticism of its nosological uncertainty and low rates of therapeutic success.[32] The psychiatric discourse on the unknown is, itself, a mechanism of clinical knowledge. Diagnosis is the focus of my own analysis because it so cleanly demarcates the arena in which the play between what is known and what is not known in the clinic is routinized in practice.

❋ ❋ ❋

—She doesn't talk. I told you, I'm doing the talking.
—She may be sick, but I don't know how she's sick. That's what I have to write on the paper.

In a sustained critique of "linguistic ideology" in interpretive anthropology, Vincent Crapanzano tracks the ruses of language, including the appearance of diagnosis as mere description.[33] Crapanzano is concerned with the interpretation of communicative phenomena in the sociocultural field that can be described as either semantico-referential, in the form of propositions that convey information, or pragmatic, having an efficiency in the fields of power and desire that they reflect and create. On his account, Western social science uses only semantico-referential language to interpret both semantico-referential and pragmatic communication, with their radically different functions and orientations to truth. He argues that the dominance of the semantico-referential at the metalevel obscures these differences, generating a closed interpretive system whose pragmatic determination is constantly reinforced by the "truthful" interpretation of data that only apparently exists independent of pragmatic context. Social science thus "represses" the pragmatics of its own metapragmatics as it develops a metalanguage in the semantico-referential mode,[34] obfuscating the location of its truth claims in a field of power and desire.

The ruses by which semantico-referential claims of interpretation conceal their pragmatic determinants are often metaphors. Pivotal to Crapanzano's critique of linguistic ideology is his emphasis on the meta-phorical nature of semantico-referential metalanguage in social science and its aptness for disguising the moral questions analysis presents as epistemological questions of interpretation (if moral questions are those that could be addressed pragmatically). It is a ruse of literalism in ethnography, for example, that takes the speech of informants as true representations of their inner states—their beliefs—and thus gener-ates psychological metaphors as so many semantico-referential truth claims to comprehend their pragmatic communication in the sociocul-tural field.[35] In this way, diagnostic or symptomatic interpretations of communication are naturalized as realistic description.[36] Crapanzano intimates the possibility of a noncircular understanding of the rela-tion between communication and forms of interpretive knowledge—an analysis of the ways in which metapragmatic interpretive systems are determined within economic and political arrangements in the socio-cultural field. Yet this is not the direction he takes. His own admittedly arbitrary and ambivalent critical tactic is to select language itself as the object of his interpretation, developing an interpretive language—a semantico-referential method of interpreting the pragmatics of commu-nication—that remains safe from psychologizing metaphor.

An analysis of clinical diagnosis that neither takes for granted its ref-erential truth, nor seeks to disqualify it, would prioritize the pragmatics of communication. It would attend to what patients and therapists are doing when they talk about mental illness: the ways in which this talk produces material, social, and emotional effects; and the field of power and desire that enables and conditions this efficacy. According to this schema, communication in the clinic could be parsed into two modes. In the semantic mode, patients and therapists communicate about illness in terms of clinical diagnosis and treatment. In the pragmatic mode, the language of patients registers symptomatically, manifesting their diag-nosed illness, while the language of therapists registers rhetorically, per-suading rather than informing patients in regard to the corresponding treatment.

Consider, in this light, an encounter I witnessed at a regional health center in Thrace. Dora, a psychiatrist and the head of the Association's mobile unit at the health center, welcomed my participation in her meetings with patients. The only one whose treatment sessions were off limits to me was Stavros, whom Dora described as a "very difficult patient," one who "could not be cured." Dora avoided their sessions, herself—often, instead, holding rushed and improvised consultations with Stavros in the open vestibule of the health center where he would wait for us to arrive every other week. He knew when we were coming. He would fetch us coffee from the vending machine, and help set up the table the staff used as a makeshift intake desk, all the while assailing Dora with greetings and requests for refills on his medications. In the first such encounter I witnessed between them, Dora tried gently to put him off: *I have to see these other patients first, Stavro. They really need our help.* Stavros agreed: *I know; you're right. But I need your help, too. . . . Could you just write me this refill? And then I won't bother you again.* Dora was adamant: *We've discussed this, Stavro. You're not due for a refill on this one yet.* She pointed to the empty box of sedatives that Stavros was holding out to her. *See the date here? How come you need it now?* Stavros pocketed the box. *I took a lot of extra pills this month. I had to. I've been so upset about my father.*

That morning, Stavros had called Dora to request an appointment, saying he was desperate over his father's death the previous week. Yet Dora told me she doubted his father was dead: *At least three times this year Stavros has told me that his mother just died. But when I'd call to check on him, his mother would answer the phone. He does this kind of thing, he exaggerates his situation. It's not just to get refills, though. I think he also wants attention from me.*

Stavros was in his early twenties, tall but malnourished and losing his teeth. He took methamphetamines, Dora told me, but he had gotten addicted first to sedatives—Stedon (US Valium), Tavor (US Ativan), Hipnosedon (US Rohypnol)—while under psychiatric care for depression during his teenage years. *But it's not a straightforward case of addiction, if such a thing exists,* Dora said. *He's paranoid and pathologically dishonest. He probably has a personality disorder.* This diagnosis tended to be confirmed by the clinical evidence of his poor response to the assorted medications Dora had prescribed: not only sedatives, but also antidepressants, which had "calmed him down" without altering the nature of his symptoms. *Likely there's a history of mental illness in his family. It would help me diagnose him if I knew about his family, but I can't get a good history because he lies all the time.*

Dispatched to the corner of the vestibule that morning to wait his turn, Stavros began to argue with a fellow patient, who was complaining about his failure to "follow the rules" of the clinic. Stavros again approached Dora at the intake table, this time more determined:

> Stavros: Look, I can't stay here like this. I really need to talk to you.
> Dora: I know you want to talk to me, but I can't right now. We'll talk in a little while.
> Stavros: But can't you just write this one for me? Then I can go to the pharmacy and it's done.
> Dora: You know I can't just write you a prescription. We need to discuss your problems. It's very bad for you to take these medications without therapy.
> Stavros: But I want to talk! You're the one who won't talk.

In reminding Stavros of their past discussions, Dora asserted her medical authority through truth claims referring to the patient's illness and treatment: she agreed with Stavros that his medications were necessary, but insisted they had to be accompanied by therapy in order to do any good. Evidently seeking an exit from the encounter, she demoted Stavros's avowed "need to talk" to a mere desire, clouding the clarity of even this claim on her attention through indirect moral incriminations of Stavros's demand for drugs. The immediate presence in the vestibule of other patients more in need of help than Stavros bolstered this effort at delegitimation.

Yet Stavros was able to wield the same pragmatic tool of moralism against his doctor, pointing out the contradiction between Dora's insistence on talking as part of Stavros's treatment and her refusal to engage in it. In tone, gesture, and outright demand, Stavros performed a clinical need that rose above his desire for drugs, wresting clinical significance from Dora's own moralistic interpretation. Thus, on reflection later that afternoon, Dora admitted to me: *Even though Stavros's father is alive in reality, there's a sense in which he is dead to Stavros. He abandoned Stavros and his mother a few years ago, when Stavros was a teenager, and now he comes and goes as he pleases. But he doesn't give them any help or money. I think he's an alcoholic, and he probably has a personality disorder—so he's completely unreliable. No doubt Stavros inherited his problems from this guy.*

A pragmatic analysis of this scene would begin by identifying the factors that determine the pragmatic functions of speech, showing how communication between Dora and Stavros both advanced their desires and reflected their positioning in a dynamic of power. But—as attested by their debate over the urgency of talking—the pragmatic and the semantico-referential functions of language cannot be reliably distinguished in this scene. The psychiatric clinic is a site for the production and application of scientific knowledge; its field of power and desire is organized by this knowledge, granting an essentially pragmatic function even to the semantico-referential language in which truth claims are articulated. It is their apparent access to the scientific truth of diagnosis that authorizes therapists' power over and against patients' in this context. The truth function of language merges here with the performative, in a mode distinct from the double functionality of Austinian constatives that inform while they represent.[37] In the clinic, the performative function of truth exceeds the propositional capacity of the constative—becoming, itself, a medium of power in therapeutic negotiations.

This powerful clinical cocktail of semantic and pragmatic language is the substance of Szasz's critique of psychiatry. Szasz uses the paradigm of hysteria—a form of "indirect communication" by which a patient expresses her needs, desires, and problems through signs of the body—to argue that mental illness is not a medical disease that can be cured, but rather the negotiated outcome of a communicative game.[38] Szasz describes all communication as a metagame in which players observe and negotiate the rules of play. The criteria for skillful game-playing, he contends, are always moral, because they constitute values about how players ought to orient the power dynamic between them—as coercion, cooperation, mutual autonomy, or reciprocity.[39] For Szasz, the fact that communicative games involve a negotiation of such conflicting moral values is the great masked secret of therapeutic encounters. If the players—therapists and patients—were to acknowledge a genuine conflict between their values, this would undermine the authority by which therapists control the criteria of the game, thus "threatening the prestige and power of the psychiatric profession."[40]

In this line, though with a different end, I treat psychiatry as a uniquely pragmatic field of communication, and truth claims as strategies in a game structured pragmatically by the valorization of truth. In the clinical encounters I have observed, I have learned from therapists and patients to register the weight and the force of words uttered under such conditions, in a dynamic of power animated by the imperative to tell the truth.[41] But I have also learned, from other sources, not to adequate these potent words to clinical diagnosis. A number of anthropologists model techniques of detachment from clinical diagnosis, in ambivalent engagements with psychoanalysis that seek to capture its attentiveness to the dynamics of encounter and speech without reproducing its arguably incidental ontological hypostases of psyche and subjectivity. Crapanzano, as indicated earlier, takes language to evoke an "external vantage point" on diverse idioms of experience and knowledge relating to "'psychological' processes," including those of spirit possession and the unconscious, thereby relativizing both the interpretive position of the anthropologist and the diagnostic position of the healer.[42] Stefania Pandolfo turns to psychoanalysis not as a diagnostic device, but as a hermeneutic idiom in which to occupy an ethical stance of noninstrumental listening.[43] Katherine Ewing puts the hermeneutics of psychoanalysis in relation to those of sociolinguistics and literary criticism, crafting a heterodox interpretive approach to the "conflicts, compromises, and multiple intentions that play a key role in generating the specific utterances and actions" that emerge in anthropological interviews.[44] This approach apprehends the ways in which subjects and interviewers adopt and recast their identities in relation to one another—a dynamic process, Ewing notes, with knowing and unknowing moments for both parties.

The field of objects I examine in part 1 of this text is delimited by this dynamic process of communication, considered not only as the expression of meaning but also as the enactment of power. The work of the ethnographic scenes I present is to characterize such language pragmatically, in relation to its localized determinants. These determinants shift from scene to scene, but they achieve a loose unity in the moralism of responsibility. Diagnosis is a fundamentally moral activity here, not only because it transpires in relations of care between people unequal in power—though what constitutes this power, and who has the upper hand, is not always clear[45]—but also because it proceeds according to the rules of a game played for truth. The will to truth, as Nietzsche has it, always stages a moral ground: its rationality is based not in a desire not to *be* deceived—for "both truth and untruth constantly prov[e] to be useful" in science[46]—but rather in an injunction not to deceive others,[47] shored up by all the pieties and contingent objectives that mitigate against dishonesty. This moral injunction produces a responsibility to tell the truth that weighs on therapists and patients alike, though in different regards and measures.

If, as Crapanzano warns, psychological metaphors often disguise moral questions as epistemological problems for social science, then in analyzing the moralism that inhabits diagnosis, I attempt to address that masked moral significance directly, without speculating on the psychological motives of those who enunciate it. But I do not treat verbal speech in this text as a privileged register of communication. Instead, I interpret speech as a form of communication that collaborates or collides with nondiscursive forms, such as behavioral symptoms, which may function as strategies of countermoralism. Symptoms and speech together constitute, for patients, a language of the body that expresses a range of intentional dispositions to conscience and critique: from overt deceit, to indirect manipulation, to unwitting negativity. The moralism of responsibility that governs this communication provides the path by which my analysis diverges methodologically from clinical diagnosis, though it often takes the same communicative material as its object.

Throughout this text, I have tried to present that object—what was communicated, as it was communicated—according to a classification of its functions.[48] Speech that I reproduce verbatim appears in direct quotation. I use italics to paraphrase or recollect speech, reconstructed from detailed notes; and indirect discourse to paraphrase or recollect speech in my own interpretive voice. Finally, I employ free indirect discourse to present communication whose function exceeds the speakers' and my own interpretive voices. This mode of discourse—which Pandolfo, drawing on Gilles Deleuze, uses in her singular ethnography to voice "speech acts with many heads"[49]—calls forth a collective experience, but not necessarily the truth of that experience. Often, in this text, free indirect discourse evokes the confabulations and confusions of collective experience.

The therapists who speak here do not do so as representatives of a consensus on psychiatric diagnosis. They articulate localized fragments of an internally varied discourse, showing just how unlikely is the achievement of coherence in this context. There is no symbolization of their communication with patients that could be recuperated in a closed hermeneutic system such as psychoanalysis. Nor is their presentation in this text a mere mapping of their positions on a knowledge/power grid, for this field is dynamic, and its subject positions relational, transferable, transient, in play.

In orienting my analysis to communication, I heed the caution offered by Nikolas Rose regarding ontological precipitates of the interpretation of language. Rose takes issue with dominant hermeneutical methods that "inescapably posit the human agent as the core of sense-making activities," imagining the constitution of selves or subjects by grammar ("subjectifying the speaker"), by narrative ("storying the self"), or by communication (the "banal model" of negotiating meaning through dialogue).[50] Taking Foucault's *Archaeology of Knowledge* as a template, Rose proposes an alternative view of language as "assemblage," a set of "enunciative modalities" or "regimes of signification"[51] that do not generate stable subjects of speech, but rather a structure of intelligibility composed of relations between positions in which discrete discursive practices are performed. In the contemporary array of "psy-" phenomena, Rose critically observes the consolidation of a regime of signification in which the model of subjectivity theorized by the hermeneutics of suspicion—a subjectivity that contains a psychological interior, develops along the contours of a biographical history, and expresses itself in intentional speech—appears self-evident.

In light of this critical framework of assemblage, I trace the complex determination of communicative exchanges elsewhere than solely in the moment of clinical encounter—including the broad and multisited discursive formation of diagnosis, as well as essentially unlocalized sites like the unconscious. To the extent that this framework emphasizes and accounts for the intelligibility of discourse, however, it does not meet the demands of the communicative field in which I worked, where the regime of signification was unable to govern the discursive practices it generated. The disruptive power of ambiguity and deception in clinical encounters attests to the importance of meaningful communication to the analysis of power in this context—against Rose's insistence on a strong distinction between what language "means" and what it "does," between "inscription" and "technology."[52] The scenes of communication that I present are often unable to conclude: the speech is confused, or dishonest, or neologistic; the norms of communication are misunderstood, or broken, or exposed as arbitrary, unjust, or sterile; and the truth must be deemed rather than negotiated.

This confrontation with unintelligibility in the clinic is a situation like those Crapanzano identifies with rapid social change or social trauma, where conventions of communication are undermined, and "the negotiations of meaning and relevant context break down," producing a crisis in evidence.[53] The relevant context for evidence in the clinic is diagnostic; but the speculative and disjointed nature of diagnosis, combined with the ambiguity and duplicity of language in clinical encounters, produces a situation of uncertainty and instability in meaning. Therapists and patients in Thrace communicatively maneuvered toward truth in relation to one another, destabilized by the unreliability of evidentiary criteria and the unavailability of interpretive conventions for communication. Yet while they can be seen as strategists in pursuit of control or other clinical goods—as, for example, Goffman and Allan Young take them to be when they bracket diagnosis[54]—I see more at stake in their encounters than strategy, more than rules to follow or roles to play. What happens when these players do not perform their roles successfully: when they lie, or get confused, or contradict themselves, or say something off script? It is in the accumulation of such moments that I see *not knowing* as an integral part of the psychiatric truth game: a move that keeps this interminable game from concluding.

I do not infer, from this communicative breakdown in the clinic, a historically prior stability riven by some destructive force. And yet some difference is made by the present moment. In medical anthropology, it has frequently been observed that the experience of illness puts life into question. For Arthur Kleinman, a prominent proponent of this view, illness is a moral experience that disrupts the stability of life within its cultural web of meaning, impelling those who suffer to seek teleological narratives oriented to a transcendent purpose in order to make sense of it.[55] Beyond the sought-for coherence of such cultural "theodicy," Lawrence Cohen exquisitely elaborates the *non-sense* that emerges from such disruptions of experience when experience is already saturated with excessive meaning.[56] In this vein, as I show in the sections that follow, what is at stake in the gnosis of clinical diagnosis is not only the unstable reference of psychiatric truth claims, but also, more profoundly, the irreducibility of meaning to reference.

In an attempt to evade the gambit of standardizing and universalizing truth claims by which psychiatry realizes itself as a global science, I have restricted the sources from which I glean the rules of its truth game to the settings where I worked: views articulated in meetings, seminars, and formal interviews by senior psychiatrists at the hospital clinic and the Association; didactic texts published by these psychiatrists; and the DSM-IV,[57] regularly consulted and invoked in these settings. I identify the specific ways in which diagnosis formed an axis both of differentiation and adequation between the international discourse of psychiatry and clinical practice in Thrace. However, I also observe, throughout, a disjuncture between diagnosis, on the one hand—a formalized apparatus of knowledge that circulates, in a self-legitimating circuit, within the networks of international psychiatry constituted by pharmaceutical labs, research publications, academic departments and conferences, clinical trial sites, and treatment sites—and, on the other, the elements of specific cases that exceeded or escaped the field of intelligibility wrought through diagnosis. This disjuncture does not divide theoretical knowledge from practice, but theoretical knowledge and practice from the objects—mental illnesses, embodied in patients—that they hypostatize. In the clinic, in the interstices and the shadows of psychiatric knowledge, the profusion of doubt allows us to perceive those objects speaking back, and now and then, as Goffman has it, destroying worlds.

WHAT THE PATIENT SAYS ABOUT
HIMSELF IS MOST IMPORTANT

My introduction to the old General Hospital of Alexandroupolis coincided with its last days. It was early October and the staff were planning their belated move to a new facility that had been standing, finished but empty, for nearly two years on the southwestern edge of town. The move would ultimately take place over the Christmas holidays. In October, on one of my first days at work, I spoke about the new hospital with Thanos, a second-year resident assigned to the outpatient clinic that day. He had attended medical school in a large city, and volubly resented his forcible relocation to the backwaters of Thrace for residency. Addressing me as if apologetically, he complained that healthcare in Greece was a shambles of legislative stagnation, funding shortages, and a "narrow ethical perspective" within the medical profession: *Even young doctors like me, who start out with new ideas, and who want to change things—we're the ones who change, eventually. We adjust to the environment and we come to expect nothing.* He did not know whether moving to the new facility would discharge this fatalism, encrusted in the physical structure of the old hospital—in its dim and cramped rooms, its baffling layout, its corroded equipment. He said he suspected the problem was more a matter of "mentality" than of "space."

It was nearing one o'clock in the afternoon when Dr. Apostolou, a senior psychiatrist at the clinic, arrived to supervise Thanos. The outpatient clinic was about to close for the day, and the patients crowding around the door to the consultation office had dwindled to a resolute few. A burly man in his late twenties pushed his way through to follow Apostolou into the office. He addressed her abruptly by her first name, startling and perhaps offending her. The nurse, who had been assisting Thanos and filling out encounter forms in a large binder, turned to me and identified the patient under her breath as "Gypsy," noting his complexion, his clothing, his broken Greek, his aggressive demeanor. Between his bursts of greeting and appeal, Apostolou whispered to us that she had seen this man the previous week, when he had asked her to "clear" his psychiatric history. She had started a new chart and instructed him to return the following week for an evaluation.

Today, the nurses at the front desk had not been able to locate his new chart. They turned up many candidates—all filed, they told him, under "the same names," Turko-Quranic names inscribed in these records indifferently to the word-order signifying filiation. Apostolou knew the patient's face, but not his name, which might have been anyone's in that archive. She sent him back to the nurses to ask again, insisting over his protests that she could not see him without a chart.

The patient returned shortly with another chart. It was not the one Apostolou had started last week, but an older one, dating back nine years. Notes from the file showed that the man had reported hearing voices at that time, but had refused to be admitted for clinical evaluation. Apostolou asked him about this, but he had no recollection. *I never heard voices*, he said. *I never had mental problems—that's why I came here today, to clear my record!* Apostolou sent him back to the nurses' station to look again for his chart. When he left the room, she told us there was no question that the older chart belonged to him. She suspected he had reported hearing voices nine years ago in order to be disqualified from army duty. *And now, for some reason, he regrets it. Maybe he has children and wants to show them he's a man who can stand up. Or maybe he can't get a job, or he can't buy property, because he doesn't have a service record. He's of an age now when it's unlikely he'd be called to service even if he registers. I've seen this many times.*

The patient soon returned with both charts. Apostolou combed through them, pointing out to him all the coinciding details: birth date and place, parents' names, educational record, residence. The man admitted that the old chart might be his, but he insisted that he had never heard voices. Apostolou said—wryly, I thought—that she had no doubt about this. But to catch him in the lie she suspected he was telling now about his past, she pretended to believe the lie she suspected he had told in the past. Their exchange developed into a game of mutual dissimulation.

Apostolou's main tactic was an emphatic moral defense of her profession: *I'm here to help sick people, not to give out "papers." I can't sign a certifi-*

cate saying that you have no psychiatric history, because I know from your file that you do. Do you expect me to lie, too, and break the law? If I put my signature on this paper, it's a pledge to the state that I'm telling the truth. Do you want me to destroy that pledge? If you want me to clear your record, I'll have to see you ten more times, so that I can get to know you, and do a thorough examination, and gather information from witnesses. Only after all that can I honestly say you don't present the medical problems that got you this certification nine years ago. She told him that if he would not submit to that process here, he could try the psychiatrist just appointed to the General Hospital of Komotini, closer to his home.

With this line of argument, the doctor was articulating to the patient a bureaucratic protocol for credibility and transparency in clinical knowledge. This was, perhaps, in order to model honesty for him, and to explain her own motive for refusing his request—at the same time that she herself was lying, about both the content and the urgency of that protocol. In fact, it was well within the parameters of her professional discretion to grant his request outright; even a conservative approach would entail two or three more visits, not ten. Instead, she turned to the language of responsibility to summon an injunction to honesty that governed them both.

The patient, fuming as he shoved the scraps of his two files back into their cardboard folders, muttered: *You're a hard [σκληρή] woman—I can tell you don't have any children.* This was true, and perhaps carried for Apostolou, though she stared impassively, a glimmer of the Gypsies' legendary second sight. As the man exited, he called over his shoulder: *Death comes to everyone—but you wouldn't understand that!*

When he had gone, Apostolou wondered aloud whether the man had been threatening her. Gypsies had a reputation for uttering curses. She was chastened by his unexpected insight; he had broken the *illusio* of her bureaucratic role. She eased into a more self-critical mode, apologizing for the way she had handled the case: *I have to admit he made me angry. I always get mad when these patients lie. But it's not personal.*

The question of what is and is not "personal" in clinical encounters like this is what I will explore in the sections that follow. Encounters like this: where a patient supplicates a doctor, seeking help or recognition or certification, offering only his word to support his claim. And where a doctor meets this claim with suspicion—perhaps, as in this case, because it matches too closely a "cultural" pattern of deception. In this case, the patient perceived that the doctor thought she knew more about him than he had told her; that she saw beyond his self-presentation into a past he was trying to hide, and a trove of secret motives. But the patient knew something about her, too: namely, that there were other reasons for her suspicion—reasons that had no diagnostic or therapeutic function in their encounter.

This mutually intimate knowledge had none of the depth or texture this doctor indicated when she told the patient (dishonestly) what procedures she would have to follow to certify his health (honestly). It did not pass through a diagnostic frame that might have converted the patient's lies into symptoms of a mental illness. This knowledge instead arose almost instantaneously, in the almost anonymous space of a crowded outpatient office—making use, as Lauren Berlant typifies "intimation," of "the sparest of signs and gestures," of "shifting registers of unspoken ambivalence,"[58] whose tacit efficiency was conditioned by profound mistrust arising, first, outside the clinic. The mutual suspicion of deceit inside the clinic transformed the one-way exposure of a therapeutic relationship—in which the most secret aspects of a patient's life are revealed to a hermetic clinical authority—into a reciprocal one. If self-presentation, on the part of the patient, and diagnosis, on the part of the therapist, are distancing maneuvers by which each takes on a conventional role in the clinical encounter, then lying is the maneuver by which a more intimate, if antagonistic, relation can be recuperated from this distance.

Apostolou soon took an opportunity to get on the good side of the curse. The next patient—the last of the day—was another Gypsy man accompanied by his wife. He, too, sought to be cleared of his psychiatric history. His certified mental illness barred him from getting a driver's license, which he needed in order to help his wife with her clothing stall at the local bazaar.

Apostolou told me later that the man struck her as a little slow (χαζούλης). She interviewed his wife instead. The woman spoke well of her husband—*He has no vices, not like me! And he's so good with the children*—and she disputed the account of his illness that appeared in his file. According to the notes, which Apostolou read aloud to them, the man had been discharged from the army for narcotics use, and there were indications that he had "gone a little crazy," behaving erratically and violently in the army camp. His wife alleged that he had been harassed and beaten by other soldiers during his service, and that the sergeants had concocted drug charges because they wanted to throw him out. *He's illiterate, so he never knew what the medical officer wrote in his file. He's perfectly healthy now, and he works when he can.* Apostolou—freshly alerted by the previous encounter to her role in the bureaucratic network of discrimination that linked the key institutions in these cases: the hospital, the army, the welfare office, the bureau of motor vehicles—was disposed to sympathize. She questioned the woman for a few minutes more, and the couple left soon after with a certificate of mental health.

Exchanging Truth for Control

In his implacable critique of psychiatry, proceeding from *The Myth of Mental Illness* in 1961, Szasz delivered a severe dual diagnosis: on the one hand, of psychiatric science as a "tissue of lies,"[59] and on the other, of lying as an essentially normal, nonpathological practice. The lies and counterlies that characterize therapeutic relationships, in his view, mark a pragmatic mode of sociality pervasive not only in but outside the clinic—a strategy for managing the social and emotional risks of interpersonal relations that, on a foundation of deception, may develop into gratifying functional collusions: "The value of lying derives not so much from its direct, communicative meanings as it does from its indirect, meta-communicative ones. By telling a lie, the liar in effect informs his partner that he fears and depends on him and wishes to please him: this reassures the recipient of the lie that he has some control over the liar and therefore need not fear losing him. At the same time, by accepting the lie without challenging it, the person lied to informs the liar that he, too, needs the relationship and wants to preserve it. In this way, each participant exchanges truth for control, dignity for security. Marriages and other 'intimate' human relationships often endure on this basis."[60]

This section is about lying, and the forms of ambivalent intimacy it fosters in clinical encounters—about the paradoxical dynamic it inaugurates of knowing and not knowing, of stabilizing and destabilizing communication. Lying has engaged some version of this dynamic in psychiatry and psychology for as long as clinical care has depended on unreliable accounts from patients about their own experience and behavior. Psychoanalytic theory in particular has developed a preoccupation with lying, understood as an expression of the play between unconscious motives and conscious intentions that defines the discursive material to be worked through in therapy[61]—and that attests, Lacan contended, to an "ethical" rather than an "ontic" status for the unconscious.[62] The analytic relation, as Michel de Certeau renders it, is a mutual process of lying that, in due course, qualifies the patient as an ethical subject. The "tact" of the analyst, engaged in a pretence of knowing the patient's hidden truth, "is the art of slipping the gamble of words' meaning into their own chain so that the analysand unearths a signifier (a 'small bit of truth' in Freud's words), like a bone deposited by the past, from which he now fashions his speech, that is, the (ethical) act of upholding alone his desire in the very language of the trickery imposed on him by his history." [63]

Without presupposing any such psychical theory of lying—or any objective clinical truth against which lying as such could be gauged— I aim to trace *suspicions* of lying, by patients and therapists, across the terrain of clinical diagnosis in Thrace. In this section, interspersed with the story of a patient suspected of lying at the hospital clinic in Alexandroupolis, I present a condensation of psychiatric conjecture about unreliable speech: a set of loosely articulated principles for registering, qualifying, and responding to the suspicious claims and demands made by patients. The uncertainty of their motives, further clouded by their ambiguous communication, derails the diagnostic procedure and calls for a strategic response on the part of psychiatrists. The conjecture I record here describes some of their key strategies in playing this game of diagnosis. [64]

A word on the method of condensation. The formal interviewing I had conducted in other psychiatric settings in Greece, before I settled in Alexandroupolis, had yielded little beyond clichéd portraiture of doctor-patient relations, and medical information on psychiatry and mental illness that I found explained, with greater breadth and clarity, in textbooks: a confounding combination of self-presentational bluster with what Bourdieu calls "native theory," [65] an articulation of norms that obscures the structural determination of their social functions—an *interested*, though not necessarily deliberate, obfuscation. And so, for a long time, I evaded invitations to conduct interviews with the clinical staff in Alexandroupolis, though it seemed to be understood in these settings that interviewing was the kind of activity I ought to be pursuing.

I conducted the interviews excerpted in this section in the weeks before my final departure from Alexandroupolis, with a handful of clinicians whom I had come to know well over the course of more than a year. During that time I saw them nearly every day, talked with them in many capacities and tones about professional and personal issues, and spent hundreds of hours observing and interacting with them in staff meetings, outpatient consultations, individual and group therapy sessions, seminars, administrative affairs, and social occasions outside the clinic. As I prepared to leave the city, I wanted to offer these people, to whom I felt a range of attachments and responsibilities, an opportunity to articulate their knowledge in the way that they wanted me—a student, an observer, a specialist on a different track, a particular kind of foreigner, a peculiar kind of friend (for some)—to hear it, even if it meant exposing that knowledge to critique.

In the event, these interviews elicited indeed partial and interested accounts of this knowledge that contained, in my judgment, indications of clinical moralism. So I present these excerpts for the specific purpose of reconstructing that moralism, whose precision, ambition, and function were inevitably disrupted, complicated, and contradicted, not only by the experience of patients but also by the experience of those whose "official views" are recounted here. These views focus on a range of deceptions wrought by patients in clinical encounters. They show that what subjects say about themselves has a central but thoroughly enigmatic status in psychiatry, as it does in ethnography. As Dr. Michailidis suggested at the conclusion of our ninety-minute interview, when he told me, having just described his procedure for telling when a patient was lying: "What teaches people isn't words, it's practices—we don't learn anything from words!"

My task, then, is not to determine and moralize the referential truth of the speech I record here, but rather to discern the dynamics of suspicion through which that truth comes into question. It is to these dynamics that I account the continuity of therapeutic relationships even when treatment seems futile. The variegated suspicions of deception at play in clinical encounters recur to implicit knowledge of a *secret* between therapists and patients—intimate knowledge that has no proper clinical function, but that inhabits and fortifies these relationships.

What's Inside the Package

Dr. Lamberakis, a senior clinician at the hospital and professor of psychiatry at the University of Thrace, described to me two modes of diagnosis in contemporary psychiatry that in practice are often mixed, though not systematically, and contingently on the training of the therapist. One, he said, is the *psychodynamic procedure*, which "takes a lot of clinical experience to master, and an investment in the specific case at hand."

Psychodynamic diagnosis involves perceiving signs transmitted by the patient's body and speech, which take their meaning from the unique but hazy context of his or her individual experience, development, and address to the therapist. The other method, Lamberakis explained, is *statistical diagnosis*, which focuses on symptoms generic enough to seem comparable across cases. This method, typified by the DSM, does not project etiologies of disorder, but aims merely to describe them. However, as Lamberakis described it, the statistical description of symptoms has not reached anything like a consensus in the field of psychiatry. For him, it was a grave weakness of psychiatry that it had not achieved consistency even in statistical diagnosis: *We say that in psychiatry, the same ten symptoms signify the entire range of possible mental disorders. The diagnosis is always a matter of probability, not certainty.*

I asked whether, given the uncertainty of diagnosis based on manifest symptoms, clinicians try to take into account what patients said about themselves.

> Lamberakis: What the patient says about himself is very important, *most* important. We also get information about him from his environment—his family, coworkers, etc. The patient may not say anything about himself at all. In those cases, it's crucial to have a lot of contact with the patient, even when he's not talking, because you learn things from his body language and also, gradually, you can develop a relationship of trust. Sometimes a patient may not *want* to tell you certain things. On the first meeting, he may not even look at you, but maybe the next time he'll open up a little, and maybe he'll begin to talk.
>
> EAD: How can you tell how reliable the information is that a patient gives you? Don't patients sometimes lie?
>
> Lamberakis: Psychiatrists see many patients who lie. There are those who *show* that all they want is a disability certificate or medication. But there's no scientific way to know if someone is lying—only ways to "sense" it. You just get a feeling that you're being deceived.

In a later interview, Dr. Michailidis, a codirector of the hospital clinic, fleshed out this "sense" of deception—but not before he addressed its epistemology. (It is significant that Michailidis was not in any way psychoanalytically inclined; his training in the "old system," as he called it, conferred on him the title of "neurologist-psychiatrist.") Acknowledging that patients frequently lied, and that this was a "big problem" for psychiatry, Michailidis said that it was very difficult to fathom a patient's purpose (πρόθεση)—so difficult, in fact, that he felt uncomfortable explaining this issue to me from what he called a "psychiatric point of view," preferring to discuss it "philosophically." From a "philosophical perspective," he said, distinguishing truth from lies was a matter of distinguishing the essential (ουσιώδες) from the nonessential. When it came to patients, the essential problem was to determine what the patient wanted. He invited me to imagine the therapeutic encounter, and the opacity there of the patient's words, in terms of a package:

> Michailidis: The conversation begins. You're given a big package and it has a first layer of wrapping, and a second, a third. By the end of the conversation, you try to find out what's inside the package.
>
> EAD: What's inside is what the patient wants?
>
> Michailidis: No, it's not what the patient wants, but what he was able to reveal to the other [να ανακαλύψει στον άλλον]. We can't always unwrap the whole package. Sometimes you tell yourself: maybe I *shouldn't* unwrap another layer.
>
> EAD: But isn't that the goal of therapy?
>
> Michailidis: No, the goal of therapy is the equilibrium of the patient. So if you open the package all the way . . . (trailing off).

For Michailidis, what the patient wants was essential, but this desire could not be characterized according to diagnostic criteria. He had developed the metaphor of the package for my sake—not because he faced the therapeutic encounter this way himself, but because I had asked how he *could* (that is, "philosophically") know when and why patients lied. In his view, the psychiatrist's basic obligation was not to know what the patient wanted, but to match medications to symptoms in order to give the patient the most help while doing the least harm: "With experience, a psychiatrist can see immediately whether a patient is lying. You can read his nonverbal expression: maybe his glance darts around, or his hands tremble, or he stutters. Those kinds of nonverbal signs tell the truth much better than speech." Michailidis gave the example of a young schizophrenic man who he could tell had stopped taking his medication, though the patient denied it. And of a woman he had once diagnosed with depression, who returned to him for treatment two years later and admitted that she had concealed from him the traumatic event that had driven her to seek help the first time. "I knew as soon as I saw her that she was hiding something, but I couldn't get the secret out of her right away."

During these interviews, when I broached the problem of lying, Michailidis and Lamberakis both inclined at first toward a distinction that we elaborated together as we continued the conversation: the distinction between a patient's concealment of symptoms or environmental stressors that could help the psychiatrist understand the case clinically, and a patient's deliberate lying to get something he or she wanted from the psychiatrist—something other than the help the psychiatrist was disposed to give. This distinction is oriented to the problem posed generally to diagnosis by the unreliability of patients' speech, rather than to the symptomatic genres of unreliability attributed to patients with certain diagnoses, which I delineate below. The discrepancy between these two kinds of problems did not constitute an impasse; but articulating them together raised the possibility of contradiction among the explanatory powers of diagnosis. I was the one who raised that possibility explicitly, "philosophically"—it was, as per Bourdieu's logical taxonomy, the kind of question that never arose in practice.

1. Delusions Are Not Lies

During a regular staff meeting at the Association, Andreas, a psychiatrist on the Alexandroupolis treatment team, instructed a younger therapist on how to manage the incipient relapse of a psychotic patient she was treating. This patient had begun to express again, after a long period of disinterest in the subject, the belief that the skin on his arms was dead. He would repeatedly touch the skin and was always surprised to feel sensation there. In the past, he had undergone dermatological and neurological exams to confirm that his skin was normal, yet he continued to believe it was dead. Andreas told the young therapist that this patient was *not lying* and warned her that it would be dangerous, therapeutically, to oblige the patient to see the conflict between reality and his belief in the dead skin as a question of truth: *His error has to be handled delicately. If you reject his reality, or suggest he's dishonest, it will convince him that you're his enemy. This will destroy the therapeutic relationship and it might precipitate a relapse.*[66]

Delusion and hallucination have historically constituted the core symptoms of psychosis, and they continue to demarcate its narrowest parameters. Delusion is defined in the DSM as a thought disorder, marked clinically by the false propositions uttered by the patient. These propositions are considered false because they transparently represent "erroneous beliefs" held by patients. The erroneous nature of such beliefs is difficult to evaluate, however, because they often develop in order to account for patients' experience of perceptual hallucinations that, while in a complex relationship to reality, cannot be said to be false.

This question of error is specified by the diagnostic procedure, elaborated in the DSM, for determining the presence of schizophrenia—arguably the most severe and certainly the most commonly diagnosed form of psychosis.[67] According to this procedure, delusions alone suffice to diagnose schizophrenia only if they are "bizarre." Otherwise—if the delusions are "non-bizarre"—a combination of other positive symptoms (hallucinations, disorganized speech, disorganized behavior) and negative symptoms (flat affect, diminished speech, lack of will) must be present to indicate schizophrenia.

According to the DSM, the bizarreness of delusions characterizes schizophrenia, yet this quality remains "difficult to judge."[68] Bizarre delusions describe beliefs that are neither plausible nor comprehensible, and that bear no resemblance to "ordinary life experiences." They carry much greater diagnostic weight than non-bizarre delusions, which are plausible but nevertheless false beliefs. The manual counsels clinicians to gather information from a patient's family members, coworkers, or other doctors to determine whether non-bizarre beliefs are actually delusional. In neither case, however, does the DSM mention lying in connection with delusion. There is no discussion in the text of psychotic patients' intentions or awareness regarding their delusions. None of the clinicians I interviewed considered delusion relevant to the clinical problem of lying.

In her work on community-based psychiatry in France, Livia Velpry explores the role of delusion in the conflict between conceptions of patients as either "rational and narrative actor[s]" or as subjects of pathological thought.[69] She notes that, since "what a patient says may be considered a symptom of mental illness" instead of information on a par with what therapists say, the disqualification of delusional speech—including "covertly delusional" speech[70]—is a crucial method for determining patient responsibility.[71] By virtue of this suspicious orientation to patients' speech, Velpry finds in community-based psychiatry a "privileged setting" for studying the active construction of "the patient's view" as a technique of diagnosis and treatment.[72]

Lying, however, is a more radically destabilizing object of negotiation than delusion in community-based care. Dishonest speech on the part of patients may not be adequated to a symptom of a mental illness; or, if taken as a symptom, it may not be redressed by treatment. Rather than reinforcing clinical authority, as delusional speech does in Velpry's account, deception by patients instead may come to undermine that authority.

Circulation

It was late August the last time I saw Smaro. She was waiting in the vestibule of the hospital clinic; due to the blockade following Martina's suicide the previous weekend, she could not get to the nurses' station to inquire about her appointment. Alexandra, the resident assigned to her (as to Martina), had told her to come to the clinic early that morning, but the weekly staff meeting had run long past the time of their appointment. Smaro had been waiting more than an hour already. I watched as Alexandra passed by and brushed her off.

Smaro was in an evening dress and heavily made up. She told me she was "in a state": *Things are a mess* [χάλια] *at home. I've been sleeping a lot, I have no energy to go out. Every day I take three Tavor* [US Ativan]. *It's twice my normal dose, but it's not helping.* Anxiously, morbidly, she mined me for information about Martina's suicide. *Everyone's talking about it. Is it true they found her body broken on the ground?*

By this time, I had known Smaro for almost a year. She visited the hospital clinic every few weeks for regular supervision by her doctors. Three times that year she had been admitted for periods of a few weeks or more. She often came when her father had kicked her out of the house, or when a "romantic disappointment" (a clinical term) had driven her to despair. Though she lived in a village some forty minutes from Alexandroupolis, she came to the city frequently; I often saw her around town. *I have a few boyfriends down by the harbor,* she told me, and she liked to go out. She said that, as a woman in her forties and a mother of two grown children, it made her happy and even proud to "circulate" (κυκλοφορεί) — a term that she knew Alexandra, among others, had used to disparage her sexuality as a pathology. It was the essential point of conflict with her parents, her doctors, other patients. She treasured it; she endured it.

Smaro had been admitted to the clinic at the end of October, when it was still located at the old hospital — to her a very familiar place. According to the charge nurse, she had arrived on her own, agitated, demanding protection from witches who were chasing her down the street. She said she was afraid she would die if she went to sleep. The nurse administered a sedative to calm her, and later determined that Smaro had been off her antipsychotic medication for nearly two weeks. At the next staff meeting, Dr. Blastos, a psychiatrist who had treated Smaro for twenty years, noted that her physical complaints—irregular heartbeat, back pain, headaches—seemed "hysterical," but that she was also "desperately afraid" and had "serious problems" in her relationships. These features were consistent with her diagnoses of bipolar disorder and borderline personality disorder.

Blastos proposed to hand her case over to Alexandra, a new resident who at that time had a month of experience at the clinic. He said he hoped a new therapist would elicit a different "performance" from Smaro: *In all my years as a doctor, I've never dealt with such a bad patient!* He told us that Smaro had been spreading lies about another patient at the clinic, a man she was attempting to seduce. He had been admitted for hallucinations and severe insomnia, which had plagued him since he had quit drinking the week before. He and Smaro had visited the snack bar in the main hospital building together one morning; later that day, perhaps in response to a rebuff, she started telling people that he had drunk some *retsina* there.[73] He denied it, and his blood work showed no indications of alcohol. Blastos took this as proof of Smaro's difficulty as a patient: *She's a malicious liar. I've had enough.*

This was before I met Smaro. She was the first patient I interviewed privately, and I was warned by several doctors before I approached her that I should not get involved: Smaro had a reputation for manipulating and exhausting people, and she was often hostile toward young women like me. She formed "strong attachments" to her male therapists and was likely to perceive me as a threat.

When I consulted her medical records, I found a diagnosis of "bipolar psychosis," along with occasional notations of personality disorder. The file was thick with lab results—some routine blood work to test for lithium levels, but also endocrines and hormones, and X-rays (jaw, chest): a trail of the inconclusive pursuit of her "hysterical" complaints. In our first interview, Smaro described her illness to me: *It's a disorder with my emotions [συναισθήματα]. When I'm sick, I feel these emotions rising up in my chest, anxiety [άγχος] and worry [στενοχώρια].* Months later, during another admission, she told me that she had never been given a "psychological" diagnosis: *No, it's a medical problem.* This time, she had complained to Alexandra of pain, numbness (μούδιασμα) in her legs and hands, and dizziness (ζαλάδα). She had demanded neurological and thyroid tests, but Alexandra refused, insisting that Smaro's previous tests had shown that her problems were "psychological." The next time she wanted to stay at the clinic, Smaro came at night. She was admitted by a new resident who did not know her, and who immediately ordered the battery of blood tests she requested.

The diagnosis "bipolar psychosis" cannot be found in the DSM, though a subtype of bipolar disorder listed there carries the qualifier "with psychotic features." But an authoritative account of Smaro's diagnosis appears in a psychiatric textbook published by Panayiotis Sakellaropoulos, the former director of the hospital clinic. Following the French tradition of his own psychoanalytic training, Sakellaropoulos describes "manic-depressive psychosis" as a mood disorder, distinct from schizophrenia and other subtypes of psychosis. The "madness" (τρέλλα) indicated by *psychosis* in this diagnostic label is associated with the manic facet of the mood disorder. According to the text, this mania is typified by elevated and labile mood, "unbridled instincts," "flight of ideas," insomnia, logorrhea, psychokinetic anxiety, jocularity. In manic-depressive psychosis, the "thought disturbances" characteristic of psychosis—especially paranoia and delusions of grandeur—count more as "caprice" than as signs of "deeper" cognitive or perceptual disorder.[74] On Sakellaropoulos's account, the manic patient does not really "believe" his or her delusions, or only to a limited extent, and indeed gives the impression that he or she "may be joking" when articulating delusional beliefs; only in rare cases does a manic crisis include truly delusional ideas and hallucinations.

Smaro's file noted such thought disorders: delusional paranoia, religious megalomania, occasional hallucinations. But her doctors mostly emphasized the prominence of affect in her presentation, expressed in symptoms of mania such as hypersexuality, excessive activity, anger and violent tendencies, general "overemotion," sensitivity, suicidality. For many years, she had taken a lithium compound, the standard treatment for bipolar disorder. During acute crises she had occasionally been treated with Largactil (US Thorazine), a first-generation antipsychotic, though it made her sick. Her current medication regime, along with the sedative Tavor (US Ativan), included Aloperidin (US Haldol), an antipsychotic, and Akineton, the standard anticholinergic prescribed to prevent the extrapyramidal side effects of antipsychotic medication. Notes in her file indicated personality disorder, which would account for her failure to respond to these medications, and for her general difficulty as a patient.

2. Patients Who Really Want Help Do Not Lie Intentionally

Drawing a contrast with the case of patients who gave him the feeling he was being deceived, Dr. Lamberakis presented a scenario of justifiable lying by patients:

> It's a different situation with patients who don't tell the truth for other reasons. Those who have genuine medical problems don't tell lies *consciously*. Why would they come to the doctor, if they didn't really want help? But they sometimes hide things because they don't trust the doctor. For example, a patient with depression may hide the fact that his father is an alcoholic. It's not that he lies about it—if he's asked, he might tell, but he won't say it on his own. Or he might diminish the severity of the thing. The truth comes out according to the patient's own rhythm. With time and persistence, the doctor can draw it out of him. We take the burden off the patient by asking questions: "Did your parents drink? How much, or how often, did this happen? Were they ever violent?"

In this scenario of a patient who legitimately wants help, the truth—clinically important information that is being concealed—will come out, ultimately, because the patient does not have the *intent* to deceive his doctor. This is clearer in the example Michailidis offered of the schizophrenic who lied about quitting his medications: "This patient had paranoid delusions, which is typical of many schizophrenics in the active phase. He was afraid that his family was trying to harm him. And strangers. And even me, his doctor. He was very paranoid about his medications: he believed they were poisonous. He couldn't admit to me that he'd stopped taking them, because he feared I would punish him, you know, confine him, and force him to take the medications. What he was feeling was the necessity to protect himself." Like many non-bizarre delusions, this one adopted the contours of the patient's objective reality rather precisely. For Michailidis, the patient's lie, based in a diagnosable delusion, circumvented the onus of truth by its pragmatic motive. There was no will to deceive here—only the will to survive. The patient still wanted help.

In such cases, as Lamberakis implied, lying is understood to be unintentional: unmotivated by a conscious will, and rooted in an involuntary reaction of fear and mistrust that the patient may not know is guiding his behavior. Lamberakis maintained that the therapist could willfully transform such reactions into a dynamic of safety and trust with the patient: a dynamic in which the truth does not carry a risk, and the patient's intention—to get help—can be harmonized with the therapist's.

And what of those other patients of whom Lamberakis also spoke, those who do not want help but seek "something else" from their therapists? By implication, the lies of such patients are conscious, geared toward the something else that they want. These patients have a will to deceive.[75]

Abduction

Each time we talked, Smaro returned, at length or by fleeting allusion, to an experience to which she accounted her illness and the persistent ferocity of her relationship with her parents, especially her father. The way she told it, it was the story of an abduction: the theft of her life, and her forcible transformation into a mental patient. She gave me versions, and not only me: the story appeared several times in her enormous file, transcribed years before in multiple hands. There might have been many more versions. The core events remained the same with each telling, but Smaro shifted details and combined them in different sequences, thwarting my attempts to locate a source, a cause. What emerged, instead, was an account charged with significance that nevertheless did not add up: an account that pointed to a crime and concealed it at the same time.

The story goes:

At the age of nineteen, Smaro had been a student at the local nursing school attached to the old General Hospital of Alexandroupolis, the same hospital where she would receive psychiatric treatment later on. She was living with her parents in the village where she had grown up, and she was engaged to be married to a local boy. *One day I went down to Drama. They were giving a seminar for nurses at the hospital there, so I went to study. But I also had a friend who lived down that way, so when I finished my classes, I went to visit her. I was walking down the highway, I couldn't find a bus. Suddenly I was kidnapped by three men in a car. They stole my purse and then dumped me by the side of the road. They would have kept me, but I threatened them with my cigarette lighter. Or: I was walking down the highway and suddenly a car pulled up next to me. The men in the car robbed me. They tried to grab me, too, but I scared them off.*

After that I kept wandering down the road, I didn't know where I was going. I walked and walked until I reached the next village. I was lost, I was scared, I had no money and no ID. But I found a family who gave me refuge. Or: A nun at the village church took me in. Or: I went to the police station. They—the family, the nuns, the police—believed me. They could see I'd been robbed. Or: They could see I'd been abducted. I spent the night at the church. But the next morning, when I was praying for God's help, some nurses showed up and took me off to the hospital. Or: The police must have called my father. He called the hospital and had some nurses pick me up at the station.

My father came down to Drama to visit me in the hospital. He didn't believe I'd been attacked, even though the police said so. He kept saying that I'd wandered off by myself, for no reason, and I wasn't well. He was the one who ordered my committal. He wouldn't say anything else to me. They put me in a straightjacket and threw me in the nuthouse (τρελλάδικο). I spent a week in the locked ward. They drugged me, I can't remember much about that time. When I got out, I quit nursing school, and I got married right after that. My family kept the whole episode a secret.

Or: I stayed in that hospital for months. I was terrified of the patients on the ward: they were really hard cases, wretched people. I wasn't crazy like they were, I didn't need to be restrained. But they restrained me anyway. I was traumatized. When my father took me home, I spent months in bed. I was really depressed, I couldn't eat or sleep. I lost half my body weight. Finally my parents called the clinic. Dr. Blastos came all the way out to my house to examine me, and he saw right away how sick I was. He admitted me and that was the first time I came to the clinic. I got better in a month's time. But I was never completely well again, after that. I've been on heavy medications ever since. I hate them, I'm really not sure they're good for me. And I've never been able to forgive my father. We used to be very close. I was his favorite child.

After I came home from the hospital, I married my fiancé. I did it for love. Or: I was already pregnant with our first child. I married him against the wishes of his parents. On the night before the wedding, they came to see me at my parents' house: this is the custom. But they weren't there to welcome me to the family. They called me a dirty whore and told me I had to break off the engagement. I went through with it anyway. But we broke up a few years later, anyway, when my second child was born.

Months after we met, Smaro told me, as she had intimated many times, that she held her mother-in-law responsible for her divorce: One night I came home—to my husband's house, I mean, his family's house—and I found earth from a tomb scattered across my pillow. This is witchcraft, you know. She put it there. It made my husband want to leave me. Or: That's what caused my illness. And my illness made my husband angry. He tried to kill me many times! And then he abandoned me.

Later, Smaro told me that she had begun seeing a psychologist at the hospital clinic in Alexandroupolis long before her episode in Drama. She would meet with the therapist once a week, "just to talk"; she had never needed medication until after the trauma of her involuntary committal. Had there been a predisposition, then, to emotional instability—a portent of the illness that would show itself fully for the first time in Drama? Her story did not work that way. Smaro said she had needed the psychologist's support to handle her divorce and the difficulty of raising two small children on her own. But her divorce had followed several years after the episode in Drama. The narrative turned in on itself.

3. Intentional Lies Signify Personality Disorders

Wanting to raise explicitly the association between lying and certain clinical diagnoses, I asked Dr. Lamberakis, "Isn't there a theory that with some disorders, lying is part of the illness—that some patients lie symptomatically?" He agreed: "It's not a theory; [lying] is really a symptom. Whether a patient lies like this is one of the ways of diagnosing a personality disorder. Personality disorders have other symptoms, too—there are many disorders, not just one. Symptoms like hypersexuality, antisocial behavior, inability to form close bonds with others, and so on."

The DSM classifies mental illnesses along two axes. Axis I designates clinical disorders, among them the psychoses, mood disorders, and a variety of impulse-control disorders. Axis II designates personality disorders. According to the text, personality disorders share some features with clinical disorders—including "distress or impairment" and "deviation from cultural norms"—but have a distinct temporal course. They are defined as "pervasive" and "enduring pattern[s] of inner experience and behavior" that emerge early in life, typically by adolescence, and remain "stable" and "inflexible" over time.[76] By contrast, schizophrenia, arguably the most severe clinical disorder, bears a typical "age of onset" of the mid-twenties in men and late-twenties in women.[77] Therapists I knew described schizophrenia as an illness that emerged suddenly, dividing the patient's life into a "before and after," while other clinical disorders, such as bipolar, would come and go during a patient's life.

The DSM is designed to aid clinicians in the "multi-axial assessment" of their patients, who may present symptoms of clinical and personality disorders as well as other medical conditions at the same time. These diagnoses are thus by no means mutually exclusive. Yet in practice, therapists in Thrace often associated the axes with different types of patients. Those considered "heavy" (βαριά) cases were typically diagnosed with psychoses, or acute mood disorders such as severe depression and bipolar disorder—all belonging to Axis I. If personality disorders were also diagnosed in these patients, it was generally without implications for their treatment. According to Lamberakis, patients with a primary diagnosis of personality disorder were not often admitted to the clinic, since they could usually be managed as outpatients. Outpatient treatment was also preferred because these patients tended to disrupt the normal functioning of the clinic with their incessant complaints, noise, and aggression toward other patients. *These people are more difficult than sick*, he said.

In the DSM, this "difficulty" is delineated in ten personality disorders, sorted into three descriptive clusters: (1) the "odd or eccentric" cluster of paranoid, schizoid, and schizotypal personality disorders; (2) the "dramatic, emotional, or erratic" cluster of antisocial, borderline, histrionic, and narcissistic personality disorders; and (3) the "anxious or fearful" cluster of avoidant, dependent, and obsessive-compulsive personality disorders.[78] Lying is symptomatic of all these subtypes. According to the text, patients of the paranoid, avoidant, and dependent types may cultivate restraint or aloofness, hiding their thoughts and feelings out of fear and mistrust. The borderline and histrionic types evince a different kind of dishonesty, distinguished by the attention-seeking exaggeration of pain or need, including self-destructive behavior.

The most deceitful type of personality disorder in this taxonomy, however, is the antisocial. The Feighner criteria for clinical diagnosis, on which the third edition of the DSM was based, specify "persistent and repeated lying" as a defining "manifestation" of antisocial personality.[79] According to the DSM-IV, a person with this type of personality disorder, unlike others, is often deliberately manipulative in pursuit of desired objects (money, sex, drugs), and may engage in "criminal" deceit, such as theft or malingering.[80] The "external incentives" of "personal gain" that would otherwise permit a clinician to distinguish a malingerer from a symptomatically dishonest patient are thus at work in antisocial personality disorder; indeed, the manual counts malingering as a diagnostic criterion for the disorder.[81] What distinguishes symptomatic deceit in antisocial personality disorder from the nonsymptomatic deceit of malingerers is thus not the absence of external incentive, but the impulsiveness and compulsiveness by which the incentive motivates the deceit,[82] and the "maladaptive" persistence of deceit despite the functional impairment and distress it causes for the patient.[83]

In his interview with me, Lamberakis concurred with the DSM that patients who perform these sorts of dishonesty are behaving symptomatically. But pathology does not account for the "difficulty" of patients with personality disorders as compared with clinical disorders. What patients with these disorders really wanted when they lied was often unclear to therapists, he said: their dishonesty seemed intentional but lacked any obvious motive, and often thwarted the patients' own requests for help. As another psychiatrist explained it to me: *These patients have no regard for truth, but no real reason to lie, either.*

This tangle of desire and difficulty may be unraveled through a digression into a pathology that the DSM designates "factitious disorder."[84] This is classified in the manual as a clinical disorder rather than a personality disorder, though it is associated with borderline personality. According to the DSM, people with factitious disorder "intentionally" feign or produce symptoms of mental or physical illness "in order to assume the sick role." Factitious disorder is distinguished from malingering by the unconscious motive it entails. Malingering is defined as the intentional feigning of illness in order to achieve "a goal that is obviously recognizable when the external circumstances are known"—for example, avoiding military service. Malingerers are thus intentionally dishonest and conscious of their motives. Those with factitious disorder, on the other hand, though also intentionally dishonest, are not conscious of their motives, which the DSM characterizes as "psychological needs" that can be recognized as such by the "absence of external incentives."

If what patients with personality disorders "really want" can be likened to the "psychological needs" of those with factitious disorder, then patients with personality disorders can be conscious of their lying without being conscious of their motives. What is at stake in their "difficulty," then, is not their deceit as such, but their obscure and dogged motives.

Keeping Secrets

When I first met Smaro, she spontaneously, perhaps defensively, offered me a self-characterization: *I've never caused trouble, I've never been violent with other people. I'm not a bad person. But when I'm sick, I'm drawn sometimes to death. I've made ten suicide attempts in my life.* I saw her again in the clinic many months later, just after the Easter holidays. It had been a trying time for her; both of her children had come home to visit, and she found herself deeply upset, crying all the time. They were impatient with her and treated her roughly. *They don't understand that I'm fragile and I can't tolerate the racket. Their voices are like daggers in my ears.* Her mother made the situation worse, she said, chiding Smaro for the demands she placed on her children. Over the course of Easter week, her legs and hands had gone numb; her head was buzzing, and she began to forget things. She would confuse the digits of a phone number, and forget to fetch her laundry from the line. And then: *One night I took too many pills. Normally I take half a Xanax, half an Akineton, and half an Aloperidin in the mornings; and I take whole one of each at night. But that time, I took two of each. I wasn't confused; I wanted to die. My daughter was the one who brought me the pills, but she didn't say anything about the dosage.* I understood that Smaro was accusing her daughter of acquiescing to her suicide. But when I asked whether her daughter knew the correct dosage, Smaro said she thought maybe not. *I told her after I took the pills, and she panicked. My mother came running. She was furious. She said I was going to give my father a stroke with all this drama.*

After she took the pills, Smaro called Dr. Blastos and told him what she had done. *He told me to get myself to the clinic right away. But I took a long time to pack my things, and I missed the next bus. By the time I got to the clinic, it was evening. Blastos had already left. He's mad at me now. Since I got here, he's been so rude, he barely says hello to me in the hallway before he rushes off.*

Two months later, a few days into another admission at the clinic, Smaro found me in the corridor and pulled me into a consultation room. She whispered that she was in a terrible state. *My parents did it to me. They think I'm crazy. I wanted to go out a few nights ago, and they stopped me. My mother tied me down and my father beat me. I've got bruises all over the back of my head, my chest, my arms, my face.* She raised her shirt to show me the welts he had made, but I saw none. She indicated places on her face where she had been hit, stroking the corners of her mouth where her skin had been torn by a gag, seeming vexed that the wounds had already faded.

My parents are really violent with me. They tie me down to keep me at home. And then they hit me to stop me from crying. It all started after I got sick the first time, in Drama. I never told you about it before because I didn't know you well enough, I didn't know if I could trust you. It's a secret. But the next time it happens, I'll go public. I'll go to the police right away so they can see the evidence on my body. This time, she told me, after her parents left her alone, she had dressed in long sleeves and pants to hide her wounds and gone out against their wishes. She came to the clinic on her own the very next morning to be admitted. *The doctors saw the marks on me — how could they not believe me?*

When I asked Alexandra, Smaro's junior therapist, about the incident later that day, she told me she doubted that Smaro had been beaten as she claimed. *It's true that she doesn't get along with her parents. They have vicious quarrels. But Smaro has a tendency to exaggerate when she wants attention. Once she's calmed down and she's back on her medications, she'll go home again, willingly enough.* Smaro had said as much to me: she could not keep a job and had no means to support a household of her own, so she was resigned to living with her parents, no matter how badly they treated her.

In a psychological assessment questionnaire placed in her file very early in her psychiatric history, Smaro described herself as a "sensitive and honest person": she sought "open communication" with others, but wanted them to "keep her secrets." Perhaps she was delusional about the beatings and the abduction. Perhaps she was lying. Perhaps she did want to die. To what could one appeal for the truth? Physical evidence that vanished; witnesses who did not notice or stood indifferent; reports from the parties involved, all of whom had good reason to lie. In any case, a true account of what really happened was never at stake in Smaro's treatment, which always returned — perhaps by her own refusals — to the basics: medication, restabilization, home. The truth of her stories and symptoms might have pressed more on her doctors if Smaro had won their sympathy; she might have imparted some sense of what she wanted from them, without telling. But she had mistreated them, and not only them; she had lost their trust. Her deployment of the truth as a means to justice — her assumption of the role of complaining witness to her own trauma — was irrevocably undermined by her intent to deceive.

4. Patients with Clinical Disorders Suffer More

The axial distinction made in the DSM between clinical and personality disorders connotes more than the DSM attempts to explain. Dr. Politis, head of the Association in Thrace, observed in an interview with me that patients with psychoses and severe mood disorders (that is, clinical disorders) "suffer much more" than those with neuroses. Dr. Filalithi — a senior psychiatrist at the hospital clinic, and professor at the University of Thrace — likewise used the term *clinical* to denote that field of suffering toward which Lamberakis had gestured as well when he described patients with personality disorders as "more difficult than sick." In an interview with me, Filalithi described the trouble of assimilating personality disorders into the diagnosis of mental illness:

> It is very difficult [to make such a diagnosis] because these disorders don't comprise clinical symptoms that make the patient suffer. When someone is suffering, OK, you always know that he has some real problem. Or when there are symptoms and it's absolutely clear [that] a month ago he was just fine, and then suddenly, something appeared. By contrast, personality disorders have features that will follow the patient around throughout his life. And most often these features are types of behavior—for example, a person is very timid, or very violent, or he needs a lot of order in his environment. And precisely because it's this, it's not symptoms but more like elements of his character . . . it's extremely difficult to discern where the normal ends and the pathological begins. Because each of us judges the other according to our own presumptions.

Filalithi drew an equivalence here between illness and suffering. In severe mental illness, she suggested, there is a moment when suffering begins, and a hope that it may end with proper treatment. In personality disorders, on the other hand, suffering is more diffuse and entrenched. The symptoms are always present, as if exuded by the person's character, revealing what the person is rather than signifying what the patient has. Filalithi thus complicated Lamberakis's assertion that lying is symptomatic, showing the metaphorical valence of its relation to illness: people with personality disorders are like sick people, but their unreliability is dislodged from the material domain of real pathology and legitimate suffering. In this light, dishonesty appears as a moral defect rather than a symptom.

Given the ambiguous role of mental pathology in personality disorders, it is not surprising that doctors should find them nearly impossible to address clinically. Lamberakis drew a connection between the difficulty of treating people with personality disorders and their difficulty as people:

> These patients are the least liked by psychiatrists. They're considered the most difficult, because it's much harder to see the results of treatment—compared with schizophrenia, for example. Some people think that long-term psychotherapy, including psychoanalysis, may have re-

sults with personality disorders of the antisocial or schizoid types — but it would have to be very long-term.

Patients with personality disorders do take psychiatric medications, but they're less effective with these disorders. They're given to control the symptoms, but they don't deal with the underlying problem — symptoms like depression, or violence. The same drugs are more effective for other disorders than they are for personality disorders. For example, lithium, which might be prescribed for violent symptoms in a personality disorder, is much more effective at managing mania in bipolar disorder.

In the hospital clinic and at the Association, ineffectual clinical encounters between patients with personality disorders and their therapists often took the shape of irresolvable conflicts between people who did not like each other. Unlike other mental illnesses, these disorders resisted medication and therapy, and — perhaps *because* — they were permanent and inflexible features of character.

The clinicians I interviewed articulated, in the register of scientific knowledge, substantial doubt about the pathological nature of these disorders; and in the register of personal emotion, deep ambivalence about the patients who presented them.[85] Yet their doubt and ambivalence did not translate into provisional or experimental therapeutic approaches. Nor did these therapists often entertain the prospect of rescinding clinical purview over these patients. Despite their explicit acknowledgment that diagnosis was vexed, and that treatment was unlikely to work, clinicians routinely diagnosed their difficult patients with personality disorders, prescribed them medications, and attempted to engrain them in regular counseling.

The "common sense" that these disorders can and should be addressed within the biopsychiatric framework of clinical care required much effort to sustain on the part of these therapists.[86] Several explained to me that it was their responsibility as therapists to suppress the moral judgment these patients excited in them. Nevertheless, many of the patients they diagnosed with personality disorders perceived both their moralism and their bad faith in disavowing it. For some, like Smaro, this was enough to impugn the honesty and reliability of their therapists, and to ground a counterdeception.

Fishing

A year after our last encounter, when I returned to Thrace for a visit, Smaro was back on lithium and back at home, taking care of her father while her mother was hospitalized for knee surgery. It was the same three-room house where she had grown up, at the southern end of the only road in her village. They had open fields for a backyard, where they kept a melon patch and some chickens. I had wanted to see her there, outside the hospital for once, and I had wanted to meet her father.

He looked just like Smaro: short and sturdy, with dark, deep-set eyes and a lopsided smile. He was hard of hearing and easily winded; he had recently quit smoking "for health reasons," he said, but he did not begrudge Smaro her cigarettes, which she chain-smoked as we all talked in the living room. Later, he rested while we fixed lunch in the kitchen. At one point, he called out something unintelligible to Smaro from the next room. When she asked him to repeat it, he said, "It's going to rain tomorrow!" She explained that he always said this when she did not understand him; it was a joke between them, one of countless gestures of mutual affection I thought I witnessed that afternoon.

As we ate, Smaro's father—knowing I had met her in the clinic, but not, likely, the nature of my own relationship to psychiatry—told me that she was "just fine" so long as she took her pills. *Like now, for instance: she's doing really well. She hasn't been admitted to the clinic in months. But when she goes off her medications, she gets upset and out of control. Suddenly we're to blame for everything. And she always winds up in the clinic. Those times are hard for everyone: for me, for my wife, who's sick. And for Smaro, of course. It's always been that way.*

After lunch, Smaro wanted to get some air, so we took a drive in my rental car. Her demeanor changed the moment we hit the road. In the house, she had seemed to me cheerful, efficient, relaxed. Now, she turned to me urgently, on the point of tears. *I'm so lonely! I need a real companion* [σύντροφος]. *It's not good for me to be living with my parents in that tiny house, in this cursed village. I need to be in the city!* When I pressed her, she admitted she was getting along better with her father now than the year before. But that was no answer.

She directed me down a rambling dirt road to the border, where we could watch trucks coming over from Turkey and get a coffee at the station cantina. To reach the crossing, we had to pass through a security checkpoint, manned by a lone and very young soldier who politely required our IDs when Smaro began flirting with him. More men appeared as we got closer to the crossing. The cantina was filled with truck drivers and border guards on break. I remarked on Smaro's strategy in choosing this place for coffee, and she seemed pleased that I'd noticed her "fishing" (να κάνει το καμάκι) — that I "understood."

Her manipulation, being aired, was tamed. But the theme of duplicity guided our subsequent conversation. Smaro told me about her new boyfriend, a man she had met years ago at the clinic and reencountered there recently. He was an alcoholic and drug addict and, unlike her, she said, too fragile to "make it on the outside": now nearly forty years old, he was only able to live at the clinic or in the home of his overprotective, domineering mother. *The old hag doesn't care for me at all. She pretends to like me when I visit him at home, but behind my back she's plotting against me, telling him that I'm a bad influence. He told me so.*

Smaro discovered treachery as well in Alexandra, her junior therapist at the hospital clinic. She had recently overheard Alexandra discussing her case with Blastos — who had, himself, "betrayed" her by refusing to see her during her last admission. How could she trust Alexandra if she was conspiring with Blastos? When I reminded her that Alexandra was a resident in training and therefore required to consult a senior psychiatrist about all her cases, Smaro did not believe me: *If she's not a real psychiatrist, then why does her stamp say "psychiatrist"? I see that stamp on all my prescriptions.* I could not convince her, and my efforts earned me some of that surging suspicion.

Smaro ordered a second coffee, blaming her exhaustion for her foul mood. She had awoken very early that morning from a bad dream and had not been able to get back to sleep. *It was the kind of dream that comes true. I have those sometimes. Like the day my husband ran me down with his motorcycle. The night before, I dreamed he was stabbing me and I woke up soaking wet, as if covered in blood. He put me in the hospital for real a few hours later.*

This morning, I saw a group of old people in my dream. I recognized them but I didn't know their names. I was happy to see them, I greeted them as friends. But they scolded me. They said, "If you laugh now, you'll cry later." Even though I was in a dream, I understood that if I laughed in front of the old people, something bad would happen later today, when I was awake — something to make me cry. But I laughed anyway. Now I'm dreading what's going to happen.

Back at her house, Smaro showed me dozens of photographs, dating to her infancy and showing her movement through life in this cramped old house — as a little girl, then a young mother, then a patient, aging too quickly from heavy medications. There were a few of her with Blastos, posed in front of a fountain in Dublin, where they had attended an international mental health conference together years before. On leaving, I took several new photos of Smaro, hearty and smiling, with and without her father, still awaiting something to make her cry.

THE PRISM OF PSYCHOANALYSIS

In the previous section, I showed that for therapists in Thrace, the moral threshold crossed by "difficult" patients was marked by their conscious intention to lie. Therapists read their patients' intentions as signs of either clinical or personality disorders, a moral distinction by which they valorized and rationed suffering. Motives, on the other hand — "what patients want," as Michailidis put it — were "essential" to understanding their clinical presentation, but fundamentally difficult to know and to diagnose as symptoms of mental disorders. Lamberakis proposed a diagnostic procedure for determining whether patients wanted help; but wanting *something else* was announced by intentional lies, which undermined patients' claims to suffering, regardless of what motivated them. Motives thus opened a moral scene in clinical encounters that — as with Smaro's accusations, dating back twenty years — could not be concluded clinically.

Considered this way, "motive" might seem commensurate with "desire" in psychoanalytic theory — especially given these therapists' own occasional invocation of this theory, and the reticence of the biopsychiatry they practiced to propose etiologies for symptoms. But this commensurability is only apparent, for psychoanalysis was not institutionally available to furnish clinicians in Thrace a consistent framework for interpreting patients' motives. The extent of psychoanalytic practice in these settings was limited; it circulated as a prestigious but peripheral expertise. What psychoanalysis did for these therapists was to authorize their suspicion of patients' intentions, and their belief in unknown motives. It shaped a mythology of patient subjectivity, and a disposition to register the moral valence of symptoms, but no systematic instrument for diagnosis or therapy.

The classic psychoanalytic division between psychosis and neurosis, though it has been abandoned in DSM-style nosology, is unmistakably the historical source for its contemporary categories of schizophrenia and mood or personality disorders, respectively. Clinicians in Thrace frequently used the term *neurotic* in a generic way to refer to patients who did not suffer from "heavy" illnesses. This loosely diagnostic division marked a distinction in practice as well: clinicians tended toward supportive counseling for psychotic patients, while they might attempt some form of psychodynamic therapy with neurotics. In this section, I show that this loose division between psychosis and neurosis turned on the value—the informational versus symbolic significance—of what patients were considered able to say and, consequently, on how what they said might come to sound suspicious.

It was not easy for me to determine the extent or orthodoxy of psychodynamic therapy practiced in the settings where I worked in Thrace. In the dozens of therapy sessions I attended at the hospital clinic, and at the Association under more restricted conditions, clinicians carried out what they called "supportive therapy": conversational counseling aimed at solving the everyday problems patients faced outside the clinic—conflicts with family members, trouble with medications, difficulty working or obtaining income. If left unresolved, one psychiatrist explained to me, such problems might generate unmanageable anger, fear, or hopelessness, and ultimately dispose patients to relapse. Supportive therapy extended beyond the clinical encounter as well: ideally, doctors would counsel family members or friends on how best to manage a patient's moods and behaviors. Social workers assigned to their cases performed much of the bureaucratic labor required to secure financial assistance and medical supervision outside the clinic. In all facets of supportive treatment, the therapeutic team relied on patients to provide factual information about their experiences, so their therapists could help them negotiate potentially disruptive challenges. The possibility that this information might be unreliable, due to patients' confusions or delusions, did not alter the informational function of their speech in this context. In cases where the information they supplied seemed unreliable, therapists attempted to close in on the truth by seeking out more reliable sources, not by interpreting the refraction of pathological psychic conflicts in their patients' speech.

Psychodynamic therapy, on the other hand, at some level always entailed the symbolic interpretation of patients' speech, assumed to be symptomatically rich and informationally oblique. This form of therapy was not practiced at the hospital clinic, nor did it form a regular part of the clinic's residency training program, which focused chiefly on pharmaceutical treatment. However, Dr. Filalithi told me that neurotic patients who met with clinic doctors at the local mental health center, instead of at the hospital, were sometimes treated "psychotherapeuti-cally." She explained to me that, years ago, when the hospital clinic had been under the direction of Sakellaropoulos, the staff had experienced a "uniformity of purpose": *I'm not sure the form of treatment he favored is better than any other—his combination of psychoanalysis and social psychiatry. But his leadership definitely increased our effectiveness as a team. We all knew what work we were doing, and why. We knew our responsibilities. Since he retired, we've taken a much wider range of approaches. It's a situation of ideological pluralism.* The new director, Dr. Liakos, had a lighter managerial touch. Like Sakellaropou-los, he was a psychoanalyst, but he was more cautious about the aptness of psychodynamic theory for public psychiatric services in Greece.

At the Association, by contrast, students in the master's degree pro-gram in social psychiatry were instructed on psychodynamic theory during seminars and personal supervisions, and psychoanalytic inter-pretation formed a large part of the discussion following regular case presentations. Yet, though I had the sense that psychodynamic therapy was being practiced with some patients there, I was not permitted to attend these sessions, nor to meet with these patients, lest my presence disrupt their therapeutic relationships. To understand psychodynamic practice in these settings, then, I have had to rely on statements made by clinicians, either to me or in published texts.

During an interview, Lamberakis pointed out to me that psychiatrists needed to undertake a special kind of training in order to practice psycho-dynamic therapy. The only psychoanalysts now working in the public ser-vices of Thrace were Liakos, the director of the hospital clinic, and Politis, the head of the Association. Lamberakis himself had a "psychodynamic orientation," he said, but did not consider the kind of therapy he prac-ticed psychotherapy, because he had never completed the training pro-cess required for certification: *Some of my colleagues might call themselves psychotherapists, but I don't.* To clarify the distinction, he explained:

> On the one hand, there is dynamic psychotherapy, which connects the current state of the patient's mental health to conflicts in his past. Through transference and countertransference, you work on material from the patient's dreams, past events. This kind of psychotherapy is practiced only by doctors in the private sector—it's not part of the Na-tional Health System.
>
> Then there's supportive therapy, which is what I practice, and what's usually practiced in the state system. In this kind of therapy, you may

appreciate the same issues as a psychodynamic therapist—conflicts in the patient's past, the function of the therapeutic relationship. But you won't work on those issues *with the patient*. It's just part of your understanding of the case. You don't necessarily work through the influence of past events on the patient's mental state today. You don't do "interpretation" [ερμηνία].

According to "classic psychoanalytic theory," Lamberakis said, schizophrenics cannot tolerate psychotherapy: due to a weak ego structure, they tend to "come apart [διαλύονται]" under analysis. Pandelis, a psychiatrist at the Association, likewise explained to me that the psychoanalytic exploration of trauma could actually provoke a psychotic break in schizophrenics, who as a rule were unable to manage their anxiety and thus easily wounded. Nevertheless, Lamberakis observed what he called a "transformation" in psychoanalytic theory, one guided by Sakellaropoulos in Greece, that made it plausible to treat psychotics psychodynamically. In this form of therapy, inspired by D. W. Winnicott's notion of "holding,"[87] the psychiatrist establishes a "safe place" for the patient—a stable setting, time, and therapist—and in this place performs a kind of "second mothering," allowing the patient to grow up again and develop a stronger ego. Such therapy would thus implicate the patient's past, but not as something about which the patient must speak.

Since the start of his career, Sakellaropoulos has publicly promoted a psychoanalytic approach adapted both generally to the Greek National Health System and specifically to the treatment of psychotics, who historically constituted the majority of patients in that system. One article on this subject, widely read by therapists at the hospital clinic and the Association, is now included in his two-volume textbook. It provides a schema of basic psychoanalytic principles that, when appropriately modified, can be legitimately applied under heterodox conditions.[88] The most important of these principles is attentiveness to patients' transference, or "projections" of past conflicts onto their relationship with therapists; and in turn, to therapists' countertransference with patients. It is in large part the recognition and management of this dynamic that constitutes what Sakellaropoulos calls the "psychoanalytic prism" through which therapists must see their patients and their own work.[89] He notes that transference potentially organizes patients' relationships with all their therapists, and he therefore advises that psychotic patients be assigned at least two therapists, both to ensure the continuity of care and to diffuse the transferential burden to a "collective" or "psychiatric group."[90] Beyond the interpretation of patients' internal conflicts, guided by therapeutic "intuition" in discerning their etiology, Sakellaropoulos proposes that a stable therapeutic setting and the *silence* of the therapist—a refusal to provide interpretation to the patient—are the key psychoanalytic methods that can be adapted to public psychiatric treatment in Greece.[91]

Sakellaropoulos's account of psychoanalytic practice with psychotic patients in public settings is orthodox in styling. It may well describe, if abstractly, the practice of some therapists working with some patients at the Association. However, therapists there and at the hospital clinic told me repeatedly that the practical constraints they faced—shortage of staff; limits on office space and hours of operation; the disorganized character and low educational level of patients—made it nearly impossible to conduct anything but basic supportive therapy with their psychotic patients. Even then, consistent follow-up was difficult to accomplish. A coterie of neurotic patients was undergoing long-term psychotherapy at the Association and the hospital clinic's mental health center, but they represented a very small proportion of the patients treated at any one time. The younger psychiatrists, some of whom had undergone training in psychoanalytic techniques, seemed quite eager to undertake neurotic cases so that they would have a chance to engage in that kind of therapeutic relationship.

Believe Me

At the Association, then, psychoanalysis informed practice, but in a fragmentary or, as Sakellaropoulos would have it, *prismatic* way. It was even less systematic an influence at the hospital clinic. The most methodical psychoanalytic training in these settings, beyond supervisions between senior and junior therapists, took place at the case presentations convened each month at the Association when Politis, who lived in Athens, visited Alexandroupolis. On one such occasion, Kiriaki, a patient who had tapped the therapeutic resources of the Association for nearly ten years, elicited radically mixed techniques of interpretation, as well as uncertain and multiple diagnoses. Her speech and its unreliability were taken to diverge into trajectories of function and value that reflected, but did not entirely obey, the conventional psychoanalytic division between psychosis and neurosis.

At the age of thirty-four, Kiriaki was the oldest of three sisters, all of them psychiatric patients. The youngest had been admitted to the hospital clinic the previous week. (Kiriaki said that her sister had "come apart" when her affair with a seventeen-year-old boy from the neighborhood had ended violently—as it had begun, she believed—with a passion ignited by witchcraft.) Politis told us that Kiriaki was the stablest child. She had married young and worked at factory jobs much of her life. She was raising two children in Komotini, where her family had their only income from a small rental property. Her husband had begun treatment for depression and alcoholism several months before.

During the presentation, Politis and Kiriaki were seated at the front of a large room used as the Association's day center, before an audience of about twenty master's students, psychiatrists, nurses, and other therapists. Prompted by Politis, Kiriaki told her story lucidly and at length, in neat chronological sequence. She dated her illness to the birth of her first child, in Germany, where she had lived until she entered elementary school, and where she had returned, from Greece, upon her marriage. *At first, I was very sad. I cried all the time. Sometimes I would start crying suddenly, with no reason. I went to many doctors—I was looking for a Greek, but I couldn't find one. The doctor I ended up with was Turkish; he was more like us, he worked in the Greek community there. He gave me medication for depression. I know now that I misunderstood how I should take it. I didn't get better and I quit after a few months.*

It was three or four years later when I was hospitalized the first time. This was right after my second child was born. My doctor said I should go, but he didn't force me. When I got there, the most terrifying thing happened. I got to the front door and all the patients in the ward were gathered together, in the waiting room, faces painted, in costumes. It looked like they were putting on a play. But when I walked in they set upon me, shouting in my face, clawing at me. Later on, I understood there had been no play. What happened was that the patients had gathered to welcome me to the ward. They were trying to entertain me. But because I was under so much stress, I got really scared by what they were doing.

As Kiriaki described this experience, Politis sat back in his chair, holding his chin in his hand. Kiriaki smiled and stopped talking. Politis leaned forward again and asked her, *Why are you smiling?* Kiriaki, just as gently, replied, *Because I know you don't believe me.* Politis sat back, eyebrows raised: *Kiriaki, there's no question of not believing you. I'm just trying to understand what happened. I can't quite see why the patients would have gathered around to greet you like that.*

Kiriaki did not respond. Her story shifted to her next admission, this time by force, to a locked ward at the same hospital. She was considered suicidal at the time, though she said now that she had never actually tried to kill herself. A year or so later she was admitted again. Politis began to question her closely on her relationships with doctors during this period.

The Turk dropped me after the first time I was hospitalized, because I hadn't taken my medications the way I was supposed to. And I didn't go to all my appointments. So then I started seeing many doctors, maybe four or five. I wanted to keep seeing them all—the more of them I saw, the better I felt. I wanted so much to get well! And I drew courage from each one. But my doctors got angry with me. They made me choose just one. . . .

A few years later, my whole family moved back to Greece. We had saved enough money working in Germany to buy an apartment in Komotini. But I couldn't take life in the city. It was so loud and dirty, it was chaos. A little later we moved to my husband's village by the sea, to live with his parents. We rented out the apartment in Komotini to make a little extra money. But that was a mistake. Our last tenants destroyed the place and ran away without paying us rent—they owed us for months. Now we're in debt and we don't have any money to repair the property, so we can't rent it out. My husband is unemployed. So we fell apart. We started fighting all the time, and I think we're going to separate. I blame myself, I have to do better. My husband told me he wishes he'd married someone else, and I take this to heart. But my therapists are always telling me I'm too severe with myself.

Having arrived in her narrative at the present day, Kiriaki was steered back to her childhood. Politis questioned her about her first memories, and good and bad recollections of her youth. He elicited the picture of a violent, alcoholic father and a distant, depressed mother who did not intercede to protect her children. Tenderly, Politis insisted on this, pointing out to Kiriaki—in the mode of interpretation—that she answered his questions about her mother with complaints about her father, denying her mother's share of the blame.

When Kiriaki was released from the session, escorted out by her psychiatrist, Politis commenced an examination of his students. He intercepted Dora as she headed out to meet with a patient downstairs. She quickly pronounced Kiriaki "very sick," contending that her delusion about the play at the German hospital indicated psychosis. But taking into account her "self-destructive behavior," Dora proposed a diagnosis of "psychotic depression." A psychiatric nurse suggested that Kiriaki, due to her sensitive condition at the time of her first admission, might simply have misunderstood a scene that actually did transpire: perhaps it was not a hallucination or delusion, but a confused reaction to a forbidding psychiatry ward populated by heavily drugged, severely ill patients who might have looked like dramatic actors. But others agreed that the scene Kiriaki had described, and her rationalization of it afterward—an imputation of motives to the other patients that referred, implausibly, to her—was characteristically delusional. Kiriaki's psychiatrist noted that, in therapy, she had presented other symptoms—for example, hearing the voice of God—that also led diagnostically in the direction of psychosis.

There was no discussion of Kiriaki's own intervention into Politis's interpretation of her story about the play: her recognition that he did not believe it. Nor did Politis discuss his reaction to this intervention—his reassurance that he did, without question, *believe* her, though he did not quite *understand*. He stipulated now that Kiriaki had really "experienced" what she described. And yet, split onstage between his therapeutic and his pedagogical personae, Politis had, in his body language and gentle challenges, shown Kiriaki doubt. And he had accounted for this lapse to her by claiming not to understand: a further expression of doubt. His lapse, though it might have been painful or disruptive for Kiriaki according to Politis's own understanding of transference, nevertheless verified that, as an interpreter, he thought she was presenting not a lie but a delusion—an experience that was real but not true, a distinction he assumed she was in no position to recognize.

A different discourse of truth emerged in the discussion of a later and cloudier moment in Kiriaki's story—again, a moment in which Politis had showed himself, despite himself. Inaugurating a discussion of countertransference, he asked Pandelis, a new psychiatrist at the Association, how he would describe the feelings Kiriaki had evoked in him during the interview. Pandelis replied that he found Kiriaki quite "passive-aggressive": *I mean, I felt aggressed. Especially hearing about her manipulative behavior toward doctors. Seeking treatment from multiple doctors is typical borderline behavior. She told us outright that they were frustrated with her, and I identified with that frustration. She claims that her motive for seeing all these doctors was to get well, but at the same time she's showing you [Politis] just how unwell she still is, after a decade of treatment. She's implying that you've failed her, just like all her other therapists in Germany and in Greece. And she wants you to know she feels that way.*

A psychiatric nurse, who had known Kiriaki for years, said, *I really liked Kiriaki in the beginning, I felt sympathy for her. But I have to admit, as the years passed and she showed no improvement at all, and she kept demanding treatment, I started to resent her. I think at some level I've blamed her stubbornness for the failure of her treatment.* These feelings of resentment recalled Kiriaki's remark that her therapists did not want her to blame herself for her marital problems. Politis had had to push her to acknowledge her mother's responsibility for her traumatic childhood, which he felt Kiriaki was *unconsciously* resisting; her therapists, likewise, were exasperated by the guilt she expressed over her husband's troubles, which they understood as an *unconsciously* self-destructive attitude. Yet it was clear that, in some unarticulated way, they found her morally responsible for her suffering. Thus when Kiriaki voiced their own condemnation of her self-punitive attitude, she alighted brilliantly on their moral ambivalence—the contradiction between their guilt and hers for the failure of her treatment— that she had provoked, as Pandelis put it, *passive-aggressively.* Politis immediately moved to suture this rift in the moral disposition of Kiriaki's therapists, obscuring the question of truth it had raised by interpreting their feelings of resentment, in a psychoanalytic register, as countertransference: *These are emotions you'll have to acknowledge and learn how to manage in your therapeutic relationships with patients like Kiriaki.*

In my earlier description of psychoanalytic practice in Thrace, I respected a loose and flexible distinction between psychosis and neurosis, and the types of therapy considered appropriate to treat them. I concluded that orthodox psychoanalytic theory informed practice in these settings to a limited extent, and could be found only in a diluted form in the treatment of psychosis. The case presentation of Kiriaki, and the interpretation of her speech that followed, complicates this picture. In orthodox psychoanalytic theory, neurosis and psychosis characterize mutually exclusive psychic structures. This is crucial to psychoanalytic interpretation of speech, especially when it comes to lying; so different in etiology are these psychical structures that Lacan distinguishes *neurotic speech* from "the psychotic statement."[92] In neurotics, conscious intentions are formed in the ego. These intentions are disrupted by unconscious motives expressed through an ontological gap between the unconscious and the ego. Psychotics, on the other hand, are unable to form conscious intentions in the same way: here, the subject's ego does not develop the requisite integrity to sustain conscious and tenable ideas about her own interest. On this reading of psychoanalytic theory, the intentional manipulation that characterizes some neuroses is impossible for psychotics.

In the case of Kiriaki—as, I venture, in Smaro's—neurotic and psychotic speech were identified by therapists in one and the same patient, but submitted to separate moral judgments. Kiriaki's story about the play staged in the German hospital called for a distinct form of interpretation from her claims about wanting to be well; the former appeared as a morally neutral (psychotic) delusion, the latter as a morally fraught (neurotic) lie. It is not psychoanalysis but the DSM, in its protocol for multiaxial assessment, that authorizes this combination of divergent moral-psychical trajectories in a single patient-subject. The DSM does not offer techniques for confronting the moral implications of multi-axial diagnosis; unlike psychoanalysis, it proposes no vision of ethical subjectivity. The diagnostic apparatus that divides delusion from lying in this heterodox setting contains, frozen within it, a moralism that cannot be addressed in its terms. Wielding this apparatus, Kiriaki's audience of therapists maneuvered their moralism about intentional lies *around* her unconscious motives, but they did not arrive at the truth.

A WOMAN IN BLACK

If diagnosis founders upon an ethical enigma when a patient intentionally lies with a pathological motive, then another kind of enigma arises when the patient in question lies intentionally but not pathologically. This section is devoted to a single therapy session with such a patient. I was invited to attend the session by Osman, one of three Turkish-speaking psychologists on staff at the Association. The son of a Turkish woman and a Pomaki man; educated in Greece, Turkey, and Bulgaria; a speaker of Greek, Turkish, Pomaki, Bulgarian, and a little Russian—Osman was remarkably flexible when it came to code-shifting in clinical encounters. He did not work in Alexandroupolis but at the mobile units in Komotini and Xanthi, his own city, where he had grown up in a Greek neighborhood bordering a Gypsy settlement. *I know their culture*, he would tell me, and his native facility in Greek and Turkish language and demeanor put him in a position to "work" them sometimes—to intimidate them or to put them at ease, to grasp their situation or to catch them in a lie. On this occasion, in Komotini, I more or less knowingly helped him "work" a patient with whom he had reached a therapeutic impasse.

Yazmi is a Gypsy, but she doesn't look it, Osman said: in her late-twenties, she was dressed in city clothes, tailored black pants and a sweater, moderate jewelry, her hair dyed blonde and pulled back in a tidy braid. He told me she had started therapy with him two years before, when she suffered from a "reactive depression" brought on by her husband's affair with a Russian woman he had met at a bar. Osman said he was certain that, at that time, Yazmi was seriously depressed and occasionally suicidal. Her treatment—antidepressant medication and biweekly counseling sessions—had progressed well, and after about a year she seemed to recover. But when she learned that her disability income would be cut off if she discontinued treatment, Yazmi began to feign symptoms of psychosis. Osman complained that her therapy had become a useless waste of time. She was lying about her illness, he said; he knew she was lying; she probably knew that he knew she was lying; yet neither of them could bring the relationship to an end. Osman told me that my presence might help to "shake things up," and encouraged me to ask whatever questions I liked. This represented a radical departure from the protocol I had discussed with the head of the mobile unit, who as yet had barely permitted me any access to patients, and had restricted my observation to a single session—during which I had, on instruction, remained silent.

Osman had warned me that Yazmi understood and spoke no Greek, so he would be translating for me throughout the session. She sat quietly across from us. Osman began by speaking gently to her in Turkish, eliciting tentative, one-word responses. Soon, he shifted tacks, addressing me instead, in Greek:

> Osman: *I told her that you're an anthropologist from America and you want to learn about her experience. What do you want to know?*
> EAD: *Can she describe her symptoms, her feelings? What's bothering her?*

He spoke with her for several minutes, then reported:

> Osman: *She says she feels asphyxiated, like she has a cord around her neck pulling her up toward the ceiling.*
> EAD: *Did this feeling start recently?*

Osman smiled at the doubt implied by this question, but he did not put it to her. Instead, he said he would ask her to tell us more about her feelings. He spoke to her, then to me:

> Osman: *She says she can't sleep. She sometimes hears voices telling her to hurt herself, or to leave the house. She says it's good that she has people around to keep her from doing these things.*
> EAD: *Who are these people? Who's living at home with her?*
> Osman (speaking with Yazmi for a few minutes): *At first, she said she*

didn't know where her husband was. Now she's saying that he sleeps at the house, but he leaves early in the morning and stays out late every night. He works, but never brings her any money. Only at Baïram, he brought them a few presents, mostly clothes, the sweater she's wearing. She has two children at the house, a thirteen-year-old daughter and a seven-year-old son. The son is going to school now, but the daughter quit school, because Yazmi needs her at home.

Osman broke off the translation at that point and again addressed me privately. He told me that Yazmi's confinement of her daughter was a "cultural thing": You see, the girl is of the age to get married. A boy from the neighborhood already attempted to "steal" her. But Yazmi wouldn't allow it, because she needs her daughter to take care of the house.

EAD: So how does her daughter feel about this?

Osman (speaking again with Yazmi): She doesn't want to go to school. But she also hates her parents. Her father more than her mother, this is what Yazmi says. The girl is always telling her how fed up she is with them.

Speaking to Osman, not for translation, I asked whether the daughter had ever accompanied Yazmi to a therapy session. He told me he had often requested this, because he thought it would help if the girl could understand her mother's illness and get some support herself, but the daughter had never come. He asked Yazmi why, and she responded quickly. Osman translated: She says the girl hates her, she'd never come. He asked again why, pressing, and got a longer response: She thinks the girl's afraid to be seen with her going to this kind of doctor. It would bring down her own standing. People would think that she's crazy too. See—it's exactly because of this fear that I want to see the daughter. I can explain that her mother isn't crazy, that she just has trouble dealing with her problems. It's a very human situation. And the daughter can learn to do better for herself, with the right support. I'd also like to see the husband, since he's at the heart of the family crisis. He came with Yazmi once last year, but he's out of reach now.

At that point, Osman abandoned the posture of the clinical interview and began talking directly to me about "the trouble" with the Gypsy community, in front of Yazmi, who continued to sit quietly. It's really a marginal community, he said. People have a lot of problems. And there's no work. That's why so many of them go to psychiatrists: they want sedatives, so they can just take pills and forget their problems. Yazmi, for instance: she just asked for more Xanax, but she says she doesn't need a refill of her antipsychotic meds. She's not taking them, obviously. As a trained psychologist, I know that patients should be given sedatives only if they're having an acute crisis, and only for a few weeks, until their other meds kick in. If the patient is really ill, he'll improve within six months; that's the typical pattern. These patients (gesturing to Yazmi) aren't really ill. Their "symptoms" never seem to clear up. But their suffering is real, and when they ask for sedatives it's hard to deny them.

Here's another way they give us a false face: they pretend to have psychosis. They know what they have to say: they hear voices, they see things that aren't there. I hear these symptoms all the time, always the same. I understand they're very poor, and they have practically no chance to improve their condition, since they're illiterate and they have no work experience. And they face so much racism in Greek society. But when they lie, when they make up an illness to get disability papers, they put me in an impossible position. If it were just a question of dispensing money, my opinion is that the state should provide welfare without restriction. If I were a social worker, I'd do everything I could to get them more resources. But I'm a therapist, and I have a responsibility to care for people with real mental and emotional problems. I can't lie about a diagnosis. I refuse to certify psychosis when I know it's false. There are limits to what I can do as a therapist for most of the people who come to me.

Abruptly Osman turned to Yazmi and asked her, in Greek, whether she understood what he had been saying. She stared and said nothing, so he asked her again in Turkish. This time, he told me, Yazmi confirmed that she had not understood a word. So much the better! Osman said. Taking this break as an opportunity to resume the interview, I asked him whether he had ever had her describe to him the voices she claimed to hear. Rather than addressing the question to her, he broke out laughing: No, you see: it's all lies! I wanted him to find out whether Yazmi would say that the antipsychotic medications he prescribed had actually reduced her psychotic symptoms. He again declined to engage her on this topic, shrugging at me and explaining that he had no idea whether she even took the medication.

EAD: Does she find that her therapy helps her?

Osman (speaking with Yazmi, then turning to me): She says that the medications really help. They calm her down, let her sleep, give her peace. If she doesn't take them, she starts talking constantly, talking to herself, getting angry and fighting with people. The medications help her not to behave this way. She'd die without them.

I had not been clear. The term therapy (θεραπεία) also means treatment, denoting medication. Yazmi's response to my question, expressing the extent of her need for sedatives, might have arisen from this ambiguity.

EAD: *So what about the talking part of therapy? Does it help her to talk about her problems with you?*

Osman (speaking with Yazmi): *Yes, she says it really helps her. My words stay in her ears for weeks.*

Once more, Osman turned to me and reiterated the impasse with Yazmi. *Lately she's been refusing to see me more than once a month, which is the minimum for her to keep her disability status. She arrives at the health center, and I have to sit with her, ask her questions, listen to her describe her symptoms, write her prescriptions. I'm doing this even though I don't believe her symptoms are real.*

It was a cynical situation, then, for both of them. I had seen Osman, like many clinicians, raise his voice to patients who he believed were manipulating him, and who frustrated his attempts to expose their manipulation. Occasionally he simply refused to see them at all. Yazmi elicited a different response, but it was not clear to me why, or whether Osman understood why. Perhaps he did see something pathological in her need and her persistence; or perhaps he wanted to preserve the therapeutic tie that had developed in the beginning, when Yazmi was seriously ill. From the point of view of this predicament—this enigmatic attachment—it was a forceful maneuver on Osman's part to invite me to the session, to disrupt their impasse, and to derail the mutually fraudulent trajectory of their dialogue. Yet he hesitated when it came to posing the questions of mine that might have advanced that work most directly.

At last Yazmi asked Osman if she could leave. Startled, he apologized (he told me) for subjecting her to our conversation, and she gracefully assured him that she had not been bothered. He translated her parting words to me: *She thanks you, and wishes you a long life.* She left without once looking directly at me. Later, I read through her file and found detailed there the shift in symptoms to which Osman had alluded earlier. According to the notes, Yazmi had made several serious attempts at suicide early in her treatment: once with a knife, once with pills, and she kept returning to the roof of her building in order to jump. For a time, she had also abused her two children. During the first year of therapy, her depression seemed to lift; she stopped beating her children and once again took up the management of her household. But soon she began talking to Osman about seeing "a woman in black" who followed her everywhere. She reported that someone had attacked her one night, when all was pitch dark, though her husband insisted no one was there. At this point, in addition to her regular regime of antidepressants and sedatives,

Yazmi was prescribed antipsychotic medication—evidently legitimating her symptoms of emerging psychosis. Yet her diagnosis was amended from depression to "personality disorder." Her apparent delusions were taken as lies.

THE SECRET ENCOUNTER

In part 1, I have observed the use of language by all the parties to clinical encounters—therapists, patients, family members, even myself—both to deliver information and to maneuver toward other goals. Patients placed demands on their therapists without specifying what they wanted; therapists tried to determine whether such demands were claims for help, and excluded as illegitimate those that seemed not to be. Lying, which signified by concealing the unknown motives behind illegitimate demands, exposed the absence of a psychiatric language for naming what patients wanted when they did not want help. In their confrontation with unreliable speech, clinicians perceived patients' intentions in the domain of consciousness, while their secret motives were exported to the unconscious.

The unconscious thus functioned in these clinical settings as a site of the unknown. It is one of many in contemporary Greek psychiatry—including the brain chemistry of mood, neural networks of behavior, and genes—that partially formalize speculation about the causal mechanisms at work in mental illness and treatment. While these other unknowns are projected into the future, their imagined solutions proving that psychiatry has been advancing all along toward an ever more humane and effective neuroscience, the unconscious appears to be a conceptual technology of the past—the ghost of an obsolete model of psychological subjectivity. Yet it continues to perform important hermeneutic work in the clinic. Anticipated advances in the bioscience of psychiatry depend on the meaning generated in clinical encounters, but deception in those encounters—which undermines or distorts that meaning—is not addressed as a scientific problem. The unconscious, in its mysterious dominion over intentional speech, carries the moral freight of deception in the clinic, authorizing suspicion as well as a clinical means of accounting moral responsibility to patients. The way that psychiatry is played as a truth game in these particular "heterodox" settings is thus crucial to the way the moralism of responsibility operates within it.

This game—which unfolds in treatment sessions, staff meetings, encounters in passing, and negotiations extending from the clinic to the welfare office, from patients' homes to the police station—is composed of unreliable speech. The truth of a patient's affliction may be deemed by those authorized to speak it, in the paradigmatic form of diagnosis, but that truth does not necessarily effect a resolution to the case. Suspicions of deception mark not only what is unknown but also what is unresolved in clinical encounters.

The truth of mental illness wrested from these suspicions depends on the mystification of the pragmatic determinants of deception on the part of both patients and therapists. I have therefore traced the pragmatic as well as the semantic functions of speech in these encounters. In theory, the semantic conventions of communication in the clinic—by which patients achieve transparency, and their efforts at communication intelligibly express their interior motives—make it possible for therapists to diagnose dishonesty as a symptom of mental illness, and to understand their patients' motives for lying in terms of their medical needs for care. But, as in Smaro's case, lying may disrupt the clinical ambition to contain them within these semantic conventions. Deception creates a pragmatic space to depart from these conventions, to angle around the clinical exchange of symptoms for diagnosis and treatment—like the active protest effected by silence in response to a normative demand for speech.[93]

In the context of psychiatric reform in Thrace, which counts on continuous and truthful communication, deception speaks instead of an entitlement to nontransparency shared by patients and therapists. The clinic can function here as an intimate space, where ethical relations may develop indifferently to barriers of culture, class, and power. Even if they arise from these barriers, the suspicion shared by a patient and therapist that the other is lying trace the latent positivity of a secret "subjugated," as Foucault has phrased it, by the scientific discourse of psychiatry.[94]

These suspicions mark a limit of collaborative responsibility in therapeutic relationships. When patients and therapists suspect one another of lying—about the symptoms and needs of the patient; about diagnosis and treatment options; about the effectiveness of therapy; about rules and procedures; about the reliability of judgment and commitment on both sides—they counter and yet anchor the work of "responsibilization." They counter it by contesting their transparency to one other; they anchor it by securing one other in something like what Gayatri Spivak calls a "secret encounter": an ethical engagement characterized "on both sides" by "the sense that something has not got across," animated by the persistent but impossible desire to reveal that "secret."[95]

I see suspicions of deception in community-based care in Thrace as strange refractions of responsibilization through this constitutive opacity in intimate ethical relations. As against the reformist goals of increasing patients' autonomy while scaling back clinical care, these suspicions actually help to secure mutual therapeutic dependencies. In the dishonest speech by which patients are often diagnosed with personality disorders—in their unreliability, their opaque instrumentality, their mistrust and disappointment in their therapists—we can see an appeal for intimacy: a demand that therapists know them, despite their manipulations; an entitlement to place on therapists the burden of that intimate knowledge. And we can see, in their therapists' perpetuation of treatment—despite the uncertainty of diagnosis and the failed promise of therapeutic regimens—an acceptance of that burden. Patients' lives may be sustained by this relation through the bureaucratic disbursement of medication and disability income, but also through the temporality of clinical care: a temporality of expectation and satisfaction that makes a future appear out of an unlivable present. The suspicions that bind patients and their therapists in this temporality of care perhaps convey their refusal, against the incitements of (neo)liberal reform, to take full responsibility for themselves, in the interest of keeping a relation going.

❋ ❋ ❋

Thus far, I have examined lying as a communicative and psychical phenomenon, identifying diagnostic factors that determine speech as symptomatically or morally meaningful in the clinic. But this language of the psyche does not exhaust the means of accounting responsibility for mental illness in Thrace. The two scenes in part 1 featuring clinical encounters of Gypsy patients point to a further determinant of responsibility that arises outside the clinic. Culture—both as an abstract concept corresponding to a psychological narrative of human development and socialization, and as a specific array of traits and propensities attributed to discrete, especially minority, populations—helped psychiatrists in Thrace to locate the source of secret motives for irresponsible behavior that they informally relegated to the unconscious. Lying was the main focus of this conjuncture between cultures and symptoms in Thrace; but isolation, tradition, ignorance, suicidality, criminality, and a suite of other non-normative behaviors amplified the apparently pathological character of minority culture. In part 2, I address the ways in which mental illness was imbricated with culture in Thrace, through identifications and suspicions that bound Greek therapists and minority patients.

Interlude:

The Jewel of Greece

Construction of the new General Regional University Hospital of Alexandroupolis—designed and overseen by a German architectural firm, and financed in large part by European Union grants to the municipality through its "International City of Networks" program—begins in 1995 and finishes in 2001, a year behind schedule. Contract disputes and administrative formalities delay its opening for nearly another two years while the massive complex sits empty, looming indefinitely atop a slope rising from the beachfront southwest of town, set back almost a mile of scrubby lawn from the shoreline highway, its creamy slab walls and two thousand windows glinting in the sun.

The move takes place, at last, over the Christmas holidays of 2002. The new hospital opens with the new year. "The jewel of Greece," people call it. *You don't have hospitals like this even in America!* people say to me, making a joke of their pride. The new psychiatry clinic is housed in a separate one-story building extending from the front of the main hospital, connected by a sky-lit walkway and an elevator bank. Its structure is cruciform, the interior space divided into two short and two long corridors, so that all the rooms have windows to the outside. Every clinician on staff has a private office. The patients' rooms have closets and toilets. The staff meeting room is equipped with a computer and a store of filing cabinets for the newly organized archive of medical records. The ban on smoking in medical facilities passed by Parliament the previous October, and ignored by staff and patients alike at the old hospital, is adopted and enforced in this bright, uncontaminated, climate-controlled space.

It's not long before structural problems begin to announce themselves. Doors angle off their bent metal frames; sediments show in the tap water. The ventilation system rattles so loudly that it disrupts group therapy in the patients' lounge. (In group one morning, a patient who works on the outside as a contractor points to the vents in the ceiling, laughing: *That's Greeks for you! A big European Union project like this, and they pocketed the money and paid some Albanians to put in the cheapest system possible. But I'll bet it looks right on the books.*)

And then: as the first month of operation draws to a close, those living and working in the hospital clinic begin to notice graffiti on its corridor walls, inside its restrooms, in the elevators and walkways en route to the main hospital building. And then outdoors, on the cinderblock walls enclosing the hospital grounds like ramparts. And then in the bus shelter at the hospital entrance. And then on the city buses that run the hospital line. Always, the same two lines, together or separately:

Αναφισμένος ο θεός—The import of *ο θεός*, "God," is clear enough, but debate arises among the clinic staff as to the meaning of *αναφισμένος*, which they do not recognize: a neologism characteristic of schizophrenic speech, one psychiatrist suggests. The word evokes a range of meanings through the metonymic associations of phonetic resonance. The staff speculates. Perhaps it's a past participle of *αναφαίνομαι* (to appear or emerge)—meaning, then, "God (has) appeared." Or perhaps of *αναφυσώ* (to breathe or blow)—meaning, "God (is) breathed (into presence)." Or it might be a distortion of the noun *αναφυλλητό* (sob, sobbing)—meaning, "God (is) sobbing." A nurse remarks, *It's depressing for the patients to see this on the brand-new walls.* And not only for them.

ο λεξείας—The staff deems this, too, a neologism. Rooted in the feminine noun *λέξη* (word), it is transformed, with an archaic flourish, into a masculine personal noun—meaning, perhaps, *the speaker, the rhetor, the word-giver.*

Weeks later, in the dank depths of February, as graffiti accumulates inside and beyond the hospital, the culprit is identified. Anthimos, a chronic patient diagnosed with acute paranoid schizophrenia, is one of the few who could not be discharged during the move from the old hospital over the holidays. Instead, he was transferred directly: one of the originary residents of the new clinic. As many times before, he was admitted in December by compulsory order, picked up by the police for dangerous behavior in a public place. A Pontian immigrant from Georgia, he lives with his elderly father in a small Pontian settlement on the outskirts of a nearby farming town. He speaks Russian, but very little Greek. Nina, the resident assigned to his case, admits she can barely understand him. But the fact that he is speaking at all at this point indicates his emergence from an intense relapse. After two months of silence, he has found his voice. He tells Nina that when he lived in Russia, he was plagued by communists; here in Thrace, it is diabolical priests who torture him. They have split open his rib cage and forced a spirit from his body. Spiders incessantly crawl out of his chest cavity. There is a war of angels and devils taking place inside him. *He seems to be having acute pain in his chest,* Nina reports at a staff meeting, *but there's no organic reason that we can find.* She prescribes steadily increasing doses of sedatives and Leponex (US Clozaril), an atypical antipsychotic medication used only in treatment-resistant schizophrenia due to its severe side effects and the onerous requirement for weekly blood monitoring.

Anthimos reveals to Nina that he is the one writing the lines of graffiti. But he will not tell her what they mean, or why he has been writing them everywhere he goes. *It wasn't a confession,* she says to us. He has apparently been sneaking out of the clinic, making illicit trips into the city with pocket change that he collects from other patients, leaving his trail of words in specific locations. He does not ask for permission to leave, but this is an open clinic, and he comes and goes quietly; his absences go unremarked, perhaps because he is invisible even when he does stay in the clinic, hiding in his bed or a dark corner of the lounge. Nina notes that he is "less angry" now than when he was first admitted, but his hallucinations and delusions persist unabated: *There are times when I come to his bedside and he doesn't even recognize me.*

Nina is charged, that month, with supervising two young medical students on a special research project. They have been reading files for weeks while they wait to interview an actual patient. One early afternoon, as we sit together in the meeting room, discussing their project, Nina bursts in. *OK, you give it a try with Anthimos,* she says, throwing his chart down on the table. *I don't think you'll get much out of him, but it's good for you to learn what a heavy case is like. He's calm in his bed. Go ahead.*

I go with the two students; Nina suggests I might be able to help. They have prepared a questionnaire that immediately proves useless. Anthimos does not look at the students. He grunts when they ask his name, his age, his residence. He winces and slaps at the air in front of him. But he lucidly gives them the precise dates of his schooling in Georgia, his military service in Russia, and his flight to Greece as a refugee from the civil war. He tells a fragmented story, in broken Greek, about how he and his brother left their father's cabin in the woods years ago to join the army. It was cold, he says. No boots. Kars, kars—the word for snow, in Turkish.

Anthimos swats spiders as he grasps for Greek, enclosing his manifold strangeness in a pall of unintelligibility. Mute, he spoke first in writing—a cipher in his adoptive yet enigmatically ancestral tongue, signed with his tag: ο λεξείας. In the clinic, his neologistic creations signify cognitive disorder. Still, they demand sense-making on the part of his auditors, natives of the language he distends and distorts. His graffiti performs, as Michael Taussig says of "defacement," a transgressive and mystical act of unmasking and illuminating that "creates sacredness."[1] God itself materializes in these iterations of Anthimos. The battle of angels and devils taking place within his body leaves written traces on the scaffolding of the new European enterprise: development and integration of the periphery, already falling to pieces.

PART 2

Strangers

ON HYPOCRISY AND HONOR

My final meeting with Dr. Filalithi, just before her summer vacation and my departure from Thrace, was repeatedly interrupted by patients and staff seeking her attention, her counsel, her signature. Our disjointed discussion took the form of an official interview, one of the few I conducted and recorded at the clinic. She was telling me about the misunderstandings that often arose between Greek therapists and minority patients in Thrace, who did not share a language or culture. She described the special difficulty of diagnosing personality disorders in these patients, especially when it came to the "antisocial" behavior of Gypsies. A proper diagnosis in these cases, she explained, demanded a disaggregation of individual pathology from cultural norms that often appeared bizarre and immoral to therapists.

I was pressing Filalithi to consider that personality disorders called for moral judgments of character rather than clinical judgments of symptoms. Perhaps she took my probing as a sign that I did not comprehend her explanation; it would not have been the first time that my curiosity was deflected as a misunderstanding of the language. She abandoned her didactic approach, and the conversation strayed from our clinical terrain:

> OK, I'll give you a different example, which I like. Oftentimes, when I'm talking about this kind of thing here with our own people, with Greeks, they'll say they regard Europeans, northern Europeans, as very standoffish people—I mean, emotionally cold. On the other hand, if you

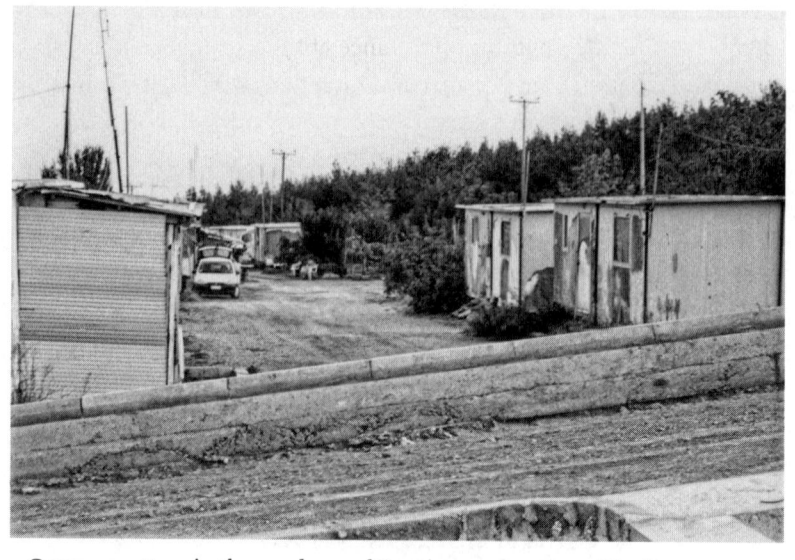

Gypsy squatters in the condemned Pontian settlement at Neo Ipsos, 2004.
Photo by Elizabeth Anne Davis

talk with northern Europeans, Englishmen or Scandinavians, they'll tell you that Greeks are very . . . put it this way: they're very hypocritical [*υποκριτικοί*]—that is, we speak with grand words, but in reality we do very little.

I believe these are both misunderstandings, owing to the fact that generally, in some regions of the Mediterranean, for various historical and other reasons, people have learned to express themselves with greater intensity. But I don't think we're hiding something by this. . . . It's simply a way of expressing feelings. People who express themselves strongly, when they see someone speak with less feeling, they don't explain it as a type of behavior; they think he has some personal mental defect. And when the others see someone who expresses himself more intensely, but what he says doesn't correspond very well to what he does, they think that it's a moral failing. But it isn't a moral failing; it's just a trait. . . . (*She starts talking louder and faster.*) That's the way it is: Greeks exaggerate when they talk!

What the doctor was offering me in this commentary on hypocrisy was a legacy of the "honor and shame" paradigm in classic Mediterranean anthropology.[1] Greeks—through the metonym of Greek men—

have been known in this anthropology for their rhetorical cunning, their voluble bravura, their public performance of "egoism" (εγωϊσμός) to advance their economic and political interests. This style of self-expression is attributed, by some, to a Mediterranean symbolics of public masculinity, according to which a "libidinized social reputation" secures advantage along with social ties between households and communities.[2] In this portrait, honesty is not a social virtue, crucial as it might be to relations of trust within the household.[3] If honesty marks the intimacy of domestic life, then dishonesty—"hypocrisy"—is the precious currency of public life.[4] It is peculiar to this interior and exterior anatomy of the Mediterranean self that it is bound by the collective morality of shame rather than the individual psychology of guilt.[5]

In view of this ethnographic burden of Mediterranean selfhood, borne quite knowingly by this ethnographically-informed psychiatrist, we can see in that example she liked so well a moment of what Michael Herzfeld has termed "cultural intimacy": a strategic performance of "rueful self-recognition," of ambivalent identification with national culture through the self-stereotyping assertion of norms, which speakers disparage and respect at the same time across different scales of abstraction and "levels of power."[6] Listening to the recording of this interview now, years later, I hear myself begin to laugh when Filalithi says that Greeks "in reality do very little." I have sensed that she is addressing me, at that moment, not as an anthropologist or a coworker in the clinic, but as a foreigner, more or less like those northern Europeans who ascribe dishonesty to the Greeks. But I do not want to talk about differences between Greeks and *foreigners*. I do not want the difference between Filalithi and myself, marked by her pedagogical address to me, to take a cultural or national form: Greek versus American. I laugh to show her that I have taken her meaning, and that if I exercise cultural stereotypes about Greeks myself, it is with sufficient irony about my position as a foreigner. She endures my laughter but does not share it. And so I insist; I tell her explicitly: "I'm not laughing for that reason!"—meaning, *you do speak with intensity, but I don't think you're lying!* I push her to address culture as a clinical problem rather than as a set of behavioral norms. I suggest that it must be difficult for patients and therapists to form a "good relation" when they approach one another from opposite sides of a cultural divide. Filalithi agrees, politely. She says, *I find that, in general, people don't try to put themselves in one another's shoes. They judge a different culture by their own values.*

Our conversation founders on this bit of potted wisdom. I take it as a refusal, and abruptly change the subject. But it occurs to me, as I listen to the recording years later, that Filalithi might have understood my laughter better than I did. Had I not, just before she began her disquisition on hypocrisy, been pressing her to acknowledge the bad faith inherent in her diagnosis of personality disorders among Gypsies? Was I not, myself, performing a certain bad faith in my refusal to identify with the cultural stereotyping she attributed to foreigners? It seems to me now that she was insisting on the impossibility for the two of us, a Greek and an American, to discuss dishonesty strictly in clinical terms. Perhaps I did observe a moral failing in her—and she, a mental defect in me. What we shared at that moment was not, then, a professional relativism about cultural difference, but rather the pretence of that common stance: a functional collusion that made it possible for our quite divergent work with minority patients to be conducted more or less harmoniously.

In such a conversation, the horizon of clarity, where irony and pragmatics are abandoned and things appear realistically as they are, recedes infinitely into the analytic distance. In the description this psychiatrist gave of the expressive culture of the Greeks, she offered an analytic puzzle to the ethnographer. She accredited the "hypocrisy" of the Greeks to a cultural context that privileges public face over private conscience, even if the clinical environment in which our encounter took place demanded that we acknowledge, as well, a psychological interior absent from this imagination of the culturally performative self. In the clinic, where lies may be interpreted first as symptoms of mental illness, the pragmatic deceptions of "Greek hypocrisy" would seem to serve as a cultural foil for pathological forms—such as those stereotypically presented by Gypsy patients with personality disorders. These cultures of deception are ethnographic artifacts; the instability of truth that troubles the clinical encounter in psychiatry likewise troubles the dialogic encounter in anthropology. The two human sciences shadow each other here, yielding a correlation between cultural difference and pathology.

Yet by asserting hypocrisy as a broader Mediterranean culture, and this regional culture as a frame of reference for our conversation, Filalithi implied a certain affinity between Greek and other cultures of deception, such as that of the Gypsies—or, in any case, a smaller distance, more narrowly and dialogically defined than it appeared in the clinical profile so often applied by Greek psychiatrists to their Gypsy patients. A "native" in both the cultural and the scientific scenarios we were discussing, the doctor was able, in this suddenly pragmatic moment of our conversation, to shift the priority of cultural over scientific reference and dismantle my suspicion of her dishonesty. In the clinic, she seemed to suggest, local cultures of deception—Greek and Gypsy—enjoy a sort of intimacy, wherein lying can be understood in terms of shared norms rather than of the distancing alterity of mental pathology.

Reflections

The predicament of personal responsibility among psychiatric patients in community-based care is painfully embodied in their ambivalent attachments to community, attachments that express both a yearning and a fear to belong and depend. What community means to these patients is shaped in part by the dream of psychiatric reformers in Greece, who imagined "the community" of community-based care, in the most abstract and idealized terms, as a healthful refuge for patients no longer (or never) to be interned in state hospitals. But it has been left to patients themselves to determine, on their own, how to belong to the communities in which they find themselves living. As I show in the sections that follow, this is a belonging beset by trouble with boundaries.

The Turkish and Bulgarian borders of Thrace—the European borders of the Muslim and Soviet worlds through the twentieth century—have long conferred on Greece a special role in constituting European identity, in both cultural and political terms. Anthropologists have variously recognized the refraction of European "border anxiety" in the governance of minority populations within Greece.[7] From a more methodological vantage, Herzfeld argues from the European borders of Greece for the special relation Greek ethnography bears to the discipline of anthropology. He traces the manifold parallels between anthropology and Greek ethnography, demonstrating the "historical artificiality of separating our own theoretical tradition from its object of study."[8] Indeed, so tightly knit together are the ethnographic study of Greek culture and anthropology as a field that only Greece, in his reckoning, in its unique position as the "internal other" of Europe, can serve anthropology as a site of internal disciplinary critique.

The central axis of this comparison relates the golden Greece of European origins to the fallen Greece of Ottoman contamination. It is a historico-theoretical comparison: the modern moment that engendered and dispatched anthropology and "romantic statism" along the same trajectory, finding the legitimation of Western civilization in a Greek antiquity irretrievably lost to its easternized modern Greek heirs, pitted the internal diversity distinctive of Europe against the homogeneity of its marginal cultures in an "international rhetorical contest" — a global game of honor and shame, whose own symbolic logic was then attributed to those cultures, especially in the Mediterranean periphery.[9] Herzfeld witnesses ethnographically the symbolism of honor and shame in Greece, and its rhetoric of "self-presentation and self-concealment" [10] — but not primarily in the sphere of sexual relations to which it has been attributed by Mediterraneanist anthropologists. Rather, he finds it operating in the theoretical relation Europe has established with Greece, which is, as the title of his book suggests, a mirroring relation.

In this critique of structural anthropology, Herzfeld takes up the symbolic oppositions of structural analysis not so much to deconstruct them as to show them at work in the dynamic between the West and its others, in the very grounds of anthropological theory, borne of colonial (and "crypto-colonial") conquest and domination. Neni Panourgiá, in her "anthropography" of mourning and kinship in Athens, turns this "classificatory device" of "othering" on its head, taking herself and her family as objects and subjects.[11] Juxtaposing the subjectifying nativity of moral bonds with the objectifying transcendence of analysis, her text verifies an alterity internal to anthropology, from a position beside rather than behind the mirror in which Greece and the West find their distorted reflections.

Taking these leads, in part 2 of this text I follow the trail of a self-reflexive and uniquely Greek dialogue between anthropology and psychiatry on the question of culture. The three main sections engage three modes of relation between patients and therapists, mediated implicitly or explicitly by cultural imaginaries in Thrace. First: a valorization of rural tradition, and its dynamics of authority and submission between doctors and patients, which seem to trump overt cultural differences between Greeks and Turks. Next: a culture of dependency on state care among Gypsies, nourished by the institutional impetus to preserve a clinical purview over pathological behavior — and, by consequence, to preserve therapeutic relations with patients whose mental illness is perpetually in doubt. Finally: a collapse of the symbolic opposition between self and other, yielding uncanny cultural identifications between Greek therapists and Pontian immigrant patients. Despite their complex heterogeneity, I interpret the mental disorders that materialize among minority patients in these therapeutic relationships with Greeks — conversion disorder, antisocial personality disorder, and paranoia, respectively—as features of ethical cultures that counter the liberal "rights culture" of personal responsibility promoted by psychiatric reform.

CONVERSION

In the summer of 2002, the Association launched a community outreach program in Komotini, a prefect capital with a large Muslim population. The program aimed to raise community awareness about the nature of mental illness and the accessibility of local psychiatric services. But the therapists who ran the program reported at their next staff meeting that the Turks of the city, like their rural kinsmen, formed a "closed community" disposed toward ignorance and shame about mental illness. The staff had set up a booth at the local bazaar, displayed the paintings of art-therapy patients, and handed out brochures. They had enlisted the help of Muslim teachers and community leaders. Even so, hardly anyone attended the information sessions they had advertised. A therapist who worked in Komotini said, *We've all witnessed the plight of Muslim patients, especially the women: they keep quiet, they're forbidden to speak for themselves or have an opinion.* The staff envisioned a long, slow process of chipping away at Muslim conservatism in the area before the new community-based psychiatric services would be able to take root.

A year after the community outreach program failed in Komotini, I worked for several weeks in the outpatient psychiatry clinic at the General Hospital of Komotini. Evyenia, a nurse who commuted there daily from Alexandroupolis to assist Dr. Karras, gave me a ride the first day. When we turned north off the interstate and entered the foothills rising to Komotini, we passed a small group of village women dressed in head scarves and long black robes, waiting for the bus by the side of the road. Evyenia told me she had once seen such a group of covered women at the beach: *All they could do was wade in up to their ankles, with their husbands calling them back to shore to watch the children!* She described the absurdity of this spectacle as a "natural critique" of the oppression symbolized and effected by conservative Muslim garb: *I pity these women. It's a terrible thing to be trapped your whole life not just inside your house but inside your clothing as well. I see this every day at the hospital. The men insist on accompanying their wives into their sessions, and the women stand silently behind them. They can't speak, even about themselves.*

Evyenia explained that sexism was not so much a Muslim religious practice as it was a custom of "traditional culture." *After all, she said, Turkish women living in Istanbul are more like Greek women today than they are like those villagers on the side of the road. Fifty years ago, Greek women used to live like that, too. My own mother was raised that way. She grew up in a suburb of Athens that was very conservative. She was supposed to be a virgin when she married. She was forbidden to leave the house without a male escort. She couldn't visit anyone but relatives or female friends. Greek husbands used to be jealous of other men around their wives— even their own friends! They're still very jealous, but the situation has changed a lot for Greek women of my generation. Mostly it's cultural influences from outside: war and tourism. The Muslim women here will have the same freedoms some day.*[12]

Later that morning, an elderly, covered Turkish woman came to Dr. Karras's outpatient office for a scheduled appointment. She was unescorted—Karras told me later that her husband, who used to come to the clinic with her, had died recently—and she communicated mainly through gestures and documentary traces: an insurance booklet, a disability certificate, flattened pillboxes. She had run out of her sedative medication some time ago, and though she had come to the hospital the previous week for a refill, she had apparently been deterred by Gypsies in the hallway, who were making such a racket that she had gotten scared and left. Karras was sympathetic. He exclaimed delightedly at the photograph of the woman stapled into her insurance booklet, taken thirty years before, at the onset of her illness. The doctor asked the patient to take off her scarf and show us what she looked like now. Hesitantly, she removed it, revealing her lined brow and long gray braids piled delicately on top of her head. Karras smiled: *You see? You look beautiful that way.*

※　※　※

Early and often during my time in Thrace, I was advised by Greek clinicians not to ask Muslim patients about their religion: *They'll be suspicious of why you're asking. They're afraid they'll be persecuted for their beliefs.* Other tactics were recommended, other questions—about traditional therapies, witchcraft and magic, herbal remedies—that might get at the same elements of difference, but indirectly. The religion of Islam would not be discussed in the clinic, guarded as it seemed to be by the silence and the sartorial concealment of covered women—remarkable precisely in contrast to the volubility and visibility of their Gypsy counterparts, who were said to be Muslims too, but "in name only."

Yet if religion was beyond discourse, a robust vocabulary of difference was available to discuss Muslim culture. Osman, Takan, and Özlem,

Turkish-speaking psychologists who worked with the Association's mobile units in the Rodopis prefecture, were the experts. Just as they shared their insight into Muslim culture with their Greek colleagues, so they took responsibility for all the Muslim patients seeking psychiatric care in these settings.

Takan often talked to me about what he called his "cultural identity." He told me he had come to embrace this identity—guiltily—when his grandfather, a devout Muslim, passed away, and Takan began to reflect on the loss. In many respects, he said, he was ashamed of "traditional Muslim culture," especially of the way it devalued women: *My mother lives upstairs from us, and she's still covered. It bothers me. It bothers my wife. This is what really exposes the hypocrisy of the fundamentalists: they insist on the veil, even though no command can be found anywhere in the Quran. But when it comes to their duty to give alms, which is spelled out in the sacred text, only then do they avert their eyes.*

Yet Takan's "cultural identity" had a proud aspect as well. He had suffered as a Greek Muslim, he told me. Years ago, when he returned to Thrace from Bulgaria, where he had earned a joint master's degree in social work and psychology, he had been unable to find work except at supermarkets and gas stations. The Association was more progressive than the state psychiatric services, where not a single Turkish translator had yet been hired, never mind a bilingual therapist. When the Association opened branches in Sapes and Komotini, Osman and Özlem were hired immediately; Takan joined the team a few years later. Still, they were overloaded with Turkophone patients, and worked in a state of constant exhaustion and frustration.

Occasionally, Osman—whose emotive vigor turned easily from boisterous conviviality to voluble tetchiness—would run into conflict with the Greek staff. *I have too many patients, but I feel like I can't give any of them to Greek therapists. See, it's a characteristic of my people to feel deep shame when they have to express their private feelings to a doctor. I have my own ways of helping them overcome their shame. Like those "cultural techniques" you were talking about.* He laughed, recalling my attempts to discuss ritual healing practices informed by the Quran. *Greek therapists don't understand this. They think I'm inappropriate with patients, that I'm too friendly and indulgent.*

An argument had erupted recently over just this issue when Iota, a psychiatric nurse, had intercepted one of his Turkish patients while he was busy writing prescriptions for someone else. She tried to defuse the patient's complaints and to give him an appointment herself. When

Osman learned of this afterward, he was furious. Iota contended that she had been trying to save him the trouble of dealing with this patient, a "whiner" (γρινιάρης) who would "eat" all of Osman's time. But he told her it was "aggressive" for her to make an assessment in his place, especially since she lacked the expertise to "read" this patient correctly. *Cultural conflicts like this are not unusual*, he told me.

The Active Position

The history of Greek psychiatric reform is also a history of cultural change, a modernization in values that would locate Greece in the developed rather than the developing world, from an epidemiological point of view. Greek reformers in the early years took, as one of their principle obstacles, the conservatism of traditional Greek culture and its penchant for stigmatizing and isolating the mentally ill.[13] As a humanitarian project, reform demanded a recession of this traditional culture and the advent, in its place, of political liberalism—or, as I often heard it called, "rights culture"—as the grounds of a superior and global morality. Resistance to this more tolerant morality was commonly attributed to cultural differences between the urban, educated psychiatrists who formed the vanguard of reform and the rural communities whose most marginal members they treated.

These reformers, in accord with Mediterraneanist anthropologists of an earlier time, contended that a traditional "culture of shame" in Greece disposed patients, especially women, to deny the psychological nature of their medical problems and to express them instead through the unwitting complaints of their bodies.[14] These conversion disorders marked the extent to which traditional culture resisted modernization. Thus, as chronically ill patients were discharged from state hospitals, the communities into which they assimilated became, themselves, objects of a different kind of reform. At the same time, therapists introduced psychotherapy into individual treatment, forging an explicit link between patients' rights and responsibilities, on the one hand, and psychological (as against somatic) symptoms, on the other—urging clinical distress out of the body and into the discursive domain of therapeutic persuasion.

According to early studies of the new community-based services in Thrace conducted by Charalambos Ierodiakonou and his team,[15] patients were slow to enter this discursive domain. Holding to their rural epidemiological profile, they typically presented physical complaints to their nascent psychotherapists, and expected laboratory tests and medications in return. Attempting to dismantle the somatic rubric of these encounters, therapists met only with mistrust and resistance, and they "gradually came to the conclusion that during the first four to five days the patient had to get what he expected, if confidence toward the doctor was to be built."[16] The "main problem" in establishing therapeutic relationships with such patients, then, was to "avoid strengthening somatization" in those early days. Gradually, the "psychogenic" theory of physical illness—explained by therapists and demonstrated by other patients whose health had improved with psychotherapy—would come to be "more acceptable," and subjects would begin to verbalize rather than somatize their mental distress.[17]

In these early negotiations, rural patients reportedly displayed a "lack of initiative" in their treatment and "dependency" on their therapists. According to psychiatrists working in Thrace, this passive disposition was nurtured by the emphasis in rural Greek society on the institution of the family. Many patients, who remained within the controlling orbit of the family and the "social superego" through which it organized rural life, presented "individuation and maturation" problems.[18] Confronted with their immature passivity, therapists were obliged at first to meet their patients' expectations and take an "active role": to gain patients' trust and cooperation by mobilizing their inclination to submit to authority. Ierodiakonou observed that therapists would need gradually to "withdraw from the active position," without provoking mistrust, and to encourage patients to assume the responsibility for their health that they had been "project[ing]" onto their caretakers.[19]

Studies on community-based care in Thrace through the 1980s document a growth in this sense of responsibility among patients. Many even began taking active part in the healthcare network, referring themselves and other patients to the outpatient clinic at the General Hospital of Alexandroupolis. During the first year of community mental healthcare in Thrace (1980–81), one local treatment team observed a 23 percent increase in the number of patients returning on their own initiative to the outpatient clinic for follow-up care, signifying "an awareness of the need for periodic reevaluation of the patient and his family."[20] During the first three months, the number of patients seeking treatment at the clinic on the advice of other patients increased by 36 percent, and that number more than doubled during the remainder of the first year. These trends indicated to reformers a "development of trust" toward therapists among the rural population, as well as a "destigmatization" of mental illness itself.[21]

These population metrics, which pervade the Greek psychiatric literature of the 1980s, do not straightforwardly represent a rise in voluntary outpatient care as against involuntary inpatient care. In fact, the total number of psychiatric patients in Thrace who received voluntary *and* involuntary treatment increased during this period. The narrative of reform that mobilizes these numbers to mark a trend toward self-directed patient care obscures the absolute expansion of psychiatric care, whose meaning to that trend is actually quite ambiguous. But it also obscures new forms of patient dependency yielded by the shift from hospital- to community-based care: the transformation of what is known as "hard chronicity" in mental illness, characteristic of custodial institutions, into the "soft chronicity" more typical in outpatient settings.[22] The documented rise in patient responsibility in Thrace thus does not necessarily index therapeutic progress. What it necessarily indexes is the proliferation of relationships between therapists and patients—even through the persistence of forms of pathology, such as conversion disorder, that are poorly suited to self-directed treatment in the community.

❋ ❋ ❋

The week I began working in the psychiatry clinic at the General Hospital of Alexandroupolis, I was asked to give an introductory presentation to the entire staff, outlining the research I planned to pursue during my time there. This was the moment when it was settled, rather without my consent, that my study of "cultural factors in mental illness" meant I would be working primarily with "Muslim" rather than "Greek" patients. After the meeting, Dr. Filalithi called me into her office to discuss a case that she said might be interesting "from a cultural point of view." She introduced me to Fazilet, a young covered woman who had been admitted to the clinic the previous day for progressive "hysterical crises."[23] Filalithi spoke to me for her, though Fazilet had finished middle school and, I discovered later, knew the Greek language well. Filalithi named her ethnic and religious affiliations, explaining that of the three main Muslim groups in the area, Fazilet was "neither Gypsy nor pure Turk." She belonged to the third group, the Pomahomadan,[24] who had "their own traditions."

Now thirty years old, Fazilet lived in the same small village where she was born, in the hills north of Sapes. She told us, intimating ambivalence about their constancy, that her husband and mother-in-law had been staying in her room at the clinic since her admission: *They're the ones who brought me here. They won't leave me.* She had apparently suffered several episodes when she "went wild" (άγρια), shrieking and rending her clothing, and then fainting. Afterward, she would remember nothing; so she, like her doctors, relied on reports from her family about these symptoms. Her file showed no organic illness or history of psychosis, though she had been admitted to the clinic once the previous year for depression, accompanied by headaches, dizziness, and numbness in her hands. Since then, she had taken Xanax but had not sought counseling with a therapist; she said it was too difficult to leave her family and travel to a health center where psychiatric services were available.

Later that morning, I attended a clinical interview with Fazilet conducted by Zevs, the resident assigned to her case. His diagnostic work turned on the portrait of her home life that he drew out with gentle questions, punctuated by unhurried lulls. He explained to me later that he usually approached Muslim women patients this way, since they were often "closed off" (κλειστές) and easily intimidated; he employed other strategies with other patients. In the interview, Fazilet told us she shared a small house in the village with her husband and two teenaged sons: *My in-laws live next door, and they're very involved in our life. My parents live nearby, too, but not as close. I've been married since I was fourteen. That's normal where I live. We had two children right away. But we decided not to have any more, for economic reasons. My older son is fifteen now. I'm so happy he'll be getting married soon. When my daughter-in-law comes to live with us, I'll finally have a girl to keep me company at home.*

When Zevs pressed her, Fazilet admitted that she sometimes felt "overwhelmed" by her responsibilities at home and was especially "distraught" (στενοχωρημέν) on account of her mother-in-law. Zevs offered to speak with the old woman about this, but Fazilet implored him not to: *She'll know I complained about her, and it'll only make things worse for me.* Instead, Fazilet asked to go home, insisting that she was well now and that her children and husband needed her. Yet she feared that she might have another "spell." *Doctor, what is this illness I have? I used to be fine. I don't understand what's happening to me.* Zevs assured her that it was nothing to be scared of: *We all have problems and worries in life. You're having trouble handling* the pressures *you face at home, and your crises are like explosions of all that bottled-up pressure.* He told her she could manage these episodes, and even prevent them, by learning how to adapt to the pressure in a healthier way.

Zevs agreed to discharge Fazilet that afternoon, so long as she promised to rest once she got home. He wanted her to avoid child care and housework for a few days, and in the future to "learn to say no" to the excessive demands her family placed on her. Fazilet promised to take it easy. She was released, the day after her admission, with an appointment for neurological exams and a checkup with Zevs the following week. He prescribed her more Xanax and a controlled hypnotic, warning that she should only take the latter when she needed to rest; he did not want to exacerbate her problems with a chemical addiction.

Fazilet's "spells" emerged from this diagnostic interview as symptoms of a classic hysterical crisis. Filalithi, who used the word *classic* to describe this case as a page out of Freud, told me that hysteria in this form was "not often seen these days," even in a place as "remote" as Alexandroupolis. The patient's social profile—female, housebound, semiliterate, rural, poor—linked her symptoms to a tradition prior to modernization, a history of mental illness before psychiatric reform. Nerves (νεύρα), depressive anxiety (στενοχώρια), and fugue; loss of motor control, consciousness, and memory: these conversion symptoms were the signs of a traditional culture whose conservatism was amplified, in Fazilet's case, by its affiliation to an isolated minority community. The doctors did not take these signs as symptoms of a discrete psychiatric syndrome that would yield to therapy, though in a different context they might have portended the onset of depression or psychosis. Traditional culture normatively shaped the conversion by which this warning was expressed—but in the clinic, the force of this culture withdrew at the threshold of modern mental disorder.

Body to Mind

At the hospital clinic in Alexandroupolis, Filalithi was the leading proponent of transcultural psychiatry.[25] The year I arrived, the training curriculum she had developed for the new cohort of residents included a textbook on the subject just published by Miltos Livaditis, a colleague with extensive clinical experience in Thrace who often gave seminars at the hospital. Remarking, in his introduction, on the unique conjuncture in Thrace of psychiatric reform and the "cultural diversity" of the population, Livaditis locates Greece downwind of a new political and cultural consciousness arising in psychiatry elsewhere:

> One of the factors that determines the quality of mental health services is the cultivation of an anthropological way of thinking among the staff. Our contemporary social context makes it incumbent on everyone involved in mental health services to recognize and accept the particular cultural-ideological identity of the person one is dealing with, and to think carefully about how this can affect his life, his behavior, and the clinical picture he presents. . . . In many societies, especially in North America and the European Union, a rich dialogue on these issues began decades ago, a dialogue that has often been critical of the prevailing ideologies and conditions [of mental healthcare]. This dialogue has imprinted itself, though only up to a point, on official psychiatric reason and its systems of classifying psychical disorders such as the DSM-IV, which underscores the usefulness of cultural factors in diagnostic and therapeutic procedures. In Greece, these issues are not often discussed.[26]

Livaditis's book, *Culture and Psychiatry*, can be read as an incitement to just such a discussion. The text outlines a psychiatric context for culture, a concept he explicitly borrows from the field of anthropology. To address what he calls "complex difficulties" in the "cross-cultural therapeutic encounter," Livaditis proposes a multifaceted program of aid and support that, in the Euro-American vein of multiculturalism, "respects" the customs and ideologies of minority communities rather than suppressing, rejecting, or assimilating them. He approaches the cross-cultural encounter in psychiatry armed with two basic "theses." First, the "subjective culture" of a patient—defined as the implicit, collective system of meanings, values, and rules internalized by a subject—must be respected and protected, and treated in the therapeutic encounter as the basis of the patient's psychical equilibrium. Second, psychological services and counseling must recognize and utilize the "level of organization of the personality" that corresponds to the patient's cultural background.[27]

To help the psychiatrist understand the patient's subjective culture and the associated organization of his or her personality, Livaditis proposes something like a differential diagnosis of culture itself. This diagnosis progresses along four axes, describing the developmental dynamic between subject and culture that gives rise to an encultured patient: individualism versus sociocentrism; horizontally versus vertically organized social relationships; strong versus weak avoidance of uncertainty; masculinity versus femininity. Within the cultural grid constructed by these four axes, Livaditis introduces several further, "microcosmic" distinctions between cultural patterns—including whether family relations are hierarchical or symmetrical, whether conceptions of self are referential or indexical, and whether cognitive and communicative modes are paradigmatic ("metaphorical") or narrative ("metonymic"). He warns that these distinctive cultural patterns may generate "misunderstandings" if conflicts arise between persons from dominant and minority cultures. Ideally, the cross-cultural encounter between dominant-culture psychiatrists and minority-culture patients should move from this initial moment of conflict toward an acceptance ("to a point") of the contingency and relativity of cultural traditions and values.

Though Livaditis draws throughout his text on international scholarship in transcultural psychiatry, citing figures from Ruth Benedict to Arthur Kleinman, his views gain their most distinctive authority from his clinical experience with minority cultures in Thrace: Turkish, Pomaki, Gypsy, and Pontian.[28] He devotes considerable attention to patients from these "sociocentric" communities—those characterized by hierarchical social and family ties, by "referential/relational selfhood," and by the indirect expression of personal experiences and emotions.[29] In his view, patients from these cultures require a conceptualization of responsibility that is invested in the group, rather than in individual subjects. He thus advises psychiatrists to orient therapy with such patients toward interpersonal relations and family dynamics, rather than toward individual "self-knowledge" and "self-governance."

In these reflections on cultural difference in the clinical encounter, Livaditis keeps to the cross-cultural approach outlined in the DSM-IV. After the first nine hundred or so pages, the text presents Appendix I, a glossary of culture-bound syndromes associated with mental pathology or dysfunction in non-Western cultures.[30] In the manual, these syndromes are counted as distinct from the local, culturally mediated expression of standard mental disorders classified in the main text of the DSM, though they might share some symptoms. The glossary of culture-bound syndromes, like the rest of the DSM, aims to be descriptive rather than prescriptive. But since many of the disorders listed here entail conversion symptoms, the glossary can be read as a corrective to the ethnocentrically prescriptive nature of the category, "somatoform disorder," presented in the main text. There, *somatoform* names a class of clinical mental disorders characterized by distress or impairment from physical symptoms not caused by a "general medical condition." This class contains a variety of disorders, such as pain disorder and hypochondriasis, introduced with the caveat: "The symptoms listed in this manual are examples that have been found *most diagnostic* in the United States."[31]

Much work in the medical anthropology of Greece has focused on somatoform symptoms more diagnostic of Greek than American patients.[32] This research has contested the status of somatic symptoms, such as nerves (νεύρα) and depressive anxiety (στενοχώρια), as culture-bound syndromes. Instead, these symptoms are presented as cultural idioms of emotional distress attributed, by patients as well as by anthropologists, to restrictive and arduous sociopolitical conditions of life. For the most part, the idioms themselves—including bodily pain, numbness, dizziness, heart palpitations, insomnia, and amnesia—do not differ cross-culturally; what differ are the normative conditions under which patients, typically poor women, put them to use in communicating their distress. The symptoms do not, in this literature, signify a distinctively Greek clinical profile, but rather a standard somatoform symptomatology, expressed in numerous and disparate cultural contexts outside the modern urban West.

Though the concept of somatization was prevalent in Arthur Kleinman's early research on neurasthenia in China,[33] in his later work he describes somatization as an "ethnocentric" term used by Western psychiatrists and anthropologists to describe the bodily expression of mental illness—ethnocentric because the "psychological" symptoms that characterize mental illness in the West are "decidedly uncommon" in the rest of the world, yet occupy pride of place in purportedly international psychiatric nosology.[34] Elsewhere, Kleinman proposes the more complex term *sociosomatic* to describe the somatic mode of symptom formation as "an idiom of interpersonal distress" that reflects patients' embeddedness in "political and social processes" foregrounding the body.[35] The study of "embodiment" in medical anthropology presaged this departure from the reductive psychomedical rubric of somatization.[36] Prominent here is the work of Nancy Scheper-Hughes, who locates the "embodiment of distress" in "somatic culture": that is, culture that "privilege[s]" the body in both phenomenological experience and interpretive meaning, constituting a way of life for many subjugated people whose bodies are inescapably the subject of their labor, the currency of their interpersonal dynamics, and the site of their suffering.[37] From the vantage of this critical medical anthropology, "nerves" are, themselves, an artifact of the psychiatric medicalization of poverty, hunger, and structural inequality.[38]

In their research on the medicalization of Greek immigrant women's experience in Montreal during the 1980s, Margaret Lock and Pamela Dunk show that a Canadian state policy of multiculturalism had the effect, in medical settings, of ascribing this sort of somatic culture to Greek immigrants. They argue that commonplace tropes of cultural difference—immigrant/host, rural/urban, traditional/modern—facilitated the diagnosis of somatoform disorders such as "nerves" in Greek immigrant women, just as it sanctioned institutional indifference to the gendered anguish of their home lives and the exploitation of their labor.[39]

Livaditis, in his textbook, takes issue with such stereotyping of "traditional" social groups and subordinate classes, especially women, in whom somatization is often viewed by psychiatrists as an index of psychological "primitiveness" or "immaturity."[40] In his discussion of conversion and somatoform disorders,[41] Livaditis presents the consistent finding of a historical decline in "classic hysteria" across Europe, from its heyday at the turn of the nineteenth century to the post–Second World War period, a trend that holds for Greece as well.[42] He observes present-day cross-cultural differences in conversion symptoms, noting that symptoms usually appear in "modern" societies only among patients with severe psychological problems, while in developing societies, they remain available to a broad range of psychologically "healthy" persons. To account for this observation, he reproduces the popular "anthropological" argument that "cultural schemas of meaning" affect both the manifestation and the interpretation of somatized symptoms, and he attributes some cross-cultural differences in somatization to the variable social "legitimacy" of "intellectual" forms of expression vis-à-vis bodily forms. However, he also credits some part of the observed discrepancy to changes or differences in diagnostic proclivities: for example, the historical shift in Western psychiatric nosology from hysteria to mood disorders, and contemporaneous cross-cultural studies that compare depression in the United States to neurasthenia in China.[43]

In an interview conducted during the final weeks of my stay in Alexandroupolis, Filalithi placed this "anthropological" view on somatization into a historical framework of cultural change. Over the course of her twenty years as a therapist in Thrace, she told me, she had observed a general shift in symptomatology "from the body [σῶμα] to the mind [νοῦς]." This was most obvious in neurotic illnesses such as depression, she said, which had replaced conversion disorders in all but a few of her patients. But she had also observed the shift among her schizophrenic patients, who showed a decrease in catatonic symptoms—lack of affect and will, twitching, stasis—and a corresponding increase in cognitive symptoms, such as paranoia and delusions. From a public health perspective, she told me, this historical change was unfortunate, since catatonic symptoms were more easily treated with medication, and they elicited less social stigma and better caregiving from family and community members. Filalithi suspected that the prevalence of catatonic over cognitive symptoms in "traditional societies" accounted for the truism in international health research that schizophrenia has a better prognosis in the developing world than in the industrial West, where Greece was now securely located.[44]

* * *

In the early winter, just before the move to the new hospital, I attended a seminar on post-traumatic stress disorder (PTSD) that Dr. Lamberakis was giving at the clinic for residents and staff. Citing the DSM, he presented what he called "new developments" in the psychiatry of trauma. He laid out for us the etiology of PTSD in discrete events of shock, as well as its neurological pathways, its affective and behavioral symptoms, and the preferred methods of psychodynamic and pharmaceutical treatment.

The following week, I met Konstandina, a Pontian immigrant in her late fifties, during one of her regular visits to the outpatient clinic. Her junior therapist, Manolis, introduced us, explaining that Konstandina had suffered from depression ever since she had fled Chechnya eight years earlier, when the war began. With the patient standing silently beside us, Manolis told me, *She was traumatized by the war, and she hasn't recovered yet.* He arranged for me to meet privately with Konstandina after her next appointment at the clinic.

Later that morning, I asked Manolis whether it might be a bad idea for me to meet alone with Konstandina. I referred to the seminar on PTSD that he and I had both attended the previous week. If Konstandina were suffering from PTSD, I suggested, she might be retraumatized by my inexpert questions about her experiences during the war and her flight from Chechnya. But Manolis dismissed PTSD, insisting that Konstandina's was a straightforward case of depression: *I thought she'd be interesting for you because of her culture, not because of her symptoms.*

And so I met with Konstandina. In our session, she was reticent and terse. I gathered that she had agreed to meet with me only to oblige Manolis. *I like him well enough,* she said, *but I really don't think I need a psychiatrist. Talking doesn't help.* Mostly she suffered from migraines, though her pain did not respond to the migraine medication prescribed by a neurologist she had seen early on, before she was referred to psychiatry. The only pills she took now were antidepressants and sedatives, which helped with her arrhythmia. *Sometimes I feel my heart pounding inside my head. My headaches are so intense that I go out of my mind. I go wandering, I don't know what I'm doing. At those moments, I'm drawn to the sea* (an idiom for suicide).

Konstandina had spent most of her life in a Greek village near Grozny. Her husband had died young, leaving her to raise their only child alone. *My family didn't give me any support. But I always felt safe in the communist system. The state took care of the people. When I left, the state was breaking down. People were losing their jobs, the buses stopped running, the violence was just beginning. I saw a lot of things.* Konstandina witnessed the Russian army enter Grozny and the masses fleeing in panic. She had come to Thrace because she knew that many Pontii were settling here; it was common knowledge that the state was offering jobs and free land to those who could demonstrate Greek ancestry. But when she arrived, she found nothing but scorn and resentment among the local Greeks. *I never learned modern Greek. In Chechnya, we all spoke Pontic at home and Russian in public. But my language is just one defect [ελάττωμα]. I'm a foreigner here.* She said the local Greeks perceived her not only as a communist—a disastrous affiliation in the wake of the Greek civil war, at least in this notoriously conservative region—but also as a throwback to the "lost people" of Ottoman Greece, tainted by Turkish rule. *I have no people here, besides the church, which is mostly elderly folks. But I don't have the will to start over again, somewhere else.*

Konstandina's somatic symptoms appeared to her psychiatrist as an archaic disguise for the mood disorder from which she was really suffering, caused in some loose sense by the traumas of war. Yet what she expressed when she spoke about her distress was not an unassimilated event of shock or violence, as trauma theory would have it, but a displacement—a tear in the communal tie of tradition that she had expected to bind her to mainland Greeks, and that should have made a homecoming out of her devastating migration to Thrace. If her headaches and fugues expressed her rupture from this tradition, they also attached her body to it, acutely and immediately. They attached her likewise to her doctor, to whose authority she continued to submit these symptoms, despite his refusals to acknowledge them. Manolis contended that her depression could be resolved with psychotherapy, if only she could learn to assimilate her experience and to accept the difficult task of adjusting to her new environment. To me, he suggested that perhaps Konstandina was "projecting" her own discontent onto the local people, who then returned it to her instead of welcoming her into the community.

Surface

Some twenty years into psychiatric reform in Thrace, I sought but failed to find a coherent framework of local beliefs and practices that might make mental illness and healing intelligible outside the medical paradigms of pharmacology and psychotherapy or the ethical paradigm of personal responsibility promoted in community-based care.[45] What I did find outside those paradigms was conversion symptoms, tracing the receding edge of traditional culture in the clinic. Traditional culture appeared in the diagnostic frame as but residual evidence of a historical change in mental illness that had yet to be completed. But psychiatric reform, as the condition of that change—in which patients learned to collaborate with doctors in their own restoration to health and freedom—at the same time reanimated a traditional moral authority among psychiatrists. Even as they struggled to liberate mental illness from bodies and channel it into speech, therapists in Thrace instrumentalized this authority to enlist patients in the project of personal responsibility, paradoxically putting the submissiveness of their patients to use in cultivating their autonomy from clinical care.

This reform has demanded from rural patients a new psychology: a faculty of subjective accountability yielded by their conscious reflection on their illness and their reasoned aspiration to the goal of responsibility. Only symptoms occurring in that subjective space could be addressed by the new forms of psychotherapy and responsible self-care introduced by reform. Yet the body, the surface of that subjective space on which conversion symptoms are written by the psyche, is not a stable entity even within reform discourse. When patients diagnosed with conversion disorder take medication to treat their bodily symptoms—vitamins, analgesics, antibiotics, anticonvulsants, beta blockers—and the medication fails to relieve them, these failures confirm their doctors' suspicions that these symptoms are erroneously corporeal expressions of problems that are fundamentally psychological in nature. But in contemporary practice, in Greece as elsewhere, the biopsychiatric imaginary of neurotransmission and genetic predisposition conceives the body as the true source and site of mental illness—even if it is expressed not in somatic but in cognitive, ideational, affective, or behavioral symptoms. In etiological terms, this biopsychiatric conception of mental illness is a complex reversal of conversion disorder. The difference consists not in a new prioritization of the biological body, but in a new relationship between that body and language: a transformation of the hysterical body, which converts psychological distress into bodily symptoms, into one for which communication and medication are coefficient means of self-regulation.

When a patient with conversion disorder enters the biopsychiatric scene in which this reordering of body and language has taken place, her disorder is intelligible only as a cultural archaism.[46] Conversion symptoms gained new legibility in Thrace in terms of the emergent discourse of patient responsibility: it was against the resistance of such "traditional" pathologies that moral and clinical reform could be accomplished, and patients weaned from their apparent dependency on the authority of doctors. Conversion symptoms appeared as refusals to psychologize, and thus to accept responsibility beyond the clinical surface of the body into a more ambiguous moral and cognitive interior communicated through speech. In their fleeting and fragmentary quality of experience, they eluded reflection; in their displacement to the body, they eluded psychological expression; and in their submission to the authority of doctors, they eluded the personal control of patients.

I take these conversion symptoms as signs of a different tradition, an alternative foundation of ethics to that of liberal "rights culture" and its moralism of responsibility achieved through reflection and decision. In patients with conversion disorder, tradition undergirds a countermoralism communicated through the mute symptoms of their bodies. In presenting their pains, their dizziness and numbness, their fugue and amnesia, rural patients put themselves in a moral relation of dependence on their doctors, recalling them to their traditional responsibility as healers of the biological and social body.

In Thrace it is rural bodies, affiliated with traditional culture, that have come to assert this dependence. The profile of conversion disorders, such as Fazilet's and Konstandina's, is shared by rural Greeks, Turks, Pomaks, and Pontii, appearing to many psychiatrists in Thrace as a symbol of their common history—an embodiment not of ethnic, national, linguistic, or religious divisions, but rather of generic conservative tradition, persisting on the margins of national modernization.

Conversion disorder thus evinces the mutual entanglement of psychiatry and anthropology in representing tradition and culture in the clinics of Thrace. When it comes to the formation, the presentation, and the treatment of psychiatric symptoms, "traditional culture" is not a domain beyond the clinic that might shed autonomous light on the local experience of mental illness in Thrace. It is, instead, an itinerant and highly adaptable clinical instrument circulating between otherwise disparate institutional spaces and fields of knowledge, enabling certain stakes to be claimed by doctors and patients in their moral contestation over who is responsible for the mentally ill.

※　※　※

The fraught position of Thrace between the Turkish and Bulgarian borders of Greece, and the radical heterogeneity of its population in ethnicity, religion, and language, confers on cultural difference a relevance to mental healthcare beyond the traditional-modern divide. Such difference often appears, there, more as a characteristic of stigmatized minority groups than of rural traditionalists. In this light, conversion disorder appears in plain contrast to personality disorder, a "cultural pathology" presented by many Gypsies in Thrace, who share the language and religion of Turks but not their rural or clinical profile. For Gypsy patients, the alienation from community and from self effected by mental illness is doubled by the clinical transformation of their culture itself into a pathological object. The conversion disorders of rural patients do not participate so obviously in this alienation; preserving the traditional valorization of somatic over mental illness, they instantiate a cultural identity as they fortify identifications between rural patients and their doctors. Personality disorders in Thrace also attain to a normative frame of culture, but the culture they represent is pathogenic rather than traditional; contestatory rather than residual. I pursue this divergence in the next section.

ANTISOCIAL

Each day at the General Hospital of Komotini, Dr. Karras would visit the pathology ward, where patients were transferred from the emergency room once stabilized. Several patients each day were hospitalized for suicide attempts—most often by drug overdose, but sometimes by more gruesome methods, such as self-mutilation. The head of the pathology department, who had served for years as the hospital's representative to the Gypsy neighborhoods of Komotini, identified suicidality, along with the drug abuse and domestic violence that seemed to provoke it, as "cultural problems" rather than medical ones. This, he told me, accounted for the much higher suicide rate in Komotini than in Alexandroupolis, which had a smaller Gypsy population.

Karras said that when he had taken up his post at Komotini, he was shocked by the number of suicides and attempts. *But I'm used to it now. Gypsies take pills like they're candy.* Psychiatric medications circulated along with narcotics in the neighborhood black markets, one reason for the suspicion with which psychiatrists greeted Gypsy patients requesting sedatives and therapeutic stimulants with high street value. But many of those patients had legitimate access to medications through their own prescriptions. The most popular were the benzodiazepines, a family of sedatives considered less addictive than the older barbiturates, but still hazardous when taken long-term or at high dosages: Xanax, Tavor (US Ativan), Stedon (US Valium), and Hipnosedon (known in the United States, where it is no longer manufactured or marketed, as Rohypnol or Rufinal—"roofies," the date-rape drug—said to have ten times the potency of Valium). In recent years, measures had been taken at the national level to control the prescription of sedatives in Greece. Doctors were now required by law to write these prescriptions on special "redline" forms, intended to alert pharmacists to the date and duration of the prescription; duplicates were kept in consultation offices so that doctors could track their chronicity. Most sedatives were supposed to be prescribed only for seven to ten days at a time, only to relieve acute symptoms of underlying illnesses that would be treated directly during the "second time" of longer-acting antidepressant or antipsychotic medications. In practice, however, sedatives were prescribed and taken for years at a time, with the same chronicity as other types of medication. Many patients were addicted to these medications; many sought them to the exclusion of other forms of treatment.

One morning during the weeks that I worked with Karras, we saw three patients in the emergency ward—all Gypsy women—who had attempted suicide the previous night. One was a seventeen-year-old who had overdosed on her tricyclic antidepressant medication after a violent fight with her parents. Another, three years married at the age of twenty, had swallowed chlorine. Her husband frequently beat her up, she said, and she had tried to kill herself as she bled from a stab wound he had given her during a fight. The third patient was a forty-three-year-old woman who had overdosed on heart medication. She, too, had a history of severe abuse by her husband, who was an alcoholic, and whom Karras interrogated after meeting his wife. All three patients were discharged from the hospital that same afternoon.

On our visit, Karras recorded the elements of these cases and made appointments with each woman to see him in the outpatient clinic the following day. He encouraged them to come, but told me later that he did not expect they would: *There's not much I can do to get them to take responsibility for their lives. Most of them will slip through the cracks. And we're really not trained to understand the social problems that lead to violence and suicide. When doctors release patients like these, they don't stop to think that they'll be returning to the same situations that drove them to suicide in the first place. The law requires us to report cases of domestic violence, but most doctors don't bother. Those of us who actually care are afraid that patients will stop coming to the hospital if their families are reported for abuse. Everyone's suspicious of everyone.*

Crazy Lady

Fatmé's file at the hospital clinic in Alexandroupolis was thin, despite her long and complicated psychiatric history. The clinic was not her primary site of treatment; she was an Association patient, and only went to the clinic on the point of death. She had twelve admissions between 1997 and 2003, lasting from two days to four weeks. Her file showed consistent diagnoses of psychotic depression and personality disorder, and treatment with a combination of antidepressants (first Anafranil, lately Effexor), antipsychotics (sometimes Nozinan [US Levoprome], sometimes Aloperidin [US Haldol], sometimes both), and anxiolytics (always Xanax). The front cover of her file identified her as a woman "of Turko-Gypsy descent" (*τουρκο-γύφτης καταγωγής*). One doctor had noted her polysemously symptomatic appearance: "rather slovenly attire, appropriate to her age, gender, culture-economic/social status [*κουλτούρα-οικονομική/κοινωνική κατάσταση*]."

During her admissions, Fatmé complained most often of physical symptoms, noted as "somatic" or "hysterical" in her file: numbness and tingling in her hands, rapid heartbeat, breathing difficulties, light-headedness. She had "episodes": *Something takes hold of me and squeezes my chest. I panic. My heart beats fast, out of control, my hands tremble. I get a knot in my throat, I can't breathe. I can't stand on my feet. I faint and fall down.*

Her doctors recorded symptoms of depression as well, which Fatmé attributed to an "ugly life": feelings of despair, helplessness, worthlessness, guilt, fear for herself and her children. She cried frequently and could not sleep. More alarming to her doctors, however, was her "prominent suicidal ideation." She had been hospitalized twice in six years for suicide attempts—overdoses on narcotics and prescribed psychiatric medications. She reported that she had made other attempts by drowning, or by drinking household cleanser.

Fatmé's suicidal thoughts coincided with "hostile wishes" toward her husband. During one admission, she confessed to her therapist that she had recently tried to kill him. She had tied his legs to the bed and started to stab him in the chest with scissors, but her younger son intervened before she could injure him seriously. She told a different doctor, during another admission: *If my husband attacks me one more time, I swear I'll kill him with his own rifle. That goes for my father, too. I want to sign a statement right now, and you can put it in my file. I'll put it in writing and sign my kids over to an orphanage.*

❀ ❀ ❀

Fatmé turned thirty-five shortly before she came again, in the depths of August, to the hospital clinic. Notes in her file reported that, at the time of this admission, she held two jobs and was also taking care of her four children and their house. Her oldest daughter had dropped out of middle school and now earned one hundred euros a month doing housework for a family in town. Her oldest son was entitled to a small monthly subsidy for his mental disability, though he did part-time construction work when he could find it. They lived in "the workers' homes," a housing development—not a Gypsy settlement—near the new hospital. Fatmé had secured a loan from the Association to move to the development and furnish the new house: one of her many debts.

(The doctor who had admitted her most recently noted that Fatmé had left a "more supportive environment"—her parents' neighborhood, where she grew up—in order to move to the workers' homes. Her new neighbors handled her illness harshly; they called her "crazy lady." She had made a lot of enemies and no friends in this new environment. The transition appeared to be the major "stressful event" disposing her to relapse. Fatmé complained to the doctor about the "enculturation" [ευπολιτισμός, the doctor's word] of her younger son, who had changed schools when they moved and was now being called "Billy" instead of his Quranic name by his Greek teacher and classmates.)

Hara, the psychiatric resident assigned to her case this time, told me that Fatmé's mental health was aggravated by a litany of privations and struggles she faced in her "home environment." The crux of all the trouble was her relationship with her husband, who was unemployed and violent—and, Hara added, "very likely mentally ill, as well." The event that "broke her nerves" and drove Fatmé to the clinic this time was a fight with him the previous night. He had smashed her cell phone, which she needed for work and could not afford to replace. She "went out of her mind" and swallowed a handful of pills: some combination of the psychiatric medications that she was taking at the time.

Fatmé was aged well beyond her years, with the slouch and impassive mien of the heavily sedated. She spoke fluid but ungrammatical Greek, quietly and only when pressed. In our conference, she told Hara and me that she had not been sleeping well for weeks. She cried all the time, and felt worn and useless. Hara asked if she cried for no reason, "without wanting to," but Fatmé said she had her reasons. During the week leading up to her admission, things had grown worse at home. *I kept hearing the voices of people I know. They were calling out my name in the middle of the night, trying to scare me. I'd get up and count my kids, to make sure nothing had happened to them.* Hara told me later that psychotic elements such as hallucinations and paranoia would arise from Fatmé's depression when she suffered unusual stress.

Now that Fatmé was away from home, she worried her children would not have enough to eat: *I love them so much. I have no one else. I'm all alone in life. My own mother never visits me—not at home, not at the hospital. I feel like a stranger when I go back to the old neighborhood. I'm not like those people.* Hara tried to persuade her not to undertake a move she was planning to Thessaloniki or Athens. Fatmé had people in both cities, she said; she would get settled and then send for her children. Though she agreed with Hara that the move would be disruptive and difficult, she insisted, *We'd all be better off somewhere else, away from my husband and this wretched place.*

When we spoke alone a few days later, Fatmé had already relinquished her ambition to move. She had been ready for discharge the previous afternoon, but fell sick again when her children called and told her their father was beating them. They needed her to come home and protect them. They often accused her of being a bad mother, and she turned the accusation against herself. *After they called last night, I fell into a spell. My* nerves are full [τα νεύρα γεμάτα], I've passed my limit [έσπασα τα όρια]. I've had so many episodes like this. I think about going to the sea. It's better than living like this.

Anomalous

When we first met, Karras encouraged me to get to know the city of Komotini while I was working with him at the local hospital. It had a "different feel" from Alexandroupolis, he said, and I might find it interesting. One of the mornings I spent with him, we left the hospital during clinic hours to visit the bazaar in the city center where, he assured me, most of his Gypsy patients were to be found that morning anyway.[47] We did see a few of them in the great mass of jostling shoppers. A few days later, Evyenia, the nurse who sometimes assisted Karras, roped a young male nurse at the hospital into escorting us to a Gypsy neighborhood in Komotini that was infamous for its poverty and crime. We wandered around on foot, greeting children playing in the street and old women cooking around open fires on the pavement, chatting with patients Evyenia recognized and admiring the neatly tended, vividly painted stoops of the tiny cement homes. The neighborhood had a brighter aspect than Evyenia had expected, she told me: Nothing to be scared of, after all!

Cultural distinctions between Gypsies, as between other Muslims in Thrace, had strong resonance in clinical settings. I often heard therapists identify Yifti (Γύφτοι), the poorest and most reviled, by comparison to the more upwardly mobile Tsiggani (Τσιγγάνοι); and both to the Katsivalli (Κατσιβάλλοι), a separate group settled on the outskirts of Alexandroupolis who were said to descend from Hungarians. According to Takan, one of the Turkophone psychologists who worked at the Association, the Gypsies of Thrace were not Turks either by name or ascription, though they were Muslim and knew Turkish. He spoke also of Christian Gypsies: They're nomadic, and they live mostly in other parts of Europe, in the west. But they have more in common with the Muslim Gypsies here than any of the Gypsies do with Greeks or Turks. Greeks and Turks share more culture with each other than they do with the Gypsies.[48] He told me the Christian Gypsies had called themselves "Roma" after the Greek word rum (ρουμ), meaning "people"—from which, ironically, was also derived the term romiotes (ρομιότες), an Ottoman designation for the minority Greek community. The Roma had converted to Christianity from "their own religion," Takan said, in order to elevate their status in European society, while others farther east, including in Greece, had been converted to Islam by the Ottomans as a strategy of imperial land reclamation. Buffeted by such external forces, Gypsies had retained their own distinctive culture, which was the same for Gypsies across the globe, from Europe to Asia to North America.[49]

Özlem was one of many therapists in Thrace to tell me that Gypsies' refusal to work was a highly visible aspect of their culture; they survived instead on welfare and the proceeds of petty crime.[50] They did not integrate, but kept "their own customs," including beggary, theft, and bride sale. *All minority communities have a tendency to isolate themselves from outsiders,* she told me, *but this race [ράτσα] is something else. Their behavior isn't just defensive — it's deviant. Even the way they observe Islam is anomalous.*

Among the patients treated at the Association's child psychiatry institute in Alexandroupolis were a number of Gypsy children, referred by school authorities for behavioral problems or chronic absences. These children constituted a large portion of the institute's patient population, but according to the staff, their parents did not bring them regularly to sessions, and few actually finished a course of treatment. Often, a social worker told me, the "Muslim" character of these patients was obvious: the father abused alcohol, or beat his wife; the mother did not speak Greek; the child did not attend school; the parents sought medication as the only form of treatment. *The history of disability certifications with these people is funny [αστείο],* the director of the institute said during a case presentation. The staff's unofficial policy was to delay writing a child's certification until his course of treatment was well underway, lest the prized "paper" eliminate the family's motivation for therapy.

In their weekly review of new cases, the institute staff sometimes identified patients who might hold this kind of cultural interest for me. One family, whom I came to know later, did not fit the pattern, and provoked speculation as to the cultural identity of the child. The patient was a five-year-old boy with behavioral problems: he was nervous, aggressive, "out of control," and refused to attend kindergarten. The therapist who conducted his intake interview observed that the mother, a dark-skinned brunette, was "probably Gypsy, or [with] Gypsy roots." The father, however, was Greek. Another staff member speculated that perhaps the mother had gotten pregnant accidentally: *It's hard to imagine any other reason for a Greek and a Gypsy to marry.* In any case, they no longer lived together "as a couple," and in fact had been legally separated for most of the boy's life. The woman said she had left her husband because he was an abusive alcoholic. Her in-laws, who she had hoped would help her with the boy after the separation, had instead become cruel, manipulative, and demanding.

The therapist was appalled by the boy's behavior during their intake session—he yelled, cursed, hit his mother—but even more by his mother's indifference to it. She displayed an "emotional flatness" that did not bode well: She knows nothing about the boy's early development. She isn't concerned at all that he doesn't play with other children. She seems more interested in assigning blame to her husband than in helping her child. The only way I can explain her attitude is that there are cultural elements that make it seem normal to her. Otherwise, there's no excuse. After all, the father shows a lot of affection and concern for the child. That's typical of Greek families. It was not held against him in this appraisal that, due to his heavy drinking, he could not take responsibility for raising the boy himself; nor that his parents, in their antipathy toward his wife, would not help her or the child.

Cultural relativism sometimes arose in clinical settings to temper such judgments. I occasionally heard it said that Gypsies had their own moral code that was simply incommensurable with the Greek code, and that they did have positive cultural traits—for example, as a psychologist at the child psychiatry institute pointed out, the family loyalty and "clan pride" they displayed when an entire kin group (σόι) would stand up for an individual member in a conflict with outsiders. Dora, a psychiatrist who worked for the Association in a town near Komotini, told me: It's hard to deny that their cultural differences lead to problems in treatment. It's a struggle to conduct sessions with these people: they have no custom of opening up, no concept of order, no respect for authority. But many of them have a good level [καλό επίπεδο], and they're able to cooperate once we've established a relationship of trust. The key was to break through the barrier of cultural misunderstanding.

A Little Bad

Fatmé told me she was a local, a Katsivalli, born and raised in Alexandroupolis. Her mother had divorced her father during the pregnancy, and he left her to marry someone else, so Fatmé was given to her grandmother to be raised. Later, her parents reconciled, and Fatmé came to live with them, but she said that her father had never truly accepted her as his daughter. She had not attended school, even primary school, and she had married at the age of fourteen to escape the house. I didn't know anything then, she said. I expected something from marriage. But I regretted it right *away.* She wanted her own children to avoid this mistake, and she took some comfort in the fact that her two older ones, a seventeen-year-old son and a sixteen-year-old daughter, were still living with her.

I had known Fatmé for some time before her admission that summer. We had met the previous autumn when I visited the Association's agricultural cooperative, which was run by a dozen patients under the supervision of a local farmer. The patients were picked up from their homes, mostly group homes connected to the Association, and driven to the farm each morning: beyond the residential neighborhoods along the northern edge of the city; through the "tin town" (τενεκεδούπολη), a large Gypsy settlement that took its nickname from the corrugated roofs of its cinder-block shacks; and into an area of carefully subdivided fields and pasturelands that extended all the way to the hills. The patients would gather inside the one-room shed at the corner of the plot, and if it was cold they would sit for coffee and cigarettes around the old iron stove while Rania, a psychologist, led them in group discussion. In the later hours of the morning, they would make repairs to the house or the well, feed the animals (chickens, rabbits, a pair of friendly dogs), collect eggs, water and weed the vegetable crops (carrots, tomatoes, lettuce, cucumbers), and pick the best pieces for sale. Those willing to lug the produce into town and sell it could keep the proceeds, but everyone, regardless of the quantity or quality of their labor, was paid a small wage for showing up. Every other week, they would get a visit from Lazaros, a psychologist at the Association entrusted with the supervision of its two cooperatives and several group homes.

It was clear on my first visit to the farm that Fatmé was the best worker among the patients. The others referred to her as "the maestro," and she admitted with quiet pride that she had learned her skills doing agricultural work as a child. She told me then that she was born and grew up in the tin town nearby; her father and siblings still lived there, though she had moved to a different village with her husband and children years ago. *I try to stay away from the old neighborhood. My folks are pushy—my father gives me trouble over the littlest thing.*

(According to her file, an argument with her father had preceded one of Fatmé's suicide attempts. Her younger children had been behaving badly, and she had visited her parents just to get out of the house. Her father had told her to beat the children when they were bad, and to look out for herself first, as he had always done. He refused to let her stay with them for a few weeks so that she could get some rest. This was the "supportive environment" Fatmé had left when she moved to the workers' homes.)

During the discussion around the stove that morning, as conversation drifted through my own introduction to the group, Fatmé kept quiet. The others, a few young and a few older Greek men, joked and offered bits of autobiography until Rania steered them toward the topic of their relationships with therapists and other patients. Fatmé, prodded out of her silence, commented on the problem of communication. *To be around other people, she said, you have to be good. You have to smile at everyone and say nice things. But you have to be a little bad as well. You have to be able to gossip and lie. You have to protect yourself. People can be jealous and mean.* Rania interpreted this observation for the group: *Yes, it's important to stand your ground with other people and not let them change your true character.* Fatmé fell quiet again, unmoved to make herself understood.

At the hospital clinic, almost a year later, Fatmé disclosed to me some details of a life that required such armor. I asked her to speak of her illness, and what emerged was hardship: her poverty, her unmet needs, the cruelty she had suffered at the hands of her father, her neighbors, her husband. She told me that she had fallen ill for the first time at seventeen and had been disabled ever since. *My kids know that I'm not well, and they try to help me at home. But my husband makes my condition worse. He's mean and lazy. He beats me up all the time.* She showed me scars on her arm, her shoulder, and the bridge of her nose where he had split the skin with his fist. *He stopped beating me when I was pregnant with our third child, our second son.* (Lazaros told me later, based on what the husband—an occasional patient of his—had said, that the man considered the younger boy their only "real" son, since the older one had "mental problems.") *For a while, after he was born, my husband was better. He got some money together and bought a cement-mixer to start a business. Actually, he bought it with my money. I'm still in debt for it.* He got sick again when he was injured in a car accident, and since then he had been nothing but a burden to her. *I've thrown him out of the house so many times, but he always comes back. He has nowhere else to go. Even his own family refuses to take him in. Sometimes, when he hits me, I fight back. But sometimes I lose myself. I tear my clothing and I run out into the street. Or I lock myself in the bedroom.*

This was what it meant to Fatmé to be "ill": fragile, edgy, disposed to breakdown. Breakdown meant losing herself, her nerves, her control, her mind. She had worried lately that her children might develop the same "psychological problems" from the deprivations and the abuse they suffered along with her. (Her younger son, aged ten, was the only one of her children attending school, but he ran into as much trouble there as he did at home. Fatmé could not afford to buy him pencils or proper shoes, and she said he was harassed by other children and often punished by his teachers for coming to school unprepared.) But although she had worried even more about the children since she had been absent from home, she wanted to stay a few more days at the clinic: *It's peaceful for me here, away from the children. It's really the guilt that makes me ill. I'm sick from my own failures with them. I can't protect them.* She said she had recently been thinking of taking her medications "all together" and committing suicide. I misunderstood, thinking she meant that she would take all her medications at once to die. But when I asked how her children would survive without her, she corrected me. What she had in mind was gathering all her children together, so that they could all "drink the pills" and die together. *I really feel like we'd all be better off that way.*

From time to time as we talked, Fatmé reported seeing double, or that a dark fog (ὀμίχλη) was clouding her vision. She had been to see an ophthalmologist: *He told me I'm not really seeing these things, they're just ideas that I have.* Hara had attributed her other physical complaints—including color bursts, swelling (φούσκωση) in her fingers and feet, a fast heart rate, faintness—not to conversion disorder but to low blood pressure. She had arranged for Fatmé to see a cardiologist that afternoon. Fatmé herself blamed these problems on her medications: *They help me sleep, but then sometimes I sleep so deeply, it's like I'm in a coma. I'm afraid I won't hear if an intruder comes into my room to cut my throat.* She actually suspected a specific person had this in mind, but she did not know who it was—her "research" into his identity had yielded nothing certain.

When I left the clinic later that afternoon, I discovered Fatmé on the same bus heading back to the city. She had been discharged, and bore a different demeanor: calm, smiling. Two Gypsy women in the back of the bus were watching her, and she seemed to know this, for she kept her voice low and did not speak to me of her illness or the hospital. She had told me earlier that she had no true friends, no one to whom she could "say everything" and trust to understand her: *There are only a few women in the neighborhood I know well enough even to exchange a few words. I told one of them once that I was thinking of taking a knife to my husband. She never came to visit again.*

Mythomania

In his textbook on culture and psychiatry, Miltos Livaditis examines the unique obstacles to therapeutic relationships between Greek psychiatrists and patients from the cultural minorities of Thrace.[51] He finds Turkish patients especially mistrustful of Greek therapists, due to "traumatic experiences of the past" and "political tensions" between Greece and Turkey. Pontian immigrants, he writes, often implicate their therapists in the grave disappointment that their host society does not measure up to the nostalgic ideal of "homeland" that enticed them to immigrate to Greece. But Livaditis insists that for Greek psychiatrists, Gypsies are the most problematic of the minority groups. Low standards of living, lack of education, criminality, drug addiction, and violence toward women and children are "common phenomena" in their community, according to the text. These pathogenic factors in Gypsy culture appear in contrast to the normative factors in Turkish and Pontian culture that disjoin these "traditional" groups from modern society. In the more pathogenic conditions of Gypsy culture, Livaditis finds an account for why therapeutic encounters with these patients are typically limited to prescribing medications and writing disability certifications.

The clinical implications of these social problems are charted in a research paper that Livaditis coauthored on psychopathology among Gypsy outpatients treated at the General Hospital of Alexandroupolis.[52] Gypsies had been chosen for the study for several reasons. According to the text, they comprised roughly 7 percent of the regional population but 60 percent of those visiting the hospital's outpatient psychiatry clinic. The Gypsy outpatient population presented "disproportionately prevalent and severe problems" of psychiatric illness and stability "independent of diagnosis," though the most common diagnoses were personality disorder and psychosis. The erratic attendance of these patients at scheduled appointments, their poor adherence to medication regimes, and their "hysterical behavior . . . and hostility" toward therapists translated into dire prognoses. In fact, data showed that the health of these patients often worsened on exposure to psychiatric care. The authors note that "very obvious cultural differences in behavior and appearance" presented by Gypsies in clinical settings often "cast doubt on their credibility."

Karras struggled with such "aggressive" and "dramatic" patients, whom he described diagnostically as "antisocial" and "psychopathic."[53] These were the patients who barged into his office, demanding attention and medication; who argued with him about disability papers; who did not follow directions or schedules; who were violent and drug-addicted—who, he said, forced him to "lay down the law" by yelling at them, refusing to see them on demand, and restricting their medications. He tried to schedule their appointments on separate days from his other patients, to protect them as well as himself—but *the psychopathics show up whenever they like!*

The diagnostic term *psychopathic* does not appear in the DSM-IV; the closest category is "antisocial personality disorder."[54] But Sakellaropoulos's influential textbook on social psychiatry, derived loosely from the French classification of mental pathologies, offers an account. This text presents the syndrome of "psychopathic personality" (ψυχοπαθητική προσωπικότητα) in a series of "pathological personalities," adding "sociopathy," "antisocial personality," and "psychopathic disequilibrium" as common glosses for this particular form of "social deviance."[55]

According to Sakellaropoulos, "antisocial" or "psychopathic" traits include instability, impulsivity, and disorientation; but this personality type can also be "charming," "persuasive," and "misleading," either by cognitive fault or by conscious pretense. His text describes the typical development of this pathological personality, beginning with a moody childhood and discipline problems that evolve in adolescence into conflict with authority figures, disruption of studies, drug and alcohol abuse, and petty crime. The adult life of this personality type is characterized by unemployment, dangerous behavior, ruses and rackets, criminal activity, egoism, emotional instability, and frequent romantic sexual entanglements and breakups.[56] Its "psychological characteristics" include explosions of destructive rage without any "working through" or thought to consequences, failure to develop authentic relationships with others, attribution of blame for one's problems to bad luck and other people, self-image as a "victim of society," incapacity to make long-term plans, and profound dysphoria and boredom underneath a "superficial" coldness or emotional "anaesthesia." Especially in women, according to Sakellaropoulos, this personality presents "hysterical characteristics" such as nervous crises, submissiveness, and transient somatization.[57] Antisocial men and women alike are entertained by "deluding" themselves and others, and given to "mythomania" in their avoidance of reality. Though in some people this personality can take destructive delight in scandal and provocation, Sakellaropoulos insists that "the psychopathic is more *amoral* than deviant" and displays, rather than malice, a "general avoidance of responsibility."[58] Patients with this type of personality disorder, he writes, do not "open up," but instead "externalize" their conflicts in behavioral or somatic symptoms. Lacking an introspective tendency, they stand incapable of honesty and moral responsibility generally.[59]

Like Karras, Filalithi largely associated this antisocial personality type with her Gypsy patients. In an interview, she offered me what she described as "speculative theories" about the prevalence of personality disorders in Gypsy communities. The *biological theory*, as she gave it, held that Gypsies, as an evolutionary breeding population, had developed a genetic disposition to aggressive behavior. The *materialist theory* proposed that the chronic social and economic deprivation suffered by Gypsies forced them to adopt antisocial behavior as a means of survival. On the *relativist theory*, which Filalithi said she preferred, the "cultural conditions" of Gypsy life were seen as a normative context for behavior that only *appeared* pathological to outsiders. She referred me to a passage from the textbook by her colleague Livaditis, highlighting this source of misunderstanding between Greek therapists and their Gypsy patients in Thrace: "Gypsies often express themselves in dramatic or aggressive ways, which the unsensitized therapist too readily judges as antisocial or dishonest behavior in the service of some strategy for seeking advantage. However, in reality, [this behavior] is often a matter of idiomatic ways of expressing distress or despair."[60]

It was on the basis of such misunderstandings, Filalithi explained, that Greek psychiatrists often made errors in diagnosing Gypsy patients. She said it was crucial to gather information about the patient's "cultural background" (she used the English phrase) before making a diagnosis. Most important in this regard was the opinion of other members of the patient's community as to whether the behavior in question was strange, crazy, or dysfunctional. In Filalithi's view, pathology was often a matter of the degree rather than the type of behavior in question. For example, in a Gypsy man who beat his wife, pathology might be identified only by the extremity and frequency of the assaults.

The concept of culture invoked in Filalithi's "relativist" theory of minority pathology attributes the disordered behavior of individuals to a moral code, and ascribes cross-cultural conflicts to incommensurabilities between such moral codes. Culture thus provides an account of mental pathology in the context of diagnosis, which may be skewed by a clinician's inadequate attention to the cultural background of the patient. This relativism, however, directly contradicts the alternative "materialist" view that Filalithi also presented—an etiological account, in which pathogenic social, economic, and political conditions are understood to cause standard mental disorders, such as reactive depression and personality disorder, which can be accurately diagnosed without reference to the patient's cultural background.[61]

It is unclear, in the relativist theory, whether the normativity of antisocial behavior in Gypsy communities entails a psychological etiology or whether its normativity is only a matter of behavioral expression. What is clear is that only some conditions are ripe for antisocial normativity.[62] These conditions are peculiarly collective: according to Sakellaropoulos, the explosive crises that occasionally erupt in the antisocial personality type can "provoke in people with similar personalities a chain reaction of irritation or aggressive rage," directed at oneself or others, as in "epidemics of suicides or self-mutilation"—which, the text reports, are "well known in communities that shelter psychopathic persons."[63] The disorder thus presents itself more as a "community problem" than a therapeutic one in such environments.[64] Filalithi confirmed this view when I asked her to compare pathological violence in an individual patient with extreme but widespread violence in that patient's community: Well, at that point, we're talking about a social problem. We can't address that with psychiatry alone.[65]

Theater

Lazaros, the supervisor of the Association's farming cooperative, was seeing less and less of Fatmé during the summer she was hospitalized. He told me he still felt a strong tie to her, and expected that she would come to him with her problems before any other therapist. He filled in for me the psychiatric history of her family, which Fatmé had not discussed with me. Her husband, he said, was indeed "very sick—much sicker than Fatmé herself." Their older son was mentally retarded; the older daughter was clinically depressed and had made one suicide attempt already; the second son, the "real" son, was now expressing a range of hysterical symptoms, including chest pains and labored breathing; and the younger daughter, aged eight, suffered from intense separation anxiety and exhibited severe behavioral problems. Fatmé had terminated many other pregnancies, Lazaros said, and now she was unable to conceive.

For Lazaros, it was important that Fatmé "admitted" she was ill, which meant that she had always "cooperated" in treatment. There were psychotic elements to her depression, he said, but they arose only under conditions of intense stress, when her fears would mutate into hallucinations. *Depression is the much greater danger for Fatmé. She's often been suicidal, and she's made several serious attempts with pills.* When I told Lazaros about the idea she had expressed to me, that she might bring her children with her when she committed suicide, he dismissed the threat as a "dramatization": *Fatmé puts things much worse than they are when she's ill. But she's not wrong to worry about the mental health of her children. They're all developing personality disorders under those conditions. Without changing the environment, there's little we can do to address this kind of illness. That's why it's so crucial to intervene with the younger children now and try to break the cycle of pathology.*

❋ ❋ ❋

In September, a few weeks after Fatmé's discharge, Martina's suicide was still a fresh shock to those in the hospital clinic. The blockade remained in force "for the patients' protection," as the director said. In this state of emergency, Dr. Lamberakis announced at the weekly staff meeting that Fatmé had been hospitalized again the night before, for a drug overdose. After her transfer to the pathology ward, she had awoken during the night, removed her IV, and sneaked out of her room. She had attempted to mount the external staircase, but was stopped by a nurse. Apparently, she had planned to jump, just like Martina—whose story Fatmé, like most patients in the orbit of the clinic, knew very well by then.

Fatmé had come to see Lamberakis in his office that morning. She knew many of the clinicians intimately, and perhaps she expected something from Lamberakis that she did not get from Angelidi, the psychiatrist in charge of her case at the time. Fatmé had told Lamberakis that she was absolutely determined to kill herself and her husband unless she found some way to get away from him. She wanted help from the doctors to find and pay for a new house.

At the staff meeting, Lamberakis told us, *Fatmé is very sick, she's a mess* [στα χάλιά της]. He agreed with Fatmé that her husband was the main source of her trouble, and felt certain that removing him from the picture would advance her psychiatric treatment as well. *I told her we couldn't solve her problems right away, all at once, but maybe we could help her make some financial arrangements, so that she and the children can leave the house.*

Lamberakis wanted to discuss this plan during the meeting. But other clinicians mobilized a different agenda. Angelidi, who was assigned to the case, said she planned to visit Fatmé in the pathology ward that morning and see for herself: *I'm not convinced she's as sick as you think she is.* Blastos, who had never treated Fatmé, agreed: *Gypsies are always doing this sort of thing — it's theater! They have these problems but they never make any attempt to manage their lives; they expect us to do it for them.* Lamberakis retorted, *That comment is inappropriate* [άτοπο]. *It's not just a question of life management* [χειριστικό] *for Fatmé. She's sick — she has a mental illness.* Angelidi tried to reconcile their positions, suggesting, *We know that poor life management is characteristic of this kind of illness. But Fatmé has been told a hundred times that she needs to leave her husband, and she keeps going back to him!* Lamberakis reminded her that Fatmé had in fact tried many times to leave her husband, including her move from the Gypsy neighborhood to the workers' houses. *She's failed because she has no support, emotionally or financially, from her family or anyone else. Fatmé is from a minority, and there are cultural differences* [πολιτιστικές διαφορές] *that make it hard for her to make good choices. In her culture, it's hard for a woman to live on her own. It's hard to raise her children without a husband and in-laws. And it's much harder for minorities to get sympathy and help from the outside. Her illness is an extra burden* [επιβάρυνση], *on top of all the rest.*

In a voice raised to meet Lamberakis's, Blastos argued, *We have no way of knowing whether this "extra burden" is real. I wouldn't call it "suffering" when she's sitting around the house waiting for welfare.* Lamberakis informed him of Fatmé's work at the farming cooperative and as a school crossing guard. Laughing, not sheepishly, Blastos parried, *If Fatmé can do all that work, then she can't be as ill as she claims! Anyway, if she has two jobs, then she's better off than most Gypsy women, who have to rely on their deadbeat husbands to support them. These Gypsies: half the men have personality disorders! It's not just Fatmé.* He described another Gypsy patient at the clinic who he thought was in much worse shape than Fatmé — though, even so, he was not inclined to help her, either. That woman's husband had moved his girlfriend into their house and had threatened to kill his wife if she left. *Now she's developed psychotic symptoms in addition to depression. Why should Fatmé get special care?*

Lamberakis declined to respond to this challenge, saying only, *I disagree with you about this case. We all have our own preclusions* [αποκλεισμές] *about Fatmé's psychopathology. Either she's at the point of violence or she's not. We'll wait and see.*

The convergence of extreme poverty and widespread mental illness in the Gypsy communities of Thrace generated a profound conflict, both epistemological and ethical, for psychiatrists disposed to reflect on it. As civil servants, they controlled their patients' access to means of survival, in the form of disability certifications that would qualify them for welfare subsidies. Therapists frequently described their Gypsy patients not as mentally disabled from labor, but as culturally reliant on welfare; as one nurse told me, *It's not illness, really; they just don't want to work.* But often, the problem was posed differently: How could the category of "reactive" mental illnesses such as personality disorders, which refused any clear distinction between medical and political-economic causes, be incorporated into the state welfare system?

The welfare system in Greece operated independently from the two semiprivate insurance systems that covered most healthcare costs, disability subsidies, and retirement pensions (s. σύνταξη) for workers. The IKA (Social Insurance Institute) granted pensions of about 335 euros per month in 2003 to people who had paid income taxes into the system for at least five years. The OGA (Agricultural Workers' Insurance Organization) granted smaller pensions, of about 150 euros per month in 2003, to farmworkers and owners of farmland. Together, these two organizations covered close to 75 percent of Greek citizens, and a number of smaller pay-in groups covered other workers in specialized industries.[66] On the other hand, benefits from welfare (πρόνοια), a fully public agency, were available to citizens who were chronically unemployed or had not been employed long enough to qualify for worker coverage. These subsidies (s. επίδομα) amounted to roughly 160 euros per month in 2003, in addition to healthcare coverage. Yet unlike retired or disabled workers, welfare recipients suffered frequent delays in their subsidies; in the spring of 2003, for example, four months passed during which patients received no welfare income at all. When payments resumed, the state made no promise to pay the arrears.

Patients with a range of medical conditions could qualify for disability certification: not just mental illness, but any medical problem that disabled them from working. Qualifying mental illnesses were not restricted by law, but many therapists told me that the state had lately been putting pressure on psychiatry departments to reduce the number of certifications (γνωματεύσεις) they issued, in order to conserve state funds. This informal national policy was not difficult to enforce locally, a social worker explained, since all posts in state hospital administration were civil service appointments, and patronage relationships ("teeth" [δόντια]) went "all the way up," connecting department heads in the hinterland to the Ministry of Health in Athens. Psychiatrists were encouraged to write certifications only for highly dysfunctional patients, which usually meant those with psychoses or severe mood disorders like depressive or bipolar disorder. To gratify their claims, or simply to silence them, many psychiatrists continued to write "papers" for patients with other disorders, postponing the moment of refusal to their encounter with petty bureaucrats in the welfare office.

Some patients found a way around this fate by feigning symptoms, chiefly symptoms of psychosis. Therapists, referring to their responsibility to distribute fairly the scarce resources of the state, routinely dismissed the claims of these patients—often Gypsies—as cunning manipulations. To the extent that they were not dismissed as outright malingerers, these patients often emerged from their clinical encounters with a diagnosis of personality disorder, rather than of more severe clinical disorders like schizophrenia or depression that would warrant full disability certification. As one psychiatrist told me, *You'd have to be antisocial to fake psychosis!*

Thus another game of negotiation, alongside diagnosis, was being played in these clinical encounters. Psychiatrists and patients found themselves either on the same side or on opposite sides of the rules governing the distribution of state resources. In making claims on these resources, patients pushed psychiatrists to decide how the state would mediate their clinical relationships. Were they bound primarily to the scientific discourse of psychiatry by which the state authorized their power to distinguish personality disorders from clinical disorders? Or did they acknowledge the state's role in the deprivations that might dispose their poorest and most marginalized patients to develop personality disorders? If so, would they distribute the resources under their control in ways unauthorized by state policy? Personality disorders in Gypsy patients forced into view the contradictions and the conflations between therapeutic and bureaucratic functions of psychiatric care in Thrace—the ways in which pathology and poverty were linked and separated by therapists in their work for the state.

For Gypsy patients, antisocial personality disorder described a similarly ambivalent relationship to the state, coupling a rejection of the norms of responsible citizenship with claims on state welfare. Symptoms took the form of disregard for the law: chronic unemployment leading to welfare fraud, evasions of compulsory education and military service, customary divorces and remarriages not recognized by civil law, and outright criminal activity. Yet it was precisely these antisocial behaviors that signified Gypsies' need for psychiatric care. In this sense, antisocial personality disorder among Gypsy outpatients in Thrace bears a robust resemblance to the "political personality" Wendy Brown has observed in liberal subjects formed through the "wounded attachments" of identity politics. These politics, she argues, are waged in paradoxical identitarian investments, in which the "marginal, deviant, or subhuman" is recast as contestatory identity, thus binding particularist "claims to injury and exclusion" to the universalist ideals from which these "marked" social identities deviate.[67] Such politics represent a foundering project of subversion and emancipation—one animated by a desire to "inscribe in the law" the "historical and present pain" of the claimants, and to seek recognition before the law in terms of that pain rather than in novel terms that might effect their liberation from oppression.[68]

Antisociality did not present a seamlessly pathological face in the clinics of Thrace; yet neither could it be dismissed as an instrumental guise or a psychical allegory for the politics of dispossession. If Gypsy patients addressed moral claims to the state through the antisocial behaviors they presented to their doctors, this does not mean that their strategy was a form of deliberate resistance to state power. The rejection of liberal citizenship embodied in these behaviors was more obviously a form of dependency on the state than of contestation.[69]

This dependency was facilitated by the clinical imagination of culture in Thrace. In the relativist sense articulated by Filalithi, culture offered suspicious clinicians a way to marshal their medical authority against the deceptive tactics of patients who addressed them as gatekeepers of state resources.[70] The diagnosis of antisocial personality disorder as a "cultural pathology" in these patients thus constituted a refusal not only to accede to these deceptive tactics and falsely certify a more severe disorder that would warrant full disability income, but also to acknowledge the deceptive tactics as such. This cultural diagnosis stood as an assertion of psychiatric purview over a broad spectrum of deceptive behaviors, from deliberate fraud to severe disability.

The refusal on the part of clinicians either to accept or to reject outright the suspected lies of their patients in antisocial cases smacks of the bureaucratic "fear of responsibility" (ευθυνοφοβία) in Greece that Michael Herzfeld has studied. He presents this "logic" of "buck-passing" as a legal principle as well as a conventional rhetoric of excuse in everyday encounters between supplicant citizens and public servants in Greece.[71] He reads the stereotypically Mediterranean attitude of fatalism in regard to bureaucracy as a "secular theodicy" by which citizens seek transcendent accountability in the state—and symbolize its failures in national stereotypes of self and other. One of the main "tactical uses" of these stereotypes, Herzfeld argues, inheres in the "ethical alibis" they offer for all parties to deflect personal responsibility.[72]

But the logic of ευθυνοφοβία offers only a partial account of the impasse I observed between Greek psychiatrists and Gypsy patients seeking prescriptions or disability papers. This impasse certainly describes a conflict of rhetorical strategies: psychiatrists presented themselves as impersonal guardians of scientific knowledge, as of the common interest of the national community entrusted to them as state employees; Gypsy patients presented themselves as the victims of medical and state neglect embodied, personally, by their therapists. Yet the conflict of these strategies was not resolved by the "ethical alibis" provided by the symbolic logic of self/other stereotyping. What is distinct about these clinical encounters, in comparison to the bureaucratic ones discussed by Herzfeld, is the irreducibility of pathologies to social dynamics. Therapists were concerned to retain a clinical purview over the antisociality of their Gypsy patients, legitimating it as a mental pathology even if they also recognized it as a pragmatic strategy. These state clinics, then, were bureaucratic institutions in which self/other stereotyping did not function only as "the idiom in which social and cultural exclusion become mutually convertible."[73] These convertible exclusions, while clearly operative in clinical encounters between Greek psychiatrists and Gypsy patients, were nonetheless secondary to the relationships generated there—relationships that were primarily and fundamentally moral in nature, sustaining as they did a mutual dependency between state welfare and supplicant citizens, between suspicious and suspect persons.

One evening in early winter, a mute and apparently catatonic patient arrived at the hospital clinic in Alexandroupolis under police escort, transferred from a local immigration detention center. Though the staff cajoled and harangued him in Greek, English, and German, the languages they had studied in school, they could not elicit any speech from him. They asked a foreign resident in cardiology to try Arabic. Turkish seemed the best candidate, but no one present actually knew the language. Finally, Dr. Filalithi consulted Aspa, a medical student completing her three-month rotation in psychiatry. Filalithi was certain that Aspa was Pontian and might know Turkish even though she spoke standard Greek fluently.

Aspa may have been disconcerted by this presumptive identification, but she readily admitted that she did speak Turkish, as Filalithi had suspected. She explained to us that the Pontic language had been forbidden for Greeks under Ottoman rule. In the nineteenth century, the Ottomans harshly suppressed Pontian culture in the Black Sea region, in response to the Pontii's participation in the Greek revolutionary war and their burgeoning self-consciousness as a nationalist Hellenic community.[74] In the postrevolutionary period, many relinquished their native language for their own protection and took up Turkish in its place. Others, migrating north to the Orthodox lands of the Caucasus, the Volga, and the Ukraine, conserved Pontic in secret but learned Russian so that they could pose as locals.[75] So today, Aspa concluded, *Pontii speak Greek or Russian as a second language, but they speak Pontic or Turkish as a native language. If they don't, they aren't Pontii!*

The sudden influx of Pontian patients into the health centers of Thrace since the early 1990s had created an urgent need for Russian-speaking therapists. Requests had been made and ignored at the Association. Thus it was a relief when Osman, a psychologist in Komotini, finally disclosed what he had known for some time: that nearly all the Pontian patients spoke Turkish as well as Russian. Osman had discovered the "secret language" of his Pontian patients only gradually. They were afraid, at first, when he addressed them in Turkish: *They thought they'd be deported if the authorities found out it was their language, too. They know about the plight of the Muslims here.* Osman tried to persuade them that their confidentiality in therapy was protected by law, and that they had the right to speak Turkish: *I swear to them I'll accompany them personally to the courthouse if they ever get in trouble for it.*

For Takan, another psychologist in Komotini, this revelation of the secret language of the Pontii—no longer Pontic now, but Turkish—was only one in a string of tragic absurdities to unfold in their relationship with the Greek state. He was the first of many to tell me that, after the fall of the Soviet empire, Greece had invited Pontian emigrants from the former republics to settle in Thrace in order to "neutralize" its Muslim vote. (A previous attempt had involved tax incentives for Greek families with multiple children, and the restriction of welfare benefits to large Muslim families. This policy, Takan said, was discarded under pressure from "the left.") The resettlement policy proved disastrous for the state. Funding to aid the Pontii ran out quickly, leaving a massive population of impoverished and traumatized immigrants in the poorest region of the country, without support. Another problem, from the point of view of the state, was that an ample number of the Pontian settlers had turned out to be Muslim, for their ancestors had converted to Islam during Ottoman rule. Their incorporation into the territory of Thrace had only increased its Muslim population.

Returns

The Asia Minor Catastrophe of 1922–23, in the wake of the First World War, was a cataclysmic event of mass slaughter and forced migration following clashes between Greek and Turkish armies in Anatolia. It was the crisis that ultimately defined the Turkish border of Greece as the eastern border of Europe. The 1 million "Christians" who emigrated to mainland Greece during the Catastrophe and its aftermath, many of whom were resettled in Thrace, spoke a variety of languages—Turkish, Pontic and other Greek dialects—and included about one hundred thousand Armenians. They were as culturally mixed as the "Moslem" population of 150,000 that remained in western Thrace, including Turks, Pomaks, and Gypsies.[76] It is a commonplace in historical scholarship of the event that the Treaty of Lausanne, which fixed the border and the terms of the population exchange between Greece and Turkey in 1923, utterly failed to produce the internal homogeneity sought by both nations. In Thrace, it yielded instead a perennial conflict between the Christian majority and the Muslim minority.

The status of Asia Minor refugees as a Christian majority in Thrace is one legacy of the Catastrophe, which continues to resound in strategies of the Greek state to protect that majority against the expansion of local

Muslim communities. By virtue of one such strategy, the ratio of these two voting blocks has recently been disturbed by the settlement in the region of Pontian immigrants—perhaps as many as thirty-two thousand people between 1989 and 2005, almost a tenth of the regional population at the time.[77] To some, the Pontii appear today as yet another wave of Greek refugees "returning" to the region—sharing with the Asia Minor Greeks of the Catastrophe their religion, their ancestry, and their history of exile.[78] They have carried with them, as well, the weight of the epic Greek struggle against imperial oppression outside the national borders.

But the landscape to which these exiles have returned has been transformed since the earlier wave. My first encounter with that landscape was afforded by Dr. Michailidis, a senior psychiatrist at the General Hospital of Alexandroupolis. He was the only "local" (ντόπιος) among the senior medical staff—many of whom commuted weekly to Alexandroupolis from a primary residence in Athens—and seemed to have a personal stake in introducing me to what he called, with a wink, the "native culture." When I returned to Alexandroupolis to stay the following year, Michailidis would vouch for me at the clinic, conferring on my work there a legitimacy that would nevertheless be perpetually if obliquely disputed—most of all by Michailidis himself, from the standpoint of what he called "modern science."

One afternoon during that first visit to Alexandroupolis, Michailidis—playing host and patron—took me on a driving tour of the countryside northwest of the city. We stopped to visit an elderly patient of his, a depressed alcoholic, who owned a small farming plot on the slopes beneath the new hospital site on the outskirts of town. The patient was not at home, but Michailidis confidently led me through the field where he was growing tomatoes, cucumbers, and melons. Most of the crops had been ruined by the late summer heat, but Michailidis selected a few ripe pieces to bring home to his wife. Displaying to me, the anthropologist, a savvy about culture as a cipher of difference that I would come to discern in his clinical work with minority patients, he explained, *These vegetables are a gift to me, according to the Greek custom. Peasants hold their doctors in great esteem. They show their appreciation in the simple ways of rural life.* Cash gifts were once common, he said, but now illegal. (In time, I would hear repeatedly the story of a senior psychiatrist at the hospital, framed by a disgruntled Gypsy patient who slipped some cash into a bag of figs that he proffered as a gift.) These days, in place of cash, patients would often bring eggs, cheese, honey, slabs of meat. Michailidis said it was a matter of respect to accept these gifts; they secured the social tie as well as the therapeutic bond between doctor and patient.

He accepted other gifts—a pot of yogurt, a sack of green peppers—later that afternoon, when we visited the village of another of his patients. This was in a Turkish village, on a steep hillside above the interstate. At the turnoff, we passed an army vehicle manned by young soldiers with machine guns, on the lookout for illegal transports from Turkey. When we arrived at the patient's homestead, we learned that he was in the mountains with his sheep. But the covered women of the house received us and served us tea. Michailidis told me, *Our visit is a great honor for them. And you see—it's proof that Greeks and Turks can be friends.* Displaying his comfort with "Muslim customs," he joked with the eldest unmarried daughter of the household that he might take her as a second wife. He arranged the family for a photograph with me before we took our leave.

As we continued west, Michailidis pointed out the names of the villages we passed through, settlements so small and scattered that most were barely visible from the road. Nea Hilli, Nea Santa, Neos Pirgos, Nea Psathades, Neo Heimonio: these "new towns" were named, he said, after the Anatolian cities that Greeks had deserted in the 1920s, during and after the Asia Minor Catastrophe. These refugees had been urban people, merchants and traders; they had never kept animals or worked the land. It was here in Thrace that they learned to be farmers and shepherds—rural folks, "like the Turks who had lived in these hills for ages," even before Thrace was claimed by "the Pashas" in the fifteenth century.

On our return to Alexandroupolis, passing along the shore through clusters of housing developments in arrested construction, Michailidis admitted that the state had preferred the Asia Minor refugees to local Turks for land grants and building permits in the postwar years. The settlers flourished in Thrace. Their children went to school, and found their way into retail and civil service jobs in the larger towns. But the Turks remained behind, in the hills, and turned east for aid. Michailidis reported the rumor that Turkey funneled great sums of money into these villages, through personal loans and municipal grants for irrigation equipment and Turkish-language school materials. Even the satellite dishes we saw on every homely cottage rooftop were provided by Turkey, retrieving to these remote compatriots the news and cultural programming broadcast there—"propaganda," Michailidis said, to ensure their political fealty. The rural way of life led by these peasants thus isolated them from Greek society and the national political community, even as it fortified their tie to the land.

When I settled in Thrace myself, I would hear these remarks of Michailidis reverberating in the explanations Greek doctors offered me of their encounters with Muslim patients. They told me that the Turks of Thrace maintained political ties with Turkey even though they bore Greek citizenship and all its entitlements. That the provision for exempted populations in the Treaty of Lausanne was supposed to create an "equilibrium" between Greece and Turkey—but while Greece had protected its Turks, Turkey had violated the peace treaty in the 1950s with its brutal treatment of Greeks living in Istanbul. That Turkey nurtured plans to take back the territory of western Thrace, a threat that compelled the deployment of half the Greek army along the Turkish border. That, though its domestic policies were resolutely secularist, Turkey actively fostered the religiosity of Turks in Thrace, in order to keep them ignorant, docile, loyal, and populous. That these peasants—who kept quiet and to themselves in their remote villages—were invisible, but not innocent. That Thrace grew more Muslim year by year.

❀ ❀ ❀

In Thrace today, descendents of the Asia Minor refugees comprise the greater part of the Greek population. As one patient told me, *We're all from over there: most of us locals [ντόπιοι] can trace our families back to Asia Minor.* I met this patient, Soula, at a rural health center not far from Komotini. Her social worker introduced her to me as a "typical case" of schizophrenia. Soula was in her early thirties at the time. She lived with her parents in a cement bungalow down the street from the health center and made a meager living as the neighborhood hairdresser. When she learned that I was a foreigner, with an interest in culture, Soula told me the story of her family. During the Asia Minor Catastrophe, she said, both her grandmothers, as young girls, had fled to Thrace and married local Greeks. *It's a common story in this area. It's how our people became farmers. But nowadays, the land is dried up. It's useless even for pasture. Irrigation is too expensive. The young people are leaving the villages to work in the cities. It's worse now than when I was a child. My father used to have three big plots that he farmed, in those days. Today, we have too many foreigners coming to Thrace. They're stealing all our land.*

Soula's file reported a "paranoid delusion" regarding the Pontii. It had apparently begun after a large pastureland on the outskirts of town, rented by locals for generations, was reclaimed by the municipality in order to build a permanent housing settlement there for Pontian immigrants. Soula grew suspicious, bitter, and depressed, shutting herself away in her room for fear of contact with "foreigners." She mutilated herself with her father's farming tools and made a number of suicide attempts. She "ranted" about the Pontii in her treatment sessions. According to her therapist, she was "fixated" on a specific Pontian patient whom she often saw at the health center. Soula said she could hear this patient whispering about her in a secret language that she did not understand.

The identity of Soula's nemesis suggests that this clinical symptom of paranoia was verging on something more or other than a medical problem. In such cases—and I saw many in Thrace—paranoia presented itself as an orientation to others on the part of patients who had good reason to be vigilant in guarding their boundaries of self and community. The minority patients in Thrace who presented the most obviously "other" face to local Greek identity—Turks, Pomaks, Gypsies—were not the only objects of this guarding. The boundary between Greeks and another "other" people, uncannily like Greeks—the Pontii—was as profoundly fraught with paranoia.

As a minority population, Pontian immigrants in Thrace were recognized for historical and cultural ties to mainland Greeks that distinguished them from other minority groups in this region. They were often derided as parasites on the state, but they were mostly not subject to the pervasive suspicion directed toward illegal immigrants cycling through detention centers along the Turkish border. On the contrary: their immigration to northeastern Greece was often discussed as a *nostos* (νόστος): a homecoming from exile. These ancestral Greeks enjoyed a singularly ambivalent reception, in which the self-image of the Greek community in Thrace—heirs if not descendents of Pontian migrants from earlier times—was intimately and ethically bound up in the conferral of state goods: citizenship, land, housing, education, social services, and medical care, on a scale unimaginable for other immigrant groups.[79] In the sections that follow, I explore that ambivalent bond between Pontii and Greeks, a bond set by the peculiar collapse of the symbolic mirroring relation between self and other.

In psychoanalytic theory, paranoia describes a relationship between self and other in which the other functions not as another subject but as a self-referential phantasm,[80] a function that is evident even in the DSM's depiction of paranoid schizophrenia. This is a pathology of boundaries:

the subject is unable to distinguish clearly between self and other, so the inside appears everywhere outside and the outside everywhere inside—pursuing, invading, possessing the self. Boundaries appear only fleetingly, in fragments, failing to protect the subject from invasion, and creating untenable equivalences between the many figures who impinge as outsiders.[81]

It is in this sense of "paranoia" that I interpret Pontian immigration in Greece during the 1990s. This is a period, Étienne Balibar notes, of "vacillation" in the borders of Europe, from the civil war in the former Yugoslavia to the increasingly violent policing of North African immigrants in France: "Borders have stopped marking the limits where politics ends because the community ends. . . . Borders are no longer the shores of the political, but have indeed become . . . *things* within the space of the political itself."[82] As a political rationality, paranoia describes that condition in which the border is a *thing* of fascination, alarm, and longing within the political community, instead of a transcendental form creating an inside and outside for that community. This condition generates continuities between categories of people excluded from full membership in the political community—such as, in the cases I consider here, Pontian immigrants and psychiatric patients.[83]

The continuity between these categories of exclusion demands that clinical paranoia in Thrace appear in the same ethnographic frame as the history of Pontian exile and return across the territorial borders of Greece. So I turn to that frame now, to the case of a Pontian immigrant patient who was diagnosed with paranoid schizophrenia. In her "delusions," she seemed to experience an uncanny identification with those she perceived as enemies. But that identification was asserted for her as a matter of responsibility by her therapists, who aimed to enlist her as a cooperative participant in the struggle against her mental illness, and thus in her movement toward full citizenship. The responsibility she bore for her mental illness was reinforced, in this way, by her tenuous membership in both the Pontian and the Greek communities of Thrace.

Seeing from the Outside

In the dying days of the Ottoman Empire leading up to the founding of the Republic of Turkey in 1923—almost a century after the birth of the Hellenic Republic—those Pontii who remained in Asia Minor were caught up in the Catastrophe and persecuted along with other subject populations. Hundreds of thousands of these ancestral Greeks were repatriated to mainland Greece under the terms of the Lausanne treaty with Turkey in 1923.[84] But the Pontii who had migrated to the Russian territories remained. Later, under Stalin, many were targeted as members of a "dangerous" national minority, and banished to central Asia.[85]

These Soviet subjects were the Pontii who "returned" to Greece in the 1990s, driven by war and economic devastation in the collapsing empire. They were Georgians, Russians, Uzbeks: refugees, foreigners who, by reputation, did not speak proper Greek and lived on welfare while they waited for their ID cards and residence permits. They were Greek Orthodox and had Greek names, but they were strangers and kept to themselves. Before they began moving to Alexandroupolis, in the early 2000s, many started out in small, isolated settlements the state had constructed for them in the uninhabited tracts of hilly country north and west of town.

The state had founded the National Institute for the Reception and Resettlement of Repatriated Ancestral Greeks (ΕΙΥΑΑΠΟΕ) in 1991 to provide assistance to the Pontii during their adjustment to life in Greece.[86] This assistance took the form of housing, stipends for living expenses, and citizenship—at least at first—but little in the way of education or social integration programs. The ΕΙΥΑΑΠΟΕ also channeled welfare funds to Pontii who suffered from medical disabilities, including mental illness. Clinicians in Thrace found that many of their Pontian patients suffered the psychological effects of trauma.

By September of 2003, ΕΙΥΑΑΠΟΕ's offices in Thrace stood empty. The ten-year funding package created for the national institute expired in 2001, and it was not renewed in the legislature. Pontii who received disability payments were redirected to municipal welfare offices. Several Pontian settlements in Thrace, where housing was deemed hazardous, were slated to be razed. Residents were asked to find apartments in local cities. A small and finite sum of rent money would be allotted to these people to aid in their new resettlement.

Anastasia was among them.

Many months before I was able to have an unguarded conversation with her—which is to say, before I was given permission to meet with her privately by her therapist, who was concerned that I might confuse the patient with an appearance of friendship and disrupt her primary therapeutic relationship—Anastasia brought me to her village. She had announced several times that she would like me to come, but insisted that

I wait until spring. The perfect day for a visit would be her birthday, she said, in April, when the chill would lift and the winds would cease tearing through her little house on the hill. Her invitation to another patient and intermittent friend, Babbis—a boisterous and ungainly middle-aged man—had been extorted by circumstance: he had overheard her speaking to me about the birthday party, and she felt obliged to include him. And so it was, on her forty-sixth birthday, that we three went on the bus to Neo Ipsos.

I had met Anastasia early the previous autumn, at the cooperative workshop where she was employed along with several other patients treated at the Association. They were paid a nominal wage to design and produce print orders, and to assemble small gift items for sale in the shop. On the day I first visited, Anastasia was occupied with stringing embroidery thread through colored paper folded into pretty shapes. When I was introduced to the group as a foreigner, she greeted me warmly and asked about my travels. She said that in addition to speaking Greek and Russian, she had studied German and English. She had toured all over Europe. Another member of the co-op described her as "cultured" (μορφωμένη).

After that first meeting, I would often see Anastasia about town: on the bus, at the post office, at the grocer's down the street from my apartment. She "got around," people said, casting aspersion. We also met at a biweekly socialization group she attended at the Association, organized by a social worker to educate patients about their mental and physical health. The therapists who knew her described Anastasia as a high-functioning, stable, and responsible patient. She was "cooperating" in a successful course of treatment for schizophrenia. She managed her own household, did her own shopping, worked a regular schedule, handled her finances, negotiated "challenging relationships" with family members and neighbors, and made "realistic" plans for her future. Beyond all this, Anastasia had overcome many practical and emotional hurdles connected to her emigration from Georgia ten years before. Pontic was her native language, but she had learned modern Greek quickly, and was generally considered "well integrated."

A social worker told me that in all that time, and despite the success of her treatment, Anastasia had never relinquished her core delusion: that she was involved in a secret love affair with a Greek pop star—an affair that she hid from her family, who she did not believe was her real family.

Several times already she had whispered to me at group meetings that she did not "agree" with her therapists, who thought she was ill. Without telling them, she would occasionally stop taking her medications, because they were not good for her and ruined her figure.

"People say I should get married, to save myself from the doctors!" she told me later on, when I knew her better. She often speculated about the life she might have led if she had married a normal man—the home she would have made in the warm ambit of financial security; the children she would have borne and raised. Plenty of men had shown an interest in her. (These men, Greek men, would ply her with cheap gifts, drinks, and sweets, attempting seduction; when she rejected their advances, they would spread rumors that she was a prostitute.) *But I'm unlucky*, she said. *I'm the kind of person who only falls in love once, and for good.* She had fallen for the pop star as a young girl. She could not marry him, because he was a Jehovah's Witness and she was Greek Orthodox, and her family would never permit it. But neither could she marry another man and lead a normal life.

Anastasia's obedience to what she expressed as her family's prohibition to marry a Jehovah's Witness—a member of a more marginal group even than the Pontii—disclosed an ambivalent affiliation to them that she disavowed in other ways, at other moments. But this prohibition was only the most concrete way in which the choice for a normal life had been stolen from her. The original theft was performed by her own character, which trapped her in both love and fidelity. She could not "save herself" from the doctors because she could not choose to marry anyone else. And yet: who would not want a secret love? The trap of emotional ties that cost Anastasia a normal life also had its pleasures. Her disposition to steadfast love disclosed her isolation from the Pontii, to whom she attributed flinty impassivity and emotional brutality; but it also opened the prospect, which she fervently pursued, of a passional private life. I took her invitation to visit her village, from which she would have preferred to exclude her fellow patient Babbis, as an appeal to see this dimension of her life—the secret, affective dimension—not enclosed within her identity as a spinster, cooperative patient, and responsible new citizen of Greece. So it was necessary that we go illicitly, breaching the protective seal of transference that had evolved between her and her therapists, and effecting a different bond: she offering up the ruined landscape of her village, I promising to see it from a different, an "educated," point of view.

Like many villages in that part of Thrace, Neo Ipsos sprung up during the 1920s, when the region was flooded with Greek refugees from Asia Minor—some coming over land from Turkey, others relocated to Thrace by the settlement commission in Athens, where they had arrived in crowded ships from the ports of Izmir and Çeşme. The settlers became farmers and later, after the civil war, factory workers. But most of the factories had closed by now. Today, Neo Ipsos was one of the larger agricultural villages north of Alexandroupolis, and it continued to grow. In the inexpensive country surrounding the town proper, middle-class Greeks from the urban south were constructing luxury homes to use during the summer or in retirement.

To reach the Pontian settlement at Neo Ipsos, we passed the grazing lands attached to large farmhouses on the low slopes of the hill; the narrow lanes winding their way up to town, lined with well-kept bungalows and gardens; and the town center, a village green resting on a shallow plateau, encircling a church, an elementary school, and the town hall. A narrow road continued north, up the steep hill, passing through a vacant tract before arriving at a dusty clearing. The settlement was a clot of one-room houses, metal frame and plywood, arranged loosely in rows, some following the crestward ridges of the hill, more along the road rising up its face. They had been erected by the state all at once, a decade before, as temporary housing for the Pontian immigrants. Anastasia told me that when she first arrived here, there had been 150 to 200 of these little shacks, and the area had been filled with people—families with young children and elderly grandparents, neighbors from towns in southern Russia, people who had started out together or met on the road. After a few years, residents had started leaving to find work in the cities. Now, nearly half of the original houses had been destroyed; we could see the rubble of collapsed buildings accumulating in a narrow valley east of the road. The little one-room school was boarded up and abandoned; Pontian schoolchildren were now being bused to the main village.

The settlement was much more peaceful now, Anastasia said. She preferred it quiet. She pointed out a tiny whitewashed church in the far distance, at the summit of the hill, which would take an hour to reach by foot: *I've heard there used to be a village up there, but the people left during World War II because they were dying of starvation.* This hamlet on the hill had been inhabited and abandoned many times. The state had been promising for years to build better housing here, so the Pontian residents could settle permanently, but Anastasia doubted this would ever take place. Despite her almost fond attachment to the hillside, she, too, was preparing to leave.

Her own house was like the others in the settlement: flimsy, dark, cramped. She plugged in a space heater when it got too cold. The main room had a small bed, a plastic table and chairs, a large television that she used to watch Russian programming. The tiny kitchen and bathroom were obscured by a plastic curtain. She had no closets or cabinets, so she had piled clothes, bags, and trinkets—a hoard of all her belongings—on her bed and chairs at the back of the room. Her walls were plastered with posters of the pop star. She played tapes of his music and offered candies and drinks while she showed me and Babbis the birthday gifts she had collected that day from shop owners she had befriended in town: a shawl, a beaded purse, a leather-bound journal.

Visitors stopped by over the span of the late afternoon. The first was Anastasia's dapper, elderly father, who lived next door with her brother. He arrived with his own older brother, Anastasia's uncle, who—drink in hand—politely interviewed me in halting Greek about my background and my work in Thrace. Anastasia tried to facilitate, interjecting and speaking for her uncle when he had trouble. Picking up the thread of "culture" that emerged from this discussion, Anastasia's father broke in, regaling me with what he called a "cultural" story about his falling out with the Orthodox Church in Russia, on the grounds of his communist commitments. As the story proceeded from a conversation with God to a tussle with a priest in the gardens of a village church, I began to understand that the men were fabulating at my expense. So I asked them about Greece instead, shifting our discourse to the scene of my own presumed authority. As Anastasia fretted over preparations in the kitchen, they spoke quietly between them in Russian. The uncle told me they were "lost people" (χαμένοι άνθρωποι)—they had fled here during the war in Georgia, compelled to abandon their homes and belongings and jobs, sacrificing everything but their lives. Georgia was a land of thieves and violence, he said. Someone like me—young, naïve, first world—would not last a day over there. As we listened to the distant rumbling of gunfire from the army camp nearby, he told me that, compared to Georgia, Greece was a peaceful refuge.

Though Anastasia asked them to stay, the two old men left when a group of three young women arrived. Anastasia introduced them as her friends from the village. They were in their early twenties, raucous, heavily made up, lots of denim. They spoke perfect, rapid-fire Greek with heavy accents. They had arrived in Neo Ipsos as children and grew up together, Anastasia told me later, though only one of them still lived here in the settlement. They were affectionate with Anastasia but roughly refused the food she persisted in offering them. They smoked and drank shots of brandy. Their minds were elsewhere. The most strident of them, called Monika, made Anastasia a gift of a silver ring with a large blue stone, which came from Georgia—*a piece of the land I brought here with me,* she said. And then she slipped into Russian, eliciting a surprised guffaw from Babbis, who had been sitting quietly by the front door. Monika began to banter with him in Greek:

> Monika: *Is my language funny? Don't worry, I know Greek, too. I know all the languages.*
> Babbis: *Say something in Russian. Say "Saturday."*
> Monika (in Greek): *Sunday.*
> Babbis: *No, "Saturday"! Not Sunday.*
> Monika: *I said Saturday! "Sunday" is how you say Saturday in Russian.*
> Babbis: *You're trying to drive me crazy!*
> Monika: *No, I think you're trying to drive me crazy.* (flirtatiously) *I know all about you. The blonde told me.*
> Babbis: *Right, the blonde! What blonde?*
> Monika: *Don't pretend. The one who works at the bar down by the harbor. She told me all about you. What happened last weekend.*

Babbis blushed and laughed, looking away from her, across the room. The girl sitting next to me warned Monika that she was a married woman and should not be flirting like this.

> Babbis: *Do I know you? I think I've seen you before.*
> Monika: *I work at the tax office. Maybe I took your money.*

Babbis laughed and shook his head, understanding that she was teasing.

> Monika: *And that one?* (pointing to one of the other girls) *She's a security guard. And the other one is a cop. Maybe you've had a run-in with them. Down at the harbor.*
> Babbis (looking away again): *You're crazy. Are you crazy?*
> Monika: *I think you must be crazy. How come you don't look at me when you talk to me? You're looking away like it's the wall that's talking to you!*

Babbis got up from his seat to stand in the doorway and laughed, doubled over. The two other girls giggled and Anastasia with them, her glance darting around the room.

> Monika (looking at the two other girls): *People say we're crazy. I don't know, though. I think "crazy" is inside us, other people can't see it.*
> Babbis: *I think it's outside. I can see it.*
> Monika: *Well, anyway, I'm crazier than you.*
> Babbis: *I have a certificate of craziness. Where's yours?*

The girl sitting next to me whispered that it was wrong for Monika to tease Babbis like this—he would "take her meaning" and be hurt. Perhaps Anastasia, a witness and refracted object of this exchange, would take her meaning as well. To the extent that Monika and her friends represented the community in which Anastasia claimed ambivalent membership, Monika's teasing threatened to identify Anastasia instead with Babbis as a psychiatric patient. Anastasia had feared precisely this identification—her hesitation to invite Babbis that day expressed this fear—and she laughed nervously at their jokes.

The association of Anastasia with Babbis was both confirmed and tempered by the appearance of another marginal figure on the scene moments after the laughter subsided. This young man, who had been hovering by the front door and singing for some time, hunched over and trembling, finally asked Anastasia for a piece of birthday cake, though he refused to come inside. The third girl muttered, *He's the really "crazy" one*, and seemed relieved when he sidled off with his cake. Anastasia said, *I pity his poor soul.*

The rhetorical terrain of madness (τρέλλα) at Anastasia's house was rich in expressive possibilities; it doubled as the topos of a different exile from that of Pontian geography. Babbis had been the one straight away to introduce the term *crazy* into his discourse with Monika, and to insist on it as the rubric for the jokes they made about themselves and each other. The hostility toward Babbis that seemed to animate Monika's subtle teasing turned, perhaps, on his identity as a Greek: when he laughed at her lapse into Russian, he exposed her own marginality as a member of the Pontian community. It was through the language of "craziness" that she addressed this discrepancy in status, articulating an image of the Pontii from without ("people say we're crazy")—an image that she resented but enlisted in her cutting wordplay with the psychiatric patient.

The girl next to me, discomfited by the exchange between Monika and Babbis, engaged this image in a different way, drawing it closer to the terrain of clinical madness. She was wearing a sleeveless top, and I noticed a series of short parallel slashes, now scarring up, across the inside of her arm. Her other arm bore a long, transecting gash. As she drank, she emerged from her polite shell. Responding to a jibe from her friend about her "sloppiness," she said: *I'm really a good person, even if I don't act so good. Give me a few drinks and I'll show you. Like last weekend. I went crazy at that club and broke a table with all the glasses on it.* She refused the cake Anastasia tried to serve her, claiming she had no appetite. She had not been sleeping either. She was "madly" in love.

As it grew darker, several older women from the neighborhood, dressed in long skirts and shawls, brought little gifts of food and sat quietly, treating the three girls to hostile stares. They spoke only Russian among themselves, and gave the impression they were conferring about the girls, audibly enough and disapprovingly. Soon the girls left, perhaps bored, perhaps troubled by the censorious performance of the older generation. They were heading to the city, to a bar down by the harbor. When they had gone, a different mood settled over the little house. The spark of spontaneous exchange died out, replaced by a gentle, consensual murmuring as Russian asserted itself as the common language, excluding both Babbis and myself. Anastasia adopted a deferential demeanor, soliciting and serving her guests, smiling politely. The community closed in on itself.

Later, as we stood at the side of the steep road, waiting for the bus that would take Babbis and me back to the city, Anastasia told me that her brother had not come to the party because he was angry with her. They had argued over something trivial a few days before, as they often did. *He's resented me since childhood, for coming between him and our father. Even though we're not really brother and sister, we were raised together as a family. But now we're like strangers. My father fights with me, too. He was being civil today, but that's unusual—maybe because you were here. He's never showed me any love or generosity. That's how I know he's not my real father.* She would tell me later that the Pontii were all like that, like her father: hard, indifferent, proud, jealous, cruel. Her affair with the pop star—which she had only very cautiously begun to reveal to me on this visit, through his posters and tapes—operated like ballast to shore up her loving nature, a nature that both marked her difference from the Pontii and attached her to them. That her

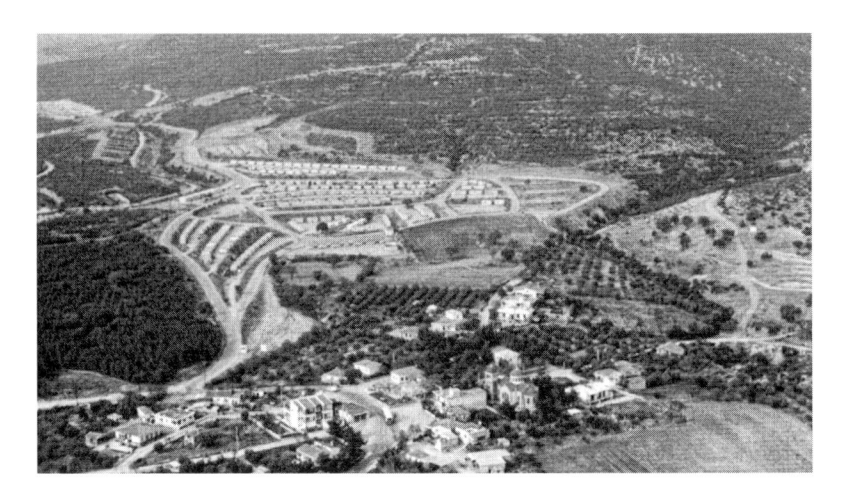

©ΕΙΥΑΑΠΟΕ, 2001

"stolen love" might appear as a delusional symptom, and trap Anastasia in her identity as a psychiatric patient, was the risk of her secret—and so she kept it from me, on this visit and for some time afterward.

Special Gifts

As I prepared to leave Alexandroupolis at the end of the summer, I met one last time with Stella, Anastasia's therapist at the Association. It was our last conversation, but our first episode of candor, for Stella finally confessed what it was that had made her resist for so long "exposing" Anastasia to me "outside the therapeutic framework." She was aware that Anastasia and I had a "special relationship," but she had tried hard to convince Anastasia that this relationship was not a friendship—that my interest in her was "professional," stemming from my research. She feared that Anastasia's interest in me, on the other hand, was "mixed up" (θόλος). She felt there was an extent to which I confronted Anastasia as an image of herself that she had lost to her illness. *You're well-educated, she said, so Anastasia is reminded that her own university studies were interrupted. You're a foreigner, so she feels an urge to travel—maybe to escape, or to go home. You're a pretty girl, so Anastasia worries about the decline of her beauty.* And yet Stella perceived signs that this was, in one respect at least, a "good identification": our association reinforced Anastasia's self-respect and her confidence as a capable, interesting, cosmopolitan person. Part of my appeal to her, Stella supposed, was that I presented her the opportunity to be that person rather than a patient. But therein lay the danger, too. We could both be misled.

※ ※ ※

Anastasia's file, dating to the year after she emigrated to Thrace, bore two surnames: one Russian, the other Greek. Her father, who accompanied her to the hospital clinic the first time, had supplied the Russian name; but Anastasia had apparently insisted on the Greek. It was her family's true name, she said; they were Pontii, after all. Perhaps, at that first moment in the clinic, she had wished to lay claim to her Greek ancestry, to reinforce her immigrant armor. Or perhaps she was seeking distance from her father and brother—a distance she measured, as well, with clinical symptoms.

In the ten years since she became a psychiatric patient in Thrace, Anastasia had only five admissions, an exceptionally small number for a patient of her socioeconomic status, especially with a psychotic diagnosis. The admissions were typically short, lasting only a few days, indicating a capacity to "come down" swiftly from relapses. Her therapists, both at the hospital clinic and at the Association, were uncertain about her diagnosis, which vacillated between paranoid schizophrenia, bipolar disorder, and "psychotic syndrome," a diagnosis often given in clinically indeterminate cases. Yet all her admissions prompted detailed descriptions of her psychotic symptoms. When I finally consulted her file, months after visiting her village, at a time when I felt I knew her quite well, I found the notes jarring. They indicated hallucinations and florid delusions whose themes were familiar to me from our conversations, but whose scope and intensity Anastasia had never intimated to me, though she had evidently been eager to express them to her therapists.

These symptoms included *delusions of influence*: Anastasia believed she was telepathic; she could read others' thoughts, and could both send and receive messages through her mind as well as her body. And *delusions of origin*: her true mother and father, who had thirteen other children—her siblings—were Eve and Christ, or Angeliki Dimitriou and Marlon Brando, or an Indian princess and Alain Delon; her true parents had given her to the people who raised her. And *delusions of grandeur*: she believed she was descended from Phillip of Macedonia and Alexander the Great; that God had given her "special gifts" and powers that others did not have; that she had traveled to another planet to help the inhabitants overthrow fascism and establish communist rule, granting justice and prosperity to everyone; that she worked in Israel and Palestine, promoting peace and averting World War III. And *perceptual disorder*: she heard the voices of other people inside her head—sometimes her relatives in Russia, sometimes her beloved, sometimes "unnatural" people who told her to listen to her doctors and to "do good."

Anastasia's file also contained a brief family medical history. After her mother had died of a heart attack at the age of sixty-two, Anastasia had immigrated to Greece with her father, an electrician, and her brother. The youngest child in the family, a sister, had married and stayed behind in Georgia. Discounting her father's alcoholism, there was no family history of mental illness.

According to the intake interview with her father, Anastasia had fallen ill for the first time at the age of twenty-six, when she was studying philology at the University of Tbilisi. After her breakdown, she had spent two months in a mental hospital in Moscow. After that, her father said, Anastasia had developed a pattern: over the course of a few weeks, she would grow listless, refusing to speak or to leave the house; and then she would swing suddenly to the other extreme, becoming talkative, excitable, excessively sociable, and spendthrift. This pattern would recur once or twice a year, and at those times he would have her admitted to psychiatry clinics in Russia. He said that, compared with that pattern, her health had actually improved when they moved to Thrace.

Soul Mate

When we finally met up to "write her story from beginning to end," as she put it, Anastasia was anxious to tell me about her family, from whom she remained deeply estranged but unliberated. She blamed her father for the way her life had gone disastrously awry. *In Georgia, I was a brilliant student. I was clever and ambitious—but I was also sensitive and kind. Suddenly one day, for no reason, I was taken to a mental hospital against my will. My parents deceived me. They told me we were going to a museum, but they took me to the hospital instead. I lost consciousness at some point. I think I was drugged. When I woke up, I was in a room with ten other people. Some of them were chained to their beds. Others were wandering the halls, weeping and yelling. The doors were locked and I thought I was in prison. That's when I got "nerves" for the first time. I'd never been ill before.*

Though Anastasia was eventually discharged from the hospital, she never returned to school. Her father would not allow it. Years later, her brother—to hurt her—told Anastasia that when their father left Georgia, he had planned to abandon her in a mental hospital if she did not agree to come along to Greece. *That's the kind of person he is—callous, pitiless. But I don't resemble him in this. Or in a lot of other ways. My real parents were great and famous people. I once heard—someone whispered to me—that I was born in a palace in Constantinople, not in Georgia, as my papers say. I inherited my majestic character from them, and my delicacy. I just don't have it in me to be indifferent toward my father. I love him, despite my will. And this makes me even more sensitive to his cruelty.*

In Anastasia's file, as in our own conversations, the fantasy that Anastasia presented, to which all other symptoms migrated or returned, and in which her alienation was condensed, was her love affair with the Greek pop star. Along with other details of their relationship recorded in her file—that, for example, they had twenty children together, all beautiful girls, whom he was raising now in Russia since Anastasia had no means—was her belief that the pop star was "like a god." He was, she said, the son of Digenis Akritas, the epic hero of eighth-century Byzantium, whose legend is celebrated to this day in Pontian folk ballads and dances. In modern Greek, the hero's epithet, "twice born" (διγενής), can denote a person bearing two sexes in one body. But Digenis embodied a different kind of duality. He was born on the Euphrates to a Greek Orthodox woman, the daughter of a Byzantine general, and a Muslim man, the son of an Arab emir taken in battle and converted to Christianity. Their son, the great hero, a warrior prodigy, spent his glorious life defending the Byzantine frontier from Arab and Turkish invaders from the east. "Twice born," bred of two peoples and two religions, Digenis materialized the border he protected. He engendered a people of his own: the Akritans, a race of border warriors, defenders of the faith and the empire, to whom the Pontii trace their ancestry. Anastasia herself bore the hero's surname, in its Greek form, and in the genitive—like all Greek women's surnames, denoting possession—and thus seemed the destined soul mate of his son. She and the pop star shared an ancestry along with an epic love.

Anastasia had met her beloved long before her first trip to the hospital. *I feel like I've known him all my life, even in childhood. We fell in love when I was nineteen, right when I entered university. I had always been a good girl and followed the rules. So I stayed pure for him after we became lovers, even though other men were always chasing me.* Most conspicuous among these other men was a professor, ten years older, who tried to seduce her while she was taking his language class. He was tall, handsome, intelligent, talented, successful—*everything a woman could want. So I was flattered by his attention, even though I refused him. The other girls in my class got jealous. They used to call me a whore, but I never gave in to him. I had no interest in anyone but my beloved.*

This professor shared all the traits of the pop star, so when Anastasia spoke to me of another, later scene of unwanted seduction, I mistook the professor for the aggressor. Instead, in this story, her beloved was the guilty party. *I came across him while I was walking in the city park. I was so naïve! I followed him into a glade of pine trees, just to talk. We were hidden back there. And he forced himself on me.* After this episode, Anastasia found she was pregnant. This was several years after her first hospitalization, during a phase in her life when she "lost time"—when the days did not pass normally, when her heart would pound in her ears and confuse her senses. Her recollection of events was not entirely clear, but she thought it was her mother who had taken her to another city to have an abortion. *I knew I couldn't have a baby in the state I was in. But I still regret it. The baby was so big when it came out of my body.* (She clasped two fists together to show me.) *I was sure it was alive. My beloved's father was a scientist, and I think he took the baby after the procedure and treated it with medicine, and then raised it as his own.*

I asked Anastasia how being raped by her beloved had affected her feelings for him. She told me she still loved him, and she did not like to think about that experience. But it had taught her something important: *Now I know what men are thinking when they follow me down the street and offer me gifts. They expect something, and they get hostile when I don't give it to them. They spread lies. They don't love me, they betray me.* She had been disturbed by male attention her whole life. She was glad to be able to take refuge in a relationship with her beloved.

Yet Anastasia blamed her chastity for the physical problems that troubled her, especially the backaches and heart palpitations of which she often complained to her doctors. *My friend told me it isn't good for a woman's health to go without relations for too long. Maybe that's why those images come to me: images of men, strangers and ones known to her, but most of all her beloved. I love seeing his image; at those moments I can sense his presence, I can feel what he's feeling. But sometimes the pleasure is too much, it's scary. When he's present with me, he can sense my feelings, too. He can read my thoughts. He controls my body. It's like he has a magical hold over me.*

The Stranger

Anastasia's longest stay at the hospital clinic in Alexandroupolis followed an "accident" in Athens three years before, and had little to do with the florescence of psychosis. According to Stella, her psychologist at the Association, Anastasia had traveled to Athens with a friend. One night in their hotel room, she had fallen or jumped from the balcony. It was several flights to the ground, and Anastasia was seriously injured with pelvic and leg fractures. She was hospitalized in Athens, and after a few weeks, her father—with financial assistance from the Association—traveled to Athens to have her discharged and transferred, by ambulance, all the way to the General Hospital of Alexandroupolis. Anastasia was admitted first to the pathology ward, but her chattering about the pop star and other odd behavior disturbed the other patients, as well as the doctors. She was eventually transferred to the psychiatry clinic for the rest of her recovery, though she presented no psychiatric symptoms severe enough to warrant admission.

At the time, Anastasia told Stella that she had been pushed off the balcony by "a stranger," who she thought must have broken into the hotel room. Stella, along with Anastasia's psychiatrist at the hospital, doubted this account. They came to believe that the presence of the stranger was either a hallucination, arising from delusional feelings of persecution, or a story Anastasia had invented to disguise her intention to commit suicide.

Anastasia gave me a different version of events. She told me that she had gone to Athens for a rendezvous with her beloved. *He was giving a concert that evening. We met up before the concert, and we made love at my hotel. Later that night, when I came back to my room after the show, I sensed the presence of a stranger. This was the one who pushed me off the balcony. I still don't know who he was, but I know I'd met him before. This man keeps coming back.*

This was the last time Anastasia had seen the pop star. *I've been chaste ever since. And even though women fall at his feet wherever he goes, I just know that he's staying as pure as I am. But it breaks my heart that he's been away for so long.* She tried to be contented with the tokens of him she had collected: tapes, posters, photos. And then there were his letters. Anastasia showed me one of these when I visited the group home in downtown Alexandroupolis where she had moved when Neo Ipsos finally closed in the summer of 2004. She kept the pop star's letters with his autographed pictures in her photo album. She took one out to show me—a greeting card with a Russian verse preprinted inside, and a personal message in blotchy red ink that read, in Greek: *To Anastasia, with love.*

❈ ❈ ❈

In working through Anastasia's story, I have come to see her secret life— her "paranoid delusion"—not as an allegory but as a beautifully precise analysis of Pontian immigration to Thrace. (I take seriously Freud's suggestion that paranoiacs are, themselves, incisive theorists of the psyche.[87]) In this story, Anastasia's main persecutors are her father and brother, who stand for all the Pontii in their disposition to wound her. Her doctors are but substitutes for these men, at a new stage of her injury: namely, her move to Greece, in which her family was deeply implicated. The most hurtful and most intimate figure in her life—a figure of her own invention, the only worthy object of her love, who recurs in her life as her lover, her rapist, her soul mate, her attempted murderer, her possessor—is a member of a persecuted minority who nevertheless achieves recognition through pop culture stardom in Greece, but who remains, for her, absent and unattainable.

Anastasia's "paranoia" is intricately wrapped up in her identity as a psychiatric patient—in the institutionalized practices of medical care through which her fantasy was diagnosed as a clinical symptom of schizophrenia. From this vantage, her story is about her exclusion from full citizenship on the basis of mental disability; about her refusal to "take responsibility" for her illness by recognizing herself as the author of her persecution, and resisting it with the aid of therapy and medication. In this, Anastasia more closely identifies with Babbis, another psychiatric patient, than she does with anyone else. Her doctors appear in this light as her persecutors: the people from whom she could be saved, if only she would get married and submit herself to domestic rather than state control. The rigid closure of Anastasia's relationship to the Pontian community is transposed here into a rigid closure of her relationship to the Greek community. The doctors stand as representatives of the Greek state; and the public medical institutions in which they treat her are places where, as Balibar puts it, the borders of the state appear when they are "no longer situated at the borders at all, in the geographico-politico-administrative sense of the term."[88] This manifestation of state borders in the medical differentiation of mental health and illness is the condition for Monika, Anastasia's young Pontian neighbor, to suggest that the Pontii "seem crazy from the outside"—but not, as Babbis insisted, as crazy as the certified mentally ill.

From another vantage—not outside the frame of this narrative, but continuous with it—that debate between Monika and Babbis about *who is crazier* shows the political rationality of paranoia working in tandem with its clinical form. From this vantage, Anastasia's story is about the constitution of community through exile and return, a repatriation that looks like immigration: a repetition with difference. This community is one in which the Pontii themselves appear, sometimes, as Muslims who speak Turkish as their native and secret language. It is plausible here for that tour-guide monologue performed by Michailidis, a self-consciously "local" Greek, to slide from the Asia Minor refugees who settled in Thrace in the 1920s, to the Pontian immigrants who repeated that settlement in the 1990s, to the Muslim peasants who had lived here for ages, operating as secret agents of Turkey. That slide—from the identification of ourselves, to those uncannily like us, to those not like us at all who are everywhere among us—describes the movement of the clinical illness of paranoia toward a political rationality, fixated on those who cross the borders of self and community: on those who "keep coming back," fearsomely and with love.

Interlude:

The Persians

In the last days of June, the story breaks in international news that George W. Bush believes "God is on his side" in the war on Iraq. He has publicly said as much to Mahmoud Abbas, the president of the Palestinian Authority. His "messiah complex" draws immediate censure from Greek politicians, and near disbelief from Alexandroupolitans I know, who speak to me about it furiously at every opportunity. A massive antiwar protest takes place a few days later in Thessaloniki. Since the war began, Athens has seen a number of demonstrations, concentrated in the zone of immunity around the Polytechnic University, down the street from the American embassy. But the march in Thessaloniki is taken by commentators as evidence that anti-American sentiment is spreading throughout the country.

Incidental to this event, and more impressive to some: several of the peace marchers in Thessaloniki vandalize and loot shops along the protest route. This "misguided violence," as newscasters call it, comes up at the Association's annual banquet that week, marking the opening of summer. Dora, concerned, turns to me: *But they shouldn't be treated like ordinary criminals! In America, don't you have a special category for people who commit political crimes?* Andreas, exhaling smoke, calmly puts an end to the conversation: *The shopkeepers should have just shot the bastards. They have the right to protect their property, don't they?*

A few days later, I attend the opening performance of Aeschylus's *The Persians* with a group of young doctors from the hospital. Over coffee beforehand, Thanos complains, as he has often done before, about the tedium and frustration of life in Alexandroupolis. He seems to take grim satisfaction from the pitiful state of the outdoor municipal theater where the play is being staged: a makeshift amphitheater with grimy concrete bleachers that most recently hosted a native folk dancing event. Nina tells me that there are beautiful, authentic, marble amphitheaters elsewhere in Greece: *You should try and see them before you go back to America!*

The play, which starts nearly an hour late, is preceded by speeches from several members of the local cultural society who have arranged for the traveling production to visit Alexandroupolis. And then by the mayor, who introduces the director of the play as "a great patriot, dedicated to preserving our civilizational heritage." This patriot, who has made a noteworthy career of modernizing ancient Greek drama, addresses the audience to establish what he calls "the schema" of the performance. *"The Persians," he says, is not a classical play. In a classical play, the plot has a predictable structure: there is a battle, the hero wins, the foe dies, and all the actors come out to take a bow at the end. The audience applauds, and it's over. The play you will see this evening, on the other hand, is very modern. It's about war, not heroism. War has no winners, and there is never an end to it—as we know all too well from current events. So in this production, the actors will not come out to take a bow. The play will be over when war itself has come to an end.*

The play is rendered in modern Greek translation and an acutely modernist aesthetic. The actors, men and women alike, are dressed in identical slim black tunics and pants. They hold their pale faces expressionless as they move in angular formations, speaking their lines directly to the audience rather than to one another.

The play commemorates, by mythicizing, the Athenian triumph over Persian invaders at Salamis in 464 BCE, from the vantage of the defeated Persians. The chorus, the bereft queen—mother of King Xerxes, leader of the naval excursion—and the ghost of her husband and Xerxes' father, King Darius, perform a relentless lamentation over the grievous loss of Persian life and honor in battle. The glory of the Greek victors is distant and muted, appearing only in contrast to the woe of the Persians, as Xerxes describes it on his return: "Painful to us, but to enemies joy."[1] To the ethereal figure of Darius, this woe is payment for the "pride and godless arrogance" that drove his son to lead the Persian campaign, despite ill omens.[2] Shamed into action by his counselors and beguiled by visions of grandeur, Xerxes literally spearheaded the invasion—and "when a man's / willing and eager, god joins in."[3] He was deceived by the gods into vainglorious optimism and given a fair voyage to Salamis, where his lords and warriors were slaughtered by the undermanned and poorly equipped Greeks. The gods were on their side.

The herald of Xerxes, portending his return, alone, to Persia, speaks of Thrace as the site of final crossing for the wounded remnants of the Persian navy. There, where they retreated across land, "there in the night a god / raised winter out of season."[4] But the godless Persian warriors supplicated that alien deity. Some were spared from the cold, and managed to cross the frozen river before daybreak, when Apollo's light melted the waters and drowned the largest part of them, burying them in the Thracian soil. Does the audience in the amphitheater that night, seated on that very soil, in that borderland where the Persians met their ruin, sense the uncanny synchrony of ancient and modern, of chosen and godless? Do these autochthonous citizens of the West achieve—as the director has instructed—sympathy and despair for those invaders from the East who would claim this land again, and again find their ruin here?

We can tell the play is coming to a close, if not an end, when the actors emerge on stage, one by one, to perform a new coda. Each advances to the front and cries out the name of a modern war and the number of its victims, sometimes wildly off count: *Hiroshima—fifty thousand! Rwanda— two hundred thousand! The Falklands!*

No applause follows the last actor from the stage. The audience remains seated for some time—tense, quiet, perhaps expecting more drama. Among ourselves, we compare the extent of dialogue we were able to understand. Nina and Zevs easily followed the play, they say, because they remember it from grade school, though Nina prefers the classical staging she saw at Phillippi. Thanos cannot say how much of the dialogue he followed; he has been paying attention instead to the wedding taking place in the open beachfront lot behind the amphitheater. He has found the music and dancing, the speeches and toasts, vastly more entertaining than our ancient-modern spectacle of fate. Playing on the staging of the occasion, he quotes Oedipus Rex to us in the ancient tongue: "Thou art blind in the mind, the ears, and the eyes."

PART 3

A System in Doubt of Freedom

THE MOST IN NEED OF OUR CARE

At the end of winter, just a few weeks after the General Hospital of Alexandroupolis had moved to its new facility, a young patient was admitted to the psychiatry clinic by compulsory order. Kleandis was notorious among the senior staff, who had been treating him for obsessive-compulsive disorder (OCD) for years. His illness had progressed to the point of danger: in a fury, he had attacked his elderly parents. In the clinic, his bouts of aggressive ranting and washing erupted in stunning contrast to his gentle demeanor, bewildering the new cohort of psychiatric residents, who were much more familiar with severe but "typical" psychotics and depressives. His admission thus proved the occasion for Dr. Filalithi to give a seminar on anxiety disorders. Noting the inadequacy of the residency curriculum to the topic, she began with a caveat: *Like other sciences, psychiatry develops theories that guide its practice: prevention, diagnosis, treatment. But there is less certainty about many theories in psychiatry than in other sciences. Psychiatry is further behind sciences like physics. Political science is even further behind. . . .*

The seminar covered four theories of anxiety disorders, which Filalithi insisted were not mutually exclusive, though they entailed divergent therapeutic techniques. According to my notes on the seminar:

> 1. Psychoanalysis conceives anxiety as a neurosis of civilization, the unconscious product of a conflict between societal laws and individual desires that causes neurotically self-punitive behaviors. Anxiety is dis-

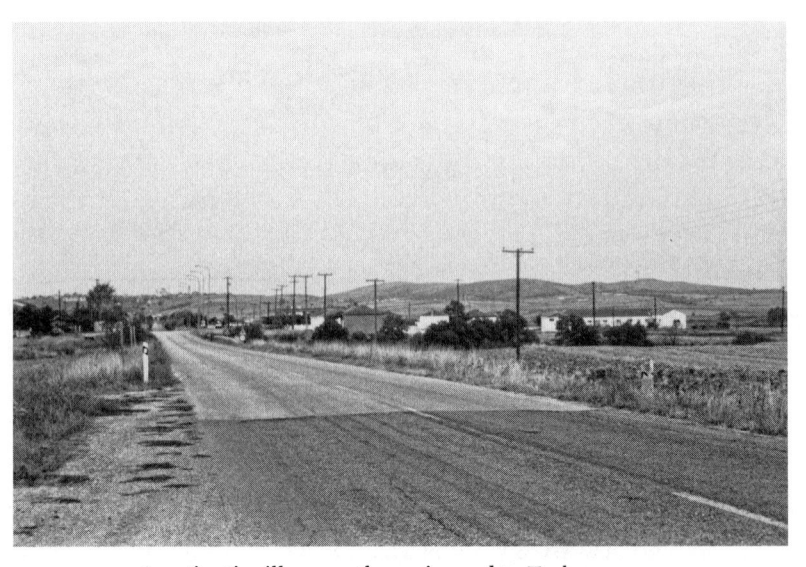

A patient's village on the main road to Turkey, 2004.
Photo by Elizabeth Anne Davis

tinct from guilt, which follows from a conscious recognition of this conflict.

2. From a biological point of view, based in ethological studies of the animal organism, anxiety is produced by operations in the limbic and reticular systems of the forebrain. The animal, faced with certain kinds of stimuli—physical threat, sex, food—experiences anxiety, which compels it to react according to the "fight or flight" pattern conditioned by the evolutionary history of the species. Medications affecting neurotransmission address anxiety at this level of autonomous arousal.

3. Cognitive psychiatry seeks a logical account of what transpires in patients' train of thought to cause anxiety. If certain thoughts are associated with certain stressful stimuli, the thoughts themselves can begin to cause anxiety. Cognitive therapy intervenes here, to create distance between patients and their anxiogenic thoughts so that they can recognize, organize, and begin to doubt them, thus reasserting control.

4. Behavioral psychiatry is closely linked with cognitive therapy. Rather than analyzing how thoughts operate in the mind, however, behavioral therapy identifies the affective consequences of behav-

iors, such as the calming effect of avoidance, and enrolls these consequences in the deliberate behavioral control of patients.

Kleandis had tried them all. He had first sought treatment at the clinic three years earlier, but his psychiatric history reached back many years to hospitals in Thessaloniki. He had taken an exhaustive array of anxiolytic and antidepressant medications, along with sedatives and certain anticonvulsants more often used to treat epilepsy and severe bipolar disorder. (The drug Anafranil, which by 2001—ten years after its market release—had achieved an international consensus as the most effective OCD medication,[1] caused Kleandis unbearable side effects and exacerbated his thyroid disease.) He had changed therapists almost as frequently, assigned to a different senior clinician with each admission. This time, it was Dr. Blastos who took the case. He prescribed Kleandis a new antidepressant and referred him to Thalia, a third-year resident, for cognitive-behavioral therapy.

Months later, after a brief and tenuous reprieve, Kleandis again found himself in the hospital clinic, overcome with anxiety and rage. At that time, Thalia reviewed his file with me. We counted nine admissions during the three years of his contact with the clinic, many lasting more than a month. Thalia told me, *I used to think of Kleandis as an ideal outpatient—the kind who can manage well in the community, partly because he's a good subject for psychotherapy. But it's becoming clear that he's actually severely ill, and he's getting worse with time. He's wearing out and giving up hope.* His desperation was marked by the radical idea, which he had frequently discussed with both of us, to stay at the monastery of Mount Athos for a few months. The last time I had seen him he had already begun preparations, growing the beard required of guests and submitting an application by way of his local priest. The ascetic life appealed to Kleandis, with its intricate rituals and its submissive devotion to a mysterious power. Thalia had reservations, but she did not intervene in Kleandis's plans: *It might be good for him to get away from home for a while—not to mention his parents. But I'm afraid the monastery might fuel his disease. And I'm not sure the monks will be able to tolerate him.*

Until recently, little attention in academic psychiatry had been paid in Greece to OCD, or anxiety disorders in general, apart from a handful of clinical studies conducted in the early 1990s at the state psychiatric hospital in Thessaloniki. While this might be explained, in part, by a low prevalence of such disorders in the Greek population, the authors of the OCD studies suggest that it has more to do with the structure of psychiatric care provision in Greece. Of the approximately two hundred patients treated for OCD between 1981 and 1991 in the Thessaloniki area, they report, "the great majority of these patients [we]re treated in private practice and not in outpatient clinics or community mental health centers" attached to state hospitals.[2] People with anxiety disorders in Greece have historically constituted a high-functioning outpatient population in the private sector, rather than being part of the much larger and more disabled population using public services.

It is the latter—especially chronic psychotics—who have formed the target population for investments and experiments in psychiatric reform. The preponderance of clinical research in Greece over the past twenty-five years has focused on such patients, especially on the efficacy and side effects of their long-term treatment with neuroleptics.[3] Some clinicians, including leaders of reform, have insisted on the enduring importance of custodial state hospitals in treating a core group of chronic schizophrenics who could not be discharged or rehabilitated, due both to the severity of their disease and to the inadequacy of outpatient care.[4] These "lost patients" remain in the obscure background of most studies, however, which attend instead to the medical and therapeutic management of "chronics" discharged from hospital settings. During the period of reform, it was to these patients that the community-based services of state psychiatry were devoted—not only because their crises were considered most urgent and disruptive to families and communities, but also because psychotic illnesses appeared to be managed well by the new medications emerging onto global markets in the 1980s.

Over the years of reform, severe mental illness itself was transformed in Greece, without receding from view. During one of his training seminars at the Association, Dr. Politis told his staff that, since the founding of the Association more than fifteen years before, he had seen the patient population change considerably: *We used to see mostly the wild [άγριοι] schizophrenics, he said*—those who had moldered away in state hospitals along with the mentally retarded, or bounced continually between penal and medical confinement. *Back then, we used to say, "Psychotics are the most in need of our care; we'll attend to the neurotics later." But now it's later, and we're beginning to see many more severe neurotics.* Politis was not pointing to a radical decrease in cases of psychosis, but rather to a shift from psychotic to neurotic in the kind of extremity presented by mental illness.[5] The profile of severe pathology was changing, and so, therefore, was the nature of therapeutic work. According to Politis, the staff would need to broaden their diagnostic criteria for accepting patients into the Association's programs. And beyond mere medication, they would find themselves practicing more and more psychotherapy.

❀ ❀ ❀

At the first staff meeting following his admission to the clinic that winter, Kleandis was introduced as a "very severe case." According to his intake therapist, the obsessive thoughts about disease and filth that plagued him even at his best moments had intensified lately, along with the cleansing rituals he had invented to repel those thoughts. He had grown increasingly desperate at home, and his parents finally sought an order for involuntary committal when his aggression toward them degenerated into outright violence. A week later, on a new medication, Kleandis was still washing up to eight hours a day, on his own count; and he had developed some new depressive symptoms as well.

At the age of thirty-one, Kleandis lived with his parents in a small farming village northeast of Alexandroupolis, along the main road to Turkey. According to his file, his psychiatric history began in his teenage years, when he suffered from "localized tremors" that spread from his hands to his neck and face. His father had experienced a similar neurological problem, for which he had sought treatment at the General Hospital of Thessaloniki. (Later, Kleandis would tell me "the real story," as he put it, one of many excluded from his file: his father was in fact a depressed alcoholic, and had checked himself into the hospital's detox facility.[6]) In his early twenties, while he was still at university in Thessaloniki, Kleandis was diagnosed with hypothyroidism, to which he attributed crippling fatigue, memory loss, and depression—and which earned him an exemption from military service. Though he was able to finish his college degree in ancient history, his depression worsened over the years that followed, and he ultimately abandoned his plans to pursue a doctorate. He was hospitalized for the first time in 1999, at the inpatient psychiatry ward of the General Hospital of Thessaloniki. It was then, according to notes in his file, that Kleandis "finally began to think that his problems were psychological" and "accepted psychiatric treatment." That admission marked the beginning of his experimentation with psychoactive medications. The file did not report his subsequent excursion to the state psychiatric hospital at Thessaloniki, where—he told me later—he was heavily sedated and subjected to electroshock treatments for three weeks.

Kleandis did not seek psychiatric care in Alexandroupolis, much closer to home, until 2001. At that time, though he complained of severe anxiety, his core problem still appeared to the staff as depression. In the course of four separate admissions to the clinic that year, his diagnosis progressed from depressive syndrome to anxiety disorder, and finally to obsessive-compulsive disorder. In the ensuing years, his condition would remit and then return with ever greater force. According to notes in his file, his poor prognosis was aggravated by his failure to "cooperate fully" with the treatment programs his therapists proposed: he made "private" decisions to quit his medications, and "colluded" with his mother's attempts to nurture his dependency on her. His doctors always hesitated to send him back into his family environment where, as he admitted himself, he had no autonomy, even in matters of bodily function: his mother fed and bathed him, and often slept in his room at night. He reported feeling guilty, ashamed, and anxious about this dependency, which he knew was connected to his rage—but he could not bring himself to "try harder on his own behalf."

THE LOGIC OF THIS LIBERAL LEGISLATION

In *Madness and Civilization*, Michel Foucault traces the modern confrontation with madness to the "great confinement" of the mad in seventeenth-century France. Not alone in their "derangement," but together with the poor, the criminal, and the disabled, the mad presented a problem for the city in their incapacity or their refusal to work—a problem that set in motion an increasingly specific, medical, and moral discernment of the mad as a special population destined for imprisonment, in the silent darkness of unreason as in the dungeons of workhouses and hospitals.[7] Psychiatric reform in nineteenth-century Europe and North America— which Foucault describes elsewhere as a movement of "moralizing sadism"[8]—yielded the new institution of the asylum and a corresponding medical science for the mentally ill. The spectacular liberation of madmen from their chains at this moment was, on Foucault's account, a false liberation: a second and more artful confinement that situated madness in an ineluctable grid of knowledge and power, with freedom glimmer-

ing through the latticework. This grid would be constructed and fortified on the modern terrain of discipline,[9] where knowledge of the mentally ill as a population—including psychiatric epidemiology, etiology,
and therapy—worked in tandem with a security apparatus of law and
police to protect society from the violent danger and moral contagion
they threatened.

This history of psychiatry offers to Foucault a precise paradigm of biopower, whose genealogy he presents as an alternative account of modern
power to the juridical history of law and its exceptions, of punishments
and entitlements, repressions and liberations—that is, of the sovereign
power of death. Biopower, the power of life, organizes itself instead as a
normative regime in which these persons are not merely objects of right
and constraint, but also subjects of knowledge and labor.

It is perhaps surprising, then, that Foucault recognizes in liberalism—precisely the "model" that "presupposes the individual as a subject of natural rights" and that makes "law the fundamental manifestation of power"[10]—something more biopolitical than a relic of sovereign
power. Liberalism, he writes, is a "framework of political rationality"
within which biopolitical problems are presented to governmental practice, a framework that requires the "respect of legal subjects" and guar-
antees the "free enterprise of individuals."[11] Liberalism on this description is not "the market" or even the theory of political economy; the
market serves more humbly as a contingent experiment to "identify the
excesses of governmentality."[12] Foucault takes liberalism instead as a
practice of posing, on behalf of society, the question of "too much government": a "form of critical reflection on governmental practice"[13] and
a principle of opposition to a governmentality that seeks ever to increase
the size and the strength of the state. It produces a distinction between
society and the state that is not apparent to governmentality itself and
that makes law the most economical form of "general intervention" into
state power by "the people."

Foucault's turn from the juridical apparatus of sovereign power to the
knowledges and technologies of biopower should not, then, be taken
as a retraction of law from the biopolitical analysis of power relations.
Rather, this turn draws attention to the relationship between that biopolitical governmentality animated by knowledge, on the one hand, and
that liberalism constituted as juridical critique, on the other.

Psychiatric reform, in its "second wave" following the Second World
War in Europe and the United States, discloses that relationship. Pre-

serving the mentally ill as a subject population, reformers have argued their civil and human rights in biopolitical terms, by way of illness-based protections and treatment-based liberations, as well as in liberal terms, by way of legal constraints on repressive policing and clinical domination. Patients' freedom—its definition and defense—is at stake in the intersection of these strategies. The most visible and controversial point of intersection is the practice of compulsory treatment, a common mode of psychiatric care in Greece—though the fact that it is no longer the *most* common mode in public services is counted as a triumph of psychiatric reform. In this section, I examine the policy of compulsory treatment in Greece to clarify the role of psychiatry there in the present formation of state power.[14]

In Greece, the authors and practitioners of psychiatric reform, concerned with the design and implementation of dispersed networks of outpatient care, have been preoccupied with the special incapacity to ethical reform, and the special danger to the community, presented by the severely mentally ill as compared with other marginalized groups. Severe pathology is thus a very sensitive gauge of the broader formation of power in which reform is undertaken. The intervention of compulsory treatment in cases of severe mental illness describes a complex mix of governmental strategies in which diagnosis functions in modalities of care and control. According to Greek law, compulsory treatment is warranted not only in cases of danger but in any case in which a patient's mental health would deteriorate without treatment. This dual pretext contains a foundational impasse in humanitarian politics regarding the mentally ill, whose very freedom is understood in urgent cases as a threat to their health.

To explore this impasse, I take as a point of departure the Italian reformer Franco Basaglia's critique of psychiatry as an essentially penal branch of medicine. He argued that psychiatry in Europe took shape historically around the legal concept of danger, and thus around a "basic contradiction" between "care of the sick and protection of the community, between medicine and law and order."[15] Psychiatry has thus always shared with law the "principles of sanction and separation," which have "defined" and "strictly limit[ed]" the development of its "medical side."[16]

The legislation of psychiatric reform in Greece was molded by the celebrated Law 180 in Italy, which—with Basaglia's influence—transformed the nature and rationale of compulsory treatment. Following the law's passage in 1978, however, Basaglia observed that European psychiatry had hardly yet begun a radical "rethinking" of its "function . . . within the social fabric,"[17] which could proceed only from the wholesale destruction of the asylum. Short of this, he warned, reform would simply reproduce obedience to the legal concept of danger, and the same contradictions that had defined psychiatry since its origins. He approved certain changes in Italian healthcare law, which now designated treatments instead of diseases, thereby detaching compulsory treatment from the diagnosis of specific illnesses, including mental illness.[18] If he did not perceive any pretext for incarceration in the patient's "right to treatment" that emerged from this redefinition of the law,[19] it is only because, in his vision of reformed psychiatry, the asylum had already been destroyed.

Needless to say, by 1995—the year the first state project of psychiatric reform officially expired in Greece—the asylum had not been destroyed. Nor had the codification of the patient's right to treatment in Greek law replaced its definition of dangerous mental conditions that warrant abrogation of the patient's right to freedom. Instead of merely reproducing the same old contradictions between security and welfare, as Basaglia had feared, psychiatric reform in Greece invented some new ones as well: between international and state law, between professional discretion and humanitarian regulation, between the right to freedom and the ethics of responsibility.

Those Having the Right

As I recounted in the prelude, the humanitarian reform of psychiatry in Greece was inaugurated with the liberation of the Greek state from dictatorship in 1974. New legislation, aiming similarly to liberate psychiatric patients from state power, emerged in this context from efforts to modernize and Europeanize the state itself. This legislation addresses the mentally ill as subjects of universal human rights, imbued with "essential dignity" and the "natural right" to freedom. The mentally ill worldwide are recognized as a special international population protected by the United Nations Declaration of Human Rights in Resolution 46/119, "Principles for the Protection of Persons with Mental Illness and the Improvement of Mental Health Care," passed in 1991. Strongly influenced by the community-care framework of psychiatric reform internationally, its third principle stipulates the right for patients to live and work, "as far as possible," in the community. Its first principle confers patients the rights, among others, to the "best available" mental healthcare; to treatment with "humanity and respect for the inherent dignity of the human person"; to protection from abuse and discrimination; and to the exercise of all civil, political, economic, social, and cultural rights belonging to other persons. All these rights obtain for all psychiatric patients— excepting those declared legally incapacitated.

Principles 11 and 16 of the resolution specify how legal incapacity can be declared in two limit cases. According to these principles, a person may be compelled to undergo psychiatric treatment without his or her consent, including by involuntary committal to a mental healthcare facility, only if a medical expert determines that the patient has a mental illness *and*

> (a) That, because of that mental illness, there is a serious likelihood of immediate or imminent harm to that person or to other persons; or
>
> (b) That, in the case of a person whose mental illness is severe and whose judgment is impaired, failure to admit or retain that person is likely to lead to a serious deterioration in his or her condition or will prevent the giving of appropriate treatment that can only be given by admission to a mental health facility in accordance with the principle of the least restrictive alternative.[20]

These limit cases represent the exception to human rights presented by mental illness, in which personal autonomy is not necessarily in the interest of the subject's health and well-being. That interest may legally be adjudicated instead by his or her legal representatives, medical caregivers, and independent review bodies.

In human rights law, broadly construed, the mentally ill are thus exposed to a conflict between their right to autonomy and their right to treatment. In the UN resolution, the responsibility for resolving this conflict is summarily delegated to the civil law of member states. The international community, represented by the UN high commissioner for human rights, is positioned to judge the performance by member states of this responsibility to protect the interests of the mentally ill as special subjects of human rights.

The onus of state responsibility, along with the state power of technocratic governance, is thus invested in psychiatry. In Greek law, the human rights of the mentally ill delineate a nominally autonomous domain of psychiatric expertise in which clinicians are entrusted with the power to protect or abrogate those rights according to their professional discretion. Even as patients' rights come into direct conflict, then, they constitute the line where law ends and medicine begins. Below, I trace the contours of this faint and irregular line.

❋ ❋ ❋

In June of 1989, the Greek Ministry of Health sponsored a national conference on Greek legislation concerning the mentally ill, or rather on its "synchronization" with international law, to which a number of prominent medical and legal experts contributed reports and commentary. Among them was Katerina Matsa, head psychiatrist of the Mental Health Association of Athens, playing the role of critic and conscience of the proceedings. In her address, she disavowed the "exoteric view" of the legislative quandary in Greece, according to which it would appear, like so many aspects of "Greek reality," as a "delayed echo" of developments elsewhere[21]—a facile metaphor linking the maturation of the Greek state in its liberation from dictatorship with the maturation of patients in their liberation from the asylum.

Yet Matsa used that exoteric view to valorize the "advances" other nations had made in their mental health legislation, showing that both the quality and the institutional framework of psychiatric care in Greece required radical change. She insisted that in the present system, "the psychiatrist cannot play any role other than that accorded to him by the state—the role, that is, of the colleague of the police . . . and the district attorney," who can only treat the patient as an "antisocial" citizen. In her view, that role contravened all therapeutic labor, for therapy must mobilize rather than "nullify" the freedom of the patient.[22]

In her address, Matsa opened a critique of law in which freedom appeared not only as a right, but also as a medical requirement of treatment. She proposed to psychiatrists the task of inventing a new political framework for safeguarding this freedom in Greece: "For all that our legislation has changed and become more liberal [φιλελεύθερη: literally 'freedom-loving'], it is not enough. We must decide what is to be the logic of this liberal legislation."[23]

Participants at the conference attempted to discover this logic, striving for a common medico-legal language that would address inconsistencies and perplexities in the extant legislation concerning the mentally ill. Much of their discussion targeted legal incapacity (δικαστική απαγόρευση) and involuntary committal (ακούσια νοσηλία) as critical disjunctures between law and medicine.[24]

The declaration of legal incapacity renders a person unable to perform legal practices, constraining him or her to act only through a guardian or legal representative. Evaluating the capacity of patients to judge "in the interest of their health,"[25] and to give or withhold consent to treatment, is a task accorded in the Greek legislation to psychiatrists. Having at their disposal no other technique for approaching it, psychiatrists might imagine this task as a matter of diagnosis. Yet the law does not require a diagnosis for the declaration of mental incapacity. Article 95 of Statute 2071, the most current Greek legislation on this issue,[26] identifies potential subjects of involuntary treatment only as "persons suffering from a mental disorder" who are "unable to judge in the interest of their health." As Maria Tziaferi pointed out at the national conference, Article 1786 of the civil code declares "legally incapacitated . . . anyone who, owing to persistent mental disease [πνευματική νόσος] that precludes the use of his reason, is unable to oversee himself and his property."[27] Legal incapacity is not attributable to any specific mental illness—and conversely, almost any mental illness could legally preclude a person from using his or her reason.

While legal incapacity is determined by medical experts, *mental deficiency (πνευματική ανεπάρκεια)* is a term used by those who are not medical experts to "avoid" psychiatric nosology in legal contexts, according to Dimitris Papasteriou, another conference participant.[28] As a legal term, mental deficiency refers to any factor that compromises a person's responsibility to perform actions with legal consequences, such as declarations of will. *Mental disease (πνευματική νόσος)* is another "avoidant" nonmedical term, related but not equivalent to the psychiatric term *mental illness (ψυχική νόσος)*. It serves the function of qualifying the legal fact of mental deficiency (as in, "mentally deficient by reason of mental disease"). This legally binding formulation makes no reference to the technical specificity of psychiatric nosology. In the view of Haritonas Fotiadis, a medical expert at the conference, such evasions of medical specificity in the legal language of mental illness can be attributed in part to the failure of psychiatrists themselves to reach any consensus on nosology.[29] As a consequence, the law tends to classify all legally incapacitated patients under the rubric of "mental sufferer" (ψυχικός πάσχοντος), without regard to the nature or treatability of the disorder actually present.

Mental incapacity must therefore be understood not as a medical condition requiring treatment, but as a legal condition authorizing incapacitation or involuntary treatment. The declaration is a legal action taken by a medical expert—the sort of action that Matsa, along with Basaglia and other internal critics of psychiatry, associate with its essentially penal function, by which the mentally ill are separated from society and maneuvered into the clinic. This function is preserved in the mental health legislation in force in Greece today, compiled under Statute 2071 ("Synchronization and Organization of the National Health System"), passed in 1992. Articles 95–98 of the statute were drafted in accordance with EEC Proposal R(3)2 ("Legal Protection of Persons Suffering from Mental Disorders Committed Involuntarily"), promulgated in 1983 by the Committee of Ministers of the European Commission, which—without formal means of enforcement—urged all member states to adopt the proposal or append it to their national legislation.[30]

Article 95 of this statute specifies two conditions, of which either one alone is sufficient to warrant involuntary committal, defined as "admission to a mental health facility for treatment without the consent of the patient." The first condition of the article requires both that patients suffer from a mental disorder that disables them to judge in the interest of their health, and that their health be likely to deteriorate without treatment. The second condition requires that patients suffer from a mental disorder for which treatment is required to prevent their "use of violence" against themselves or others.

These two conditions for involuntary committal in the Greek statute map cleanly onto the two cases specified in UN Resolution 46/119. Both formulations of the law authorize a supervention of patients' right to autonomy by their right to treatment. Yet the two cases of supervention arise from very different grounds and demarcate very different modes of responsibility. While the first condition aims to substitute expert judgment for the patient's to protect his or her health, the second condition aims to protect the community from danger, and does not require mental incapacity on the part of the patient who poses that danger. In a biopolitical vocabulary, the first condition promotes welfare, while the second promotes security.

Among Greek psychiatrists sensitized to humanitarian politics, the second condition has occasioned much more controversy in debates over national legislation. Several clinicians at the hospital in Alexandroupolis told me that it was also the more common and effective argument for involuntary committal. In an interview, Dr. Lamberakis described the two conditions this way: "That a patient may harm himself or others— that's the main reason for involuntary committal. But there's one other reason. . . . That's when a patient is not aware of his condition, and so he avoids treatment, to the point where his health will decline unless he's treated. That's what we call 'therapeutic necessity,' as opposed to the reason of 'danger to his environment.' Now, 'danger' is something very vague [στο φλου] — it isn't easily measured. It's determined by psychiatrists: you need the opinion of two doctors that a person is a danger to himself or others, just as you would to determine 'therapeutic necessity.' And you need approval from a judge. That's what the law says. In practice, of course, judges give more weight to 'danger.'"[31]

As Basaglia contended decades earlier, the problem of danger forms the crux of a long-standing conflict in psychiatry between its roles of security and welfare — its responsibilities to public safety and to patients' health and well-being. As Sakellaropoulos remarks in his textbook, the possibility that a patient being treated in the community may suffer a relapse and become "agitated" and "aggressive toward himself or others," though it occurs very rarely, is one of the few scenarios in which the psychiatrist can truly "lose" his or her patient.[32] He writes that such cases of danger provoke fear, mistrust, and a certain "coldness" on the part of the community toward psychiatric patients in general, which accounts for the recourse to custodial care still made in up to 40 percent of patients admitted involuntarily in some regions of Greece. According to Sakellaropoulos, these high rates are due chiefly to the underdevelopment of outpatient services in those regions.[33] In his view, the resolution to the problem of danger is found not in a wholesale liberation of patients from state power, but in an expansion of the state's infrastructure for effective, community-based care.

Lamberakis reinforced this view, in response to my question about how the process of involuntary committal had changed in Thrace during psychiatric reform:

> The system has changed, but not in terms of police intervention. Patients come to us now much less frequently by police escort, but not because the police procedure has changed. It's because in the areas where there are psychiatric services, the likelihood is greater that patients will already be receiving regular treatment, they will have supervision, they'll be taking preventive medications and won't have such serious relapses — so they won't get to the point where they require intervention by the police. . . . In the past, we didn't have such effective means of preventing relapses, not just because patients didn't take their medi-

cations—patients don't like taking them now either—but also for *scientific* reasons. The preventive medications were not as effective then as they are now.

But even in areas that don't have psychiatric services, people know better today when they need a doctor—there is more awareness and education among the population. Compared with what used to happen thirty years ago, I imagine people now would know to take a sick person to the psychiatrist before he gets into such a bad state.

As Lamberakis poses it here, the strategy of humanitarian psychiatry in regard to the dangerous mentally ill is not to change the legal pretext of the involuntary intercession by which psychiatry approaches dangerous patients, but rather to reduce, through better voluntary treatment, the number of cases that necessitate such intercession.

This compromise between the state's responsibility to contain danger and the state's responsibility to foster health shares its basic framework with the earliest laws in Greece concerning the mentally ill. In 1862, legislation modeled on the French reforms of 1838 was adopted in Greece, establishing its first psychiatric hospitals and regulations for the admission and treatment of mental patients. Before that time, and throughout the Ottoman period, subjects considered insane were accommodated in Orthodox monasteries and Islamic charitable institutions, or mixed in with the general population of large sanitaria or prisons.[34] The legislation of 1862 rendered the release of patients from mental institutions contingent on their cure and on the willingness of family or other advocates—"those having the right"—to take responsibility for them. It also created administrative review procedures, and established judicial authority over medical decisions regarding patient admission and discharge.

In their critical history of Greek law concerning the mentally ill, Stelios Stylianidis, an activist psychiatrist, and Dimitris Ploumpidis, a historian, trace the conflict between patients' well-being and societal risk to a "fear of responsibility" for patients on the part of the state, from the earliest legislation up to the present day.[35] More than a century passed before the first internment laws were replaced by Statute 104/73, during the dictatorship, without open debate or public disclosure.[36] As the criterion of patients' discharge from mental healthcare facilities, the new statute substituted for "cure" the "absence of danger to public order and safety." In this way, Stylianidis and Ploumpidis point out, danger was installed in the law as the "autonomous" (i.e., nonmedical) criterion of psychopathology, providing a legal foothold for administrative and judiciary control and permitting "state repression" to "short-circuit" the therapeutic project.[37]

In 1978, four years after the fall of the dictatorship, the newly elected Greek parliament attempted to liberalize this statute of 1973, introducing voluntary admission as a category of treatment and formalizing a complex system of independent reviews for involuntary committals. Yet the new legislation reiterated the requirement that patients admitted involuntarily be discharged only to "those having the right" or the "obligation" to receive them. And, for the first time, it obligated these advocates to guarantee follow-up treatment, and to bear "civil responsibility" for discharged patients, even—unconstitutionally, as Stylianidis and Ploumpidis point out—in the absence of a declaration of legal incapacity.

It is possible to discern, in more recent legislation, a shift to medical authority over compulsory treatment, away from the judicial authority established in the original internment laws. The procedure for involuntary committal is specified in Article 96 of Statute 2071, passed in 1992. The request can be made by a spouse, direct relative, or legal guardian of the patient, though in the absence of such advocates the district attorney may initiate the procedure in an emergency. The request must be addressed to the district attorney, accompanied by a medical certificate signed by two psychiatrists and referring to one or both condition(s) of Article 95: therapeutic necessity and/or danger. The district attorney, having ascertained these conditions and validated the certificate, then orders the transfer of the patient to a local psychiatry clinic or ward, either by police escort or by medical transport. Patients must immediately be informed of their rights, including the right to appeal the district attorney's decision. The facility's clinical staff is granted forty-eight hours to examine the patient thoroughly and determine whether further confinement is necessary. Involuntary treatment must be terminated when the conditions of Article 95 no longer apply to the case. The course of treatment, which the patient can appeal at any time, and which must be evaluated by a medical team at regular intervals, cannot exceed six months except by the formal decision of an independent committee.[38]

Confinement and case reviews are thus authorized, in this statute, by psychiatric expertise rather than legal judgment. But the fact that the law recognizes this expertise as such without demanding nosological specificity or "scientific proof," as Matsa and others have argued, reveals a significant discrepancy in Greek law between the *weight* accorded to psychiatric expertise and the *specificity* of that expertise. Technical knowledge, in the form of diagnosis and prognosis, does not reach the law. The 1992 legislation—including the civil and penal codes, residual portions of the 1973 statute, a ministerial order from 1979, and the European code of 1983—deploys several potentially incompatible qualifications of the danger presented by psychiatric patients that may warrant their involuntary treatment. Article 5 of a legislative decree from 1973, for example, specifies "dangerousness to public order or to the personal safety of oneself or other citizens." Article 2 of the 1979 ministerial order, however, asks only for the "*likelihood* that a patient will harm himself or others," while "dangerousness to himself or others" appears as the criterion elsewhere in the same text.[39] Article 95 of the 1992 legislation requires involuntary committal of a person "to prevent his use of violence against himself or others." As for the diagnosis of the disturbed person in question: he may be a "dangerous psychopath," "psychotically ill or diseased," "psychotic," or, in accordance with the European code, merely a "sufferer of mental disease" (διανοητική νόσος).

Instead of a coherent approach, then, Greek law and medicine *after* psychiatric reform together offer a provisional set of loose guidelines that fail to address the basic disjuncture between security and welfare—thus not only permitting but obliging a certain "anarchy" at the level of practice, as a number of participants observed at the national conference in 1989.[40] In the absence of principled directives, they found a collective ethical imperative in guarding patients against abuses of the power that remained a legal prerogative of clinicians. The law would protect patients' autonomy up to the point of psychiatric evaluation; beyond that, it was up to psychiatrists themselves, with their discrepant clinical orientations and their personal idiosyncrasies, to liberate or compel their patients—and to develop an ad hoc rationale for this judgment on the basis of their expertise.

Two basic positions emerged from the national conference regarding this "anarchic" clinical improvisation in the shadow of the law. One position urged the protection of patients by specifying as far as possible the legal language of mental illness according to psychiatric expertise. If the laws defining mental incapacity and compulsory treatment spelled out the requisite psychomedical conditions, down to the most minute diagnostic and prognostic detail, then clinical practice could be controlled by guidelines that delegitimized personal discretion and thus evacuated the potential for any abuse of power. The second and contrary position held that such rigid codification would disable psychiatrists from discharging patients who were not "in full possession of reason" when, in their expert judgment, such liberty would be beneficial to the patients' health. According to this view, "benevolent discretion" would lose sway as the law gained specificity—and clinicians must defend the therapeutic space against such encroachment of the law.

As several conference participants reminded the more idealistic partisans, however, neither strategy of protecting patients from the abuse of psychiatric power could actually materialize until a consensus on diagnostic and prognostic knowledge was reached by psychiatric experts themselves. This debate over the precision with which psychiatric knowledge should be registered in legal language demonstrates the impasse of humanitarian politics in this context. What is conceived as a legal and moral responsibility to protect and liberate patients promotes not a principled professional ethics but a pragmatic and inconsistent one. Competing imperatives—a responsibility to treat patients, a respect for their personal autonomy, and a contradictory and unstable knowledge of mental illness—determine this ethical impasse for politicized clinicians.

From their critical vantage on mental health care legislation in Greece, Stylianidis and Ploumpidis argue that if medical authority cannot decide *for the law* the key questions of danger and responsibility in mental illness, then neither can it protect the health of patients from repression by law. In their view, the laws of 1973 and 1978 that eventually made their way into Statute 2071, despite their revisions of the repressive internment legislation of 1862, represent "a social complacency and a securitarian and normalizing logic" in regard to the mentally ill, to which protestations of patients' human rights serve only as a general, abstract, and ineffective rejoinder.[41] New legislation, they argue, must address certain fundamental questions: "It is necessary to establish if dangerousness can be dissociated from the psychopathology of the subject in his social context, if mental illness is synonymous with criminal irresponsibility, if the protection of individual freedoms and the dignity of the patient can be separated from the elaboration of a therapeutic project by treatment teams."[42]

At this point of impasse, Stylianidis and Ploumpidis call on psychiatrists to reconcile penal law, which protects the community, with humanitarian law, which protects the freedom and health of patients: to bring into alignment the legal grounds of both conditions for involuntary treatment. They suggest that only a psychomedical framework, autonomous from the demands of law, can simultaneously conceptualize both a legal responsibility to avert danger and a moral responsibility to respect human liberty and dignity.

Just Well Enough

Vangelis had a history at the hospital clinic in Alexandroupolis going back twenty years. He belonged to a large extended family of psychiatric patients—all diagnosed with schizophrenia or psychotic depression; all notorious at the clinic for their intergenerational pathology, their poverty, and their violence. I had first met him in the autumn, when he was admitted to the old hospital clinic for a suicide attempt. At that time, Vangelis seemed a shadowy fixture: known to all, but mute and avoidant. Most often he could be seen sleeping on a couch in the patients' lounge. The therapists on staff, who had all treated him over the years, disagreed about the seriousness of the danger he was in. He was discharged after ten days.

I did not get to know Vangelis until the following summer, when he was readmitted to the new hospital clinic for "social reasons." It was generally agreed then among the staff that, after decades of severe mental illness, he had undergone a remarkable recovery. He became more sociable, developing friendships with other patients and seeing a girlfriend for a time. He attended group therapy regularly, and spoke with grace and dexterity about "coming out of illness." He had been admitted to the clinic this time not for urgent treatment, but because he needed a place to stay. The Association had evicted him from a group home due to the escalating violence of his conflicts with his roommates. This apartment, which housed three other men in treatment, came to be known as "the time bomb," repeatedly discussed at staff meetings both at the hospital clinic and at the Association. All four roommates were ultimately relocated.

Any other patient might have been refused admission to the hospital clinic under these circumstances, but Vangelis enjoyed a special status at the clinic. Dr. Filalithi in particular wanted to safeguard the progress Vangelis had made, and feared the relapse into drinking, delusion, and violence that might engulf him if he remained homeless. Some among the staff disputed this apparent favoritism toward Vangelis over other chronic patients who, like him, had nowhere else to go. The pragmatic priorities of individual therapists came into conflict with collective pressure to articulate a consistent policy for supporting chronic but unstable outpatients.

The first step in achieving the conditions under which Vangelis could remain well was to secure him new housing. According to state policy, housing entitlements were reserved for the growing cohort of deinstitutionalized patients whose regional number was tracked closely by reformist administrators. As it was, the Association had made a potentially illicit exception for Vangelis to live in the group home from which he had just been evicted. The hospital clinic was permitted but not funded to run its own housing program, which would therefore have to be accomplished without increasing the clinic budget; spending on other programs like the mobile units would have to be cut, and staff would have to volunteer their time. No one was willing to make these sacrifices, but the problem had been raised repeatedly when cases such as Vangelis's arose. The district attorney had informally advised clinicians to commit these patients to the state hospital at Thessaloniki, so that they could be discharged with eligibility for state housing. But Filalithi called this proposal "glib" and "countertherapeutic." Such admissions could, in any case, only be made under compulsory order, which was clearly not warranted in cases where patients had only "social" reasons for admission. And the far-off hospital in Thessaloniki was an absolute last resort for patients in this region.

I came across Vangelis one morning on his way into the patients' lounge, carrying several coffees on a tray. He smiled right at me, this man who would never meet my eyes or speak when I had approached him at the old clinic the previous fall. I introduced myself; we chatted. He asked me, using the formal mode of address, *What exactly are you studying here?* I told him I was interested in the social factors that play a role in mental illness. He leaned in. *Well, I've come through a very serious mental illness, maybe you heard about me. It was very bad, I even cut off my thumb.* (He showed me the stump.) *My whole family has these problems. If you're interested in mental illness, I know a lot about it.* I asked if he would be at the clinic a few more days; we could meet to talk. He laughed: *Oh, I'll be here. I'm staying until I find a house. I have nowhere else to go.*

When we met again, a few days later, Vangelis seemed to me more downcast than the last time we had talked, and I said so. *I took leave yesterday,* he explained. *I had company in town, and I went to spend some time with them. Coming back here was hard. It's a bad situation, now that we're locked in.* He was referring to the blockade. I did not yet know that his girlfriend was the same Martina who had committed suicide on the hospital grounds just one week earlier. Dr. Filalithi told me later that the two had known each other years ago, before Martina moved to Athens with her brother. When they met again, on her readmission to the hospital clinic, they immediately fell in love. Vangelis had apparently proposed that they find an apartment in the city and move in together. Another patient—a woman he had befriended in the clinic—got jealous and started a fight with Martina. This was just before she disappeared.

I told Vangelis now that I had been hearing a lot of complaints about the blockade. Did this make him want to leave the clinic? He paused a moment. Look, I'm homeless right now, he said. I was living in an apartment with some other people, some patients like me, you know, with psychotic illness. We had one of the apartments at the Association. But then something happened, and we were all kicked out.

Before we traveled too far down this path, Vangelis told me he would rather talk about things that had to do with my research. I don't know much, he said, but I think that every person has experiences that go along with the steps he takes in life. Like me, for example: I've taken some bad steps. Growing up was hard for me, because of my brother. I suffered a lot from him, and so did my mother. He was born that way—he's a bad soul [κακόψυχος]. Just like my brother-in-law. When I dropped out of high school, I went to work for him. He had a little shop at the market. But the man abused me—physically, mentally. Basically he treated me like a slave. Bit by bit, I was overwhelmed by melancholy [μελαγχολία]. As much as I struggled and fought, I couldn't handle it. I was about seventeen then. My mother had me picked up, and they brought me all the way to Thessaloniki in an ambulance.

I stayed at the hospital for three weeks. I met some people there; it was the first time I really had good company, people who understood me. One man I met really inspired me. He told me that I needed to live my life, not end it. I listened to him, and I believed him. When I got back here, it was hard for me, but I went out, I found company. I went to a cafeteria once, and that's where I met my wife. We got married and we had our son—he's twenty now.

In those days, I had a doctor at the hospital who would come to my house and give me injections. He tried to help me. But things didn't go well at home. I got a lot of pressure from my wife. We had a shop, selling artworks and photographic things. She expected me to take responsibility for running the whole thing and also to do all the housework, since she worked night shifts; she was a nurse. That's when I started having serious problems. I was hearing voices and seeing things. I had an episode—I heard voices telling me I had to cut my thumb off, they made me do it. That was the first time I was hospitalized here. Since then I've had a lot of relapses [υποτροπές, the clinical term]. Sometimes I'll go six months, other times two months.

After that, my wife divorced me. I didn't meet my girlfriend until later on. Back in those days, I was about twenty-five years old, I was getting sick a lot. I'd been hurt earlier in life, you know, and that's what came back to me. I would see images and hear voices, and I'd lash out. I'm trying to think how to explain it to you, so that you'll understand. See, a psychiatrist told me once that the voices I heard are guilty feelings [ενοχές]. I was abused when I was a teenager, especially by my brother-in-law, who was always telling me I was from a bad family, my parents were bad people. It made me feel like I was worth nothing. Now, all these years later, I understand that it wasn't really like that. I can see that my parents were worth loving. But I still have these bad feelings inside. Back then, I'd hear voices and see things that would bring those feelings up. Like, once I believed I was a Turkish soldier and my leg was being cut off. I used to think I was living in a different time, in the olden days, or that I was someone else. It all seemed real to me, I saw it like cinema, with the sounds and the pictures, and I'd be in the middle of it, believing it was all happening to me. I had acoustic and visual hallucinations [οπτικές και ακουστικές ψευδαισθήσεις— again, clinical terms]. But it wasn't just that, it was delusional [παραλήρημα], I really believed it was real.

So that's how I cut off my thumb. I also tried to cut my wrists with a knife. (He showed me a thick scar across the width of his inner wrist.) I did it because I couldn't stand the voices and everything. I had a moment when my reason [λογική] told me, "Look, you can't go on like this, you're better off dead." And that's when I cut my wrist. What happened was, I bled for a while, but then the blood froze and no more came out. So I walked over to the hospital. I was living in the Kalithea neighborhood then, right near the old hospital, so I had time to get there.

I don't have those problems anymore, though. I don't hear voices or see things. I would say that I'm not mentally ill anymore. But I have no home, no money, no job, no one to love me. My son doesn't want to see me. I think my ex-wife has told him all sorts of bad things about me. And it's true, I'm ashamed for him to see me like this. You know, I lost my father more than twenty years ago; he never saw me get married. And my mother—she was at my wedding, and she knew my son. But she died a while ago, from lung sickness, and she had diabetes and took insulin shots. She died in the old hospital. Dr. Filalithi gave my family some help to get her into the hospital. I visited her every day, but after a while I just couldn't handle it anymore, I stopped going because it made me sick to see her that way. My brothers and sisters were supposed to help, but I don't think they ever did. And that's how she died—alone.

Vangelis stopped. We sat in silence for a moment. I shifted tacks and asked him what he was thinking about doing when he left the clinic. He was doing so well, surely he would be leaving soon? He shook his head. *I'm not sure, I'm going to have to find work somewhere so I can pay rent. The social worker told me she found me a place to live at a good price, but I never heard anything else about it. I really don't think they'll find me a house. And I've got other problems now. My doctor ran some tests on me, and he says that I had a stroke. So maybe I won't be able to work. Mental illness . . . that's not even the point anymore. It just wasn't written [δεν ήταν γραφτό] for me to have a good life. Maybe I'm a bad soul, too.*

❋ ❋ ❋

Failing to secure state housing for Vangelis, Dr. Filalithi took up a collection among the clinic staff to finance a cheap room in the private rental market. Vangelis would be expected to get a job in order to pay a share of the rent. The clinic's social worker undertook the onerous task of finding a landlord who would rent to a psychiatric patient. Rental agreements kept falling through when Vangelis's status as a "social service client" was revealed.

During this period, when Vangelis resided in the clinic, Filalithi wrote the district attorney about his case, requesting a formal change in his legal status. If Vangelis could be "removed from the clinical framework" and placed under the aegis of nonmedical social services, she argued, then the state alone—not the clinic—would be responsible for providing him housing in addition to his welfare subsidy. This was, in effect, a reversal of the process by which a psychiatric patient gained eligibility for disability income and housing: his status as a dependent on the state would be rendered independent of his mental illness. The clinic, in turn, would be restored to its therapeutic function for Vangelis. In her letter, Filalithi suggested that Vangelis's treatment had been successful, and that he was no longer so disabled by mental illness that he could not be counted "responsible."

A month later, it remained to be seen what effect this letter would have on the district attorney's handling of the case. But by then, circumstances had already changed. According to Filalithi, who discussed the case during a staff meeting in September, Vangelis was again nearing a crisis. In a state of grief over Martina's suicide, and perhaps in frustration over his housing situation, Vangelis had left the clinic against medical advice. But he returned the morning of this staff meeting with all his belongings, demanding readmission. The charge nurse reported that he was drunk and angry, making threats. As the staff discussed him, Vangelis—who had been given a sedative to calm him while he awaited a decision—slept with his bags on the side lawn of the clinic, just outside the meeting room. *What do we expect?* said one of his former psychiatrists. *He knows we're in here, we've had a meeting Tuesday mornings at 10:00 a.m. for years. He wants us to see him homeless.*

Those attending the meeting inside tried hard not to look. Filalithi, who had seen Vangelis earlier that morning, explained that they had made a contract (σύμβαση) concerning his future treatment at the clinic: *If he's admitted this time, and he chooses to leave, he can't expect to be readmitted automatically. Each time he returns he'll be handled as a new patient, without a history of cooperation. And he'll be admitted only for treatment, not for social reasons.* Several other therapists contested the agreement. One of Vangelis's former therapists warned that he was too manipulative to be bound by it: *He knows us too well. Regardless of how sick he really is, he'll threaten suicide to get admitted whenever he wants. Or he'll beat someone up. And we'll let him in. Contracts have no power over patients like this. He's just well enough to work the system.*

Over the years, Vangelis had been admitted to the hospital clinic many times under compulsory order because he presented an apparent danger to others—usually family members, but sometimes it was his neighbors who complained, or the police picked him up on the street. Sometimes the danger he presented was to himself: he had made a number of suicide attempts, and a much greater number of threats. Some of his admissions came at his own demand; his therapists said that he wielded the threat of danger whenever he wanted to escape his life. If he was "just well enough to work the system," he was also just sick enough to need it. His "social admission" that summer, for which there was no therapeutic rationale, verified that Vangelis had achieved health but not freedom: the fate of a bad soul bound to the system. At this moment in the clinic—twenty-five years after its founding as the first open-door, short-term clinic in a general hospital in Greece, now disastrously regressing into a locked ward—the debate over "social admission" arose as a local commentary on the national reform of policy regarding involuntary committal.

Dead Ends

The passage of Statute 2071 on mental healthcare in 1992, several years after the national conference on psychiatric reform, provoked anew the debate in Greece over the meaning of "liberal" legislation on mental illness. Maria Mitrosili, a political sociologist and a contributor to a volume of interviews with psychiatric and legal experts at that moment of retrospection, reviewed the new legislation from the vantage of its "political rationality," which determined "as its limits . . . the respect for the rights of the citizen, subject of illness." She commended the protocol for involuntary committal newly specified in the 1992 legislation because it required the participation of family and other advocates, multiple independent psychiatrists, the district attorney, and the court. It therefore not only, in her view, had a higher likelihood than previous laws of "respecting the individual rights of patients," but also "attempt[ed] to rewrite the subject of 'madness' into social and legal space." This attempt appeared most clearly in the direct linkage between the medical treatment of patients, on the one hand, and their deinstitutionalization and socioeconomic rehabilitation, on the other. Yet she cautioned that psychiatry continued to bear certain legislative "peculiarities" in comparison with other branches of medicine: "Just as treatment against the wishes of the psychiatric patient remains one of the fundamental dead ends of contemporary psychiatry; and just as the capacity for logic, judgment, and will continue to define the active subject of law—so will decisions concerning specific legal issues in psychiatry remain tied to the opportunity of the moment."[43]

Mitrosili names "the opportunity of the moment" here as the contrary of basic medical principles, yet to be formulated, that could consistently guide and justify legal decisions about the mentally ill. In her view, such new principles, founded in the psychomedical freedom of the patient, could only be sought in an "absolute departure" from conventional mental institutions: "How can we attribute 'autonomy' to mental sufferers, if we do not try to determine anew the politics of the psychiatric institution?" Like Matsa and Basaglia himself, Mitrosili contests the essentially securitarian logic of psychiatry, as against other kinds of medicine—and, like them, she fails to find an alternative.

Gestures to an as yet unformulated medical framework that would underpin a more radical psychiatric politics were already prominent in the discourse of reform leading up to the legislative changes of 1992. Stephanos Orphanoudakis, a constitutional lawyer and participant at the national conference in 1989, announced a series of contradictions in involuntary committal between the European code, the Greek constitution, the current healthcare legislation, and several decisions by the Ministry of Health. He warned that if the effort toward legislative reform did not assimilate the "experiences of psychiatric science," especially on the imprecise nosology of danger, then "we will have nothing but a transition from a 'system in doubt of security' to a 'system in doubt of freedom.'"[44] Presumably Matsa, in calling for psychiatrists to find a new logic for liberal legislation, feared just such a political and moral failure.

❀ ❀ ❀

To the extent that "internationally accepted standards" for the "best available" mental healthcare are not determined independently from the human and civil rights of legal subjects, psychiatry remains sheltered from the critique of governmentality facilitated, according to Foucault, by liberalism. This conclusion is not determined in advance by some structural impasse between law and medicine, but contingently by the failure of psychiatry to define and operationalize a psychomedical conception of freedom autonomous from the legal conception tied to the penal function of psychiatry. As their commentary in this section attests, internal critics of the reform of mental healthcare in Greece have agreed that the current legislation not only does not promote the humanitarian goal of legal freedom for psychiatric patients but also fails from a psychomedical point of view to establish the criteria by which their freedom can be understood as essential to treatment. Instead, it leaves open the prospect of medical pretexts for compulsory treatment, along with the space for therapeutic discretion and improvisation.

Attuned to their own investment with, in this sense, unregulated power, the critics call for a new psychiatric politics grounded in the state's responsibility for the welfare of the mentally ill. This politics is bound to a cloudy therapeutic vision of patient freedom. Yet patients who enter therapy, even by their own consent, do not always do so equipped or willing to take on the responsibility of freedom that the law provisionally confers on them. The humanitarian politics of psychiatric reform address a subject that clinicians sometimes have difficulty finding in their patients. In the next section, I explore the relationship between the humanitarian politics of reform and the clinical ethics of practice in the "anarchic" space of therapy, where dependency—rather than freedom—may be the common end.

THE PROCESS OF PERSUASION

If "welfare" (πρόνοια) names the state's responsibility toward the mentally ill, fulfilled in community-based services that render the asylum obsolete, then "the good" or "well-being" (το καλό) of the mentally ill names the clinical dimension of that responsibility. In an interview, Dr. Lamberakis described "well-being" to me as a therapeutic goal to which the law of compulsion can lead, but which the law cannot, itself, produce:

> If a patient comes here by compulsory order, I have the obligation under the law to protect him and give him treatment by force. Medications, physical restraints, restrictions on his freedom, whatever it is. Because if I don't do that, it might mean that he would harm himself or someone else. . . . And I'm going to break the law if there's a legal order and I don't treat [the patient] because I say, well, it's against his rights. . . .
>
> When the person gets well—and there are many patients who get well after a compulsory order—I can no longer impose on him my opinion about what he should do. The law forbids me to do that. From the moment the procedure is over, it's over; I have no more legal right to intervene. It's not prison. The period of involuntary admission is limited by the law. And by me: if I discharge the patient, my ability to intervene is gone. Because at that point, my relationship with these patients changes. . . . They can take responsibility for themselves after a certain point. They may argue with me—they may say: "I don't agree with what you say, I won't follow your medical instructions," and this is their right, which I recognize, and which the state recognizes. . . .
>
> With a patient like this, I can't say: you must do this and that, and if you don't take your medications we'll force you to. And that's not just because the law says I can't—rightly so, in my opinion. I can't say it because, therapeutically, I have to work with the patient, to suggest what's best for him to do and try to persuade him. . . . We're equals in this process of persuasion. So sometimes I'm persuaded by the patient instead. It's not: *I'm the doctor and you must do what I say*. I listen to what he says, and sometimes I change *my* mind.

In this discussion of involuntary committal, Lamberakis indicated a point in the process of a patient's treatment where the law ended and therapeutic negotiation began. He suggested that even if it happened forcibly, a person restored to well-being might enter that space of negotiation in which responsibility circulated between therapist and patient. But well-being here is not a simple equivalent to responsibility; it is a medical condition that qualifies a person to judge in the interest of his or her own health. The law recognizes this condition only on the basis of medical expertise. Yet Lamberakis suggested the possibility that a patient's "healthy" evaluation of his or her own interest could diverge from the opinion of a medical expert. That divergence of opinion could only transpire beyond the scope of law, in negotiations between people who enjoy well-being.

Social psychiatry aims to draw patients into this space of negotiation, both in and outside the clinic. As Sakellaropoulos indicates in his textbook, negotiation in that space is contingent on a therapeutic recognition of the patient's "right" to judgment: "Even when the patient is lost in the chaotic world of psychotic agitation, if he is given the occasion—which is to say, if he is considered as a being with the right to his own opinion and will—the psychotic can realize his share of responsibility, and can conduct himself accordingly."[45]

Though he insists, here, on the recognition of a patient's "right to [an] opinion and will," Sakellaropoulos does not define the patient's "share of responsibility" that should emerge from this recognition. In the psychiatric settings where I worked, therapists often used the term *cooperation* (*συνεργασία*) to express that share. But this term demands some scrutiny—for cooperation, though it enables negotiation, does not necessarily imply responsibility. As Lamberakis explained to me, *responsibility* entails collaboration between equals, whereas *cooperation* describes a coercive power relation:

> Look, in my opinion, *cooperative* isn't a great term. Because it implies obedience to the therapist, a sense of superiority and inferiority. It doesn't indicate equality. But from another point of view, that meaning can be useful: when a patient sees his therapist as an authority figure, he participates more readily in treatment. . . . An element of submission is necessary. The patient must take his medications, for example, when he's particularly violent, and he doesn't understand that he needs to take his medications. If he submits to someone, it's easier than with a patient who doesn't have this feeling of obedience and respect. But generally, I don't like this word *cooperation* very much. . . .
>
> In my opinion a good therapeutic relation only happens within equality. But this isn't always so easy. Sometimes patients have a need for dependence, they need to be supported by someone, and if we give them too much freedom they get disoriented. This isn't only a matter of culture, it's a matter of psychological capacity—the capacity to be independent. And it isn't a stable thing: today you may be independent, but tomorrow you might have a relapse, and you might be feeling more agitated, and have a greater need for support, and in this case submis-

sion might be necessary. If *incapacitated* [απαγορευτικός] means that this patient has no responsibilities, that he can't be responsible for himself at all, and also that as a mental patient he's inferior to someone who is mentally healthy: that idea drives you to treat a human being like an animal. But if you take the position that this person has difficulty taking responsibility for himself, and this difficulty is 100 percent today but tomorrow it might be 30 percent; and at this moment I can only have a relationship with him like that of a father to a child and that's 100 percent of our relationship, but tomorrow it could be only 30 percent of our relationship—if you take this position, then you're able to recognize abilities in the patient that *incapacity* would exclude, otherwise. . . .

But in our everyday usage, the word *cooperative* indicates our own unwillingness to recognize the patient's equality. We should have that as our goal, even if the patient can't be equal in some phases of his illness because he needs our guidance. That's the goal. It's not only a matter of rights; it's a matter of therapy, to make the patient responsible—not to *make* him, but to help him be responsible for himself. It's a whole process that moves in that direction. . . .

I have many patients who fully participate in their therapy. . . . But it doesn't happen with all of them. You have to understand that schizophrenia is a condition that influences the psychical functions, and especially the will, to a great degree in the long term. It impedes the ability to form thoughts, and thus the ability to make agreements, and . . . thought processes generally. So you have this in mind, with schizophrenics. They can't all take part in their therapy. But that doesn't mean that none of them can. It's a matter of . . . evaluation—not your evaluation exclusively, but your mutual evaluation with the patient.

This view on schizophrenia—named as one mental illness among others that may compromise the patient's ability to participate in therapy—demarcates a psychomedical arena of needs and capacities that precedes and verges on the domain of law. In Lamberakis's formulation, the patient's equality in the power dynamic of the therapeutic relationship is tied to his or her autonomy—not, here, reducible to a legal right to consent to treatment, but a vastly more complex and obscure amalgamation of the patient's psychomedical faculties and requirements, which the therapist must be able to distinguish from the patient's legal rights even while "respecting" them. That this kind of autonomy is not possible for certain patients is not an obstacle to therapy, in Lamberakis's view, but it does present an obstacle to their achievement of responsibility.

The power dynamic of the therapeutic relationship constitutes the terrain of professional ethics for therapists under psychiatric reform. As I argued in the previous section, when it comes to protecting or liberating patients, the practice of Greek psychiatrists—though they remain, as Castel puts it, "functionaries" of the state[46]—is not wholly regulated by state policy, nor strictly overseen by state agencies. Therapists are thus oriented toward responsibility by factors other than the penal and bureaucratic roles determined for psychiatry by the state. Within a space of practice delimited but not invaded by the law—within this unregulated and improvisational space of therapy—the task of "helping patients become responsible for themselves" describes the pragmatic work of reconciling humanitarian politics with the therapeutic process. This reconciliation demands a careful harnessing of the power involved in negotiating with patients whose well-being is fragile, unstable, and unpredictable. The legal concept of danger as a *pretext* for treatment is less a priority in these negotiations than compulsion itself as a *technique* of treatment.

In addition to medications and supportive counseling, therapists in Thrace deployed a number of normative techniques to foster in patients this capacity to participate in treatment, in the ambiguous zone of responsibility beyond mere cooperation. In the remainder of this section, I explore two such techniques by which therapists attempted to bind patients to particular modes of responsible behavior. Therapeutic contracts, by formalizing the responsibilities of patient and therapist to each other, aimed to attach legalistic determinants to the negotiations taking place within the space of therapy.[47] Group therapy, on the other hand, enlisted individual patients in a collective venture of recovering from illness, in which all participants were bound to the same project of self-scrutiny and self-improvement in their lives outside the space of therapy. The objective of these normative techniques, supplementary to medication, thus seemed to be a kind of relational subject whose sociality would be grounded in personal autonomy and responsibility. Yet the foundation of these techniques on a dynamic of equality between therapist and patient often, instead, produced intractable mutual debts and dependencies.

Not Here, Not with Us

Toward the end of a long staff meeting at the Association one evening, Rania, a new psychologist, sought advice from senior clinicians about a patient whose treatment she was trying to bring to a close. At previous meetings, she had raised the trouble she was having with Zoë, a young woman diagnosed with depression and borderline personality disorder, whom Rania had been treating for six months. *She misses her appointments, habitually. But when I remind her that therapy will be terminated unless she respects the therapeutic contract, she reappears.* This month, Zoë had finally broken the habit. She missed two appointments in a row, and then skipped a third even after Rania explained that her treatment would end if she did so. *I called her mother and told her Zoë wouldn't be permitted to continue therapy. I explained it to her. I told her Zoë could call me to discuss it, if she wanted.* And Zoë did call the Association afterward, repeatedly—but not to speak with Rania. She kept telling the secretary who answered the phone that she simply wanted to confirm that she would receive no further treatment at the Association. *I recognize that Zoë is reaching out with these phone calls,* Rania said. *And I feel like I should respond. But I don't want to schedule another appointment. Wouldn't it be confusing for Zoë if we have her come to a session in order to discuss why we won't have any more sessions? Isn't that a bit sadistic?*

But Rania's colleagues on the treatment team thought a final meeting would be a good idea. One suggested that she imagine the therapeutic contract within a transactional framework: *What you need to think about, in making a decision like this, is what you would do with a patient who was paying for treatment. With a private client, you'd have to meet one last time so that she could make her final payment, and this would create an occasion for to you terminate therapy with a mutual understanding.* Another advised her: *Whatever you decide, the key is to follow through consistently. Don't change your mind because you're getting pressure from the patient or because you feel guilty. You have to make sure Zoë understands that ending therapy is not a hostile act on your part. It's about setting limits. You can't work with a patient who won't respect limits. You can encourage her to continue therapy—just not here, not with us.*

Since the earliest moments of deinstitutionalization in Europe and North America, therapeutic contracts have been used in a wide range of psychiatric treatments to define and delimit therapeutic relationships.[48] Contracts establish the time frame, setting, and nature of the therapy agreed by both parties. In private practice, they also determine the cost of therapy—no banal matter as, in theory, payment assures the neutrality of the therapist, relieving the patient of emotional debts to the therapist for listening and thus enabling the patient to enter freely into the therapeutic space. In public services, where care is provided free of charge to the patient—as it was for those treated at the Association—the therapist's neutrality is instead underwritten by the state as the guarantor of the patient's entitlement to medical care and social services.

In some psychodynamic practices, therapeutic contracts can determine what elements of a therapist's identity (or which "alternative identities") can be expressed in the therapeutic relationship, or what extent of the therapist's countertransference will be permitted to manifest behaviorally in sessions—for example, physical contact or expressions of sympathy to comfort a distressed patient.[49] But contracts in other modalities of psychotherapy have little to do with transference dynamics. In behavior modification therapies, for example, the contract binds the patient to a code of conduct: the patient might agree not to drink alcohol, or not to attempt suicide, or to take medications as prescribed, or to work toward a set of behavioral goals agreed on with the therapist during a certain phase of treatment.[50] In these cases, the explicit therapeutic aim of the contract—often enhanced by "limit-setting" and "incentives"—is to inculcate self-control and personal responsibility in the patient, whose "good faith" efforts to meet the terms of the contract are evaluated and reinforced by the therapist and/or the therapeutic milieu.[51] Contracts can also be made between therapists and the family members or other companions of the patient, who might agree not to engage in counterproductive management strategies, such as ceding to the patient's threats or indulging self-destructive behavior.

Therapists at the Association in Thrace made contracts with most of their patients. These contracts were explicitly phrased in terms of law regarding the civil and human rights of patients—law that was both *positive*, summoning the new freedom enjoyed by patients to enter and participate in treatment voluntarily, and *regulative*, protecting patients from coercion, neglect, or abuse by therapists, just as they protected therapists from blame for therapeutic blocks and failures, such as relapse or suicide. This mutual protection was strictly moral in nature, as therapeutic contracts had no legal binding power and their content was unregulated. They were negotiated in the space of therapy—which therapists in Thrace, exceedingly well-versed in psychiatric reform policy, aimed to defend from the encroachment of regulative law so as to maintain some measure of therapeutic autonomy and discretion, even as they borrowed the transactional logic of contract law to define rights and responsibilities in a metaphorical register. Contracts put these rights and responsibilities to work in a theory of therapeutic efficacy. As one therapist at the Association told me, *It's more difficult for the patient to act out and manipulate the therapist when we've established our rights and responsibilities before therapy even begins. This weakens the patient's resistance, and he's forced to confront therapy directly.*

The function of therapeutic contracts was thus privatively to limit and positively to assign moral responsibility, itself considered a therapeutic tool. In contracts between therapists and patients at the Association, the Greek state functioned as a third party to a debt relationship combining therapeutic, financial, legal, and moral responsibilities. In contracting relationships, therapists stood responsible not only to their patients but also to the state for providing care and support on behalf of the public. Patients, too, contracted indirectly with the state to earn their right to financial and social support through their efforts to function as responsible citizens. An imaginary of the welfare state was thus summoned forth each time a contract was established or invoked in therapeutic negotiations. While this imaginary was exploited by patients to insist on the responsibility that therapists bore toward them, it at the same time played the disciplinary role of motivating their responsibility to their own health.[52]

These contracts framed the ethics of responsibility for the mentally ill as the transaction of promises and the leveraging of debts between patients and therapists. In a series of pertinent papers on the transaction of organs in India and the global market, Lawrence Cohen develops a forceful critique of neoliberal bioethics discourse that focuses on such dyadic encounters between decision-making parties.[53] Under the rubric of "ethical publicity," Cohen observes the "reduction of ethical analysis to a transactional frame," in which the moral good of individual agency and the moral harm of coercion are evaluated in transactions between dyadic partners (i.e., client-middleman and doctor-patient, though rarely donor-recipient), while the conditions under which the transactions take place are pushed outside the frame of ethical consideration—conditions such as debt, gender inequity, the commoditization of bodies and their availability to surgery, all of which substantively compose the array of choices open to the partners, rather than merely determining whether the specific choice at hand is coerced.[54]

I take this style of reducing and framing ethical questions as akin to the liberal proceduralism that has pervaded debates about the rights of psychiatric patients since the 1960s. From a procedural point of view, the decision by patients to take neuroleptic medication, for example, can be ethically valorized so long as that decision is undertaken voluntarily,[55] even if it amounts substantively to patients' submission to treatment that may expose them to severe side effects, while drastically altering their sense of self and thereby their future basis for decision making.[56] For Cohen, the perpetual deferral of ascertaining whether the conditions of decision are indeed free ("if second-order phenomena can be controlled for, then an ethics is possible") is partly what permits this kind of ethical analysis to "travel light" in global debates over the ethics of organ sale and other clinical transactions.[57]

Moving toward a denser analysis of ethics than this, a more cumbersome analysis that would stick to the multilayered grounds on which patients engage in transaction, Cohen suggests that we should "keep listening" beyond their potentially "coerced or alienated speech" — beyond, that is, the opposition between coercion and agency that animates transactional ethical reasoning and eclipses any other framing of ethics — to discern the "secondary phenomena" out of which transactions are actually made.[58] For psychiatric patients in Thrace, rights-based evaluations of their health and treatment occluded the pain, poverty, estrangement, fragmentation, and desires that described (if they did not constitute) their illnesses. So I aim to "keep listening" here, beyond the moment of transaction when a patient and a therapist entered a contract. As I suggested earlier, the relationships created by therapeutic contracts were not dyadic; therapists and patients were related through the mediation of the state, which underwrote the efficacy of law in its real and imaginary functions. As Cohen points out, the bioethics of transaction presume the existence and capacity of a liberal state to regulate transactions by, in theory, securing transparent informed consent and conditions of decision making that are free from coercion.[59] The failure of the state to play this role is one of the "secondary phenomena" foreclosed from consideration within the transactional frame of bioethics.

The liberal state — a state that oversees and safeguards the ethical integrity of clinical transactions — takes law as its effective power. Therapeutic contracts are legal in form, but unregulated by state or international law, and unenforceable by any power outside the space of therapy. In this, they are unlike the civil and human rights of patients, which are theoretically enforceable in state and international courts (such as the European Court of Human Rights) and which are, themselves, tools for regulating state policy (as in the European Union's auditing Greek psychiatric reform). Patients bear rights in regard to treatment, but not in regard to therapeutic contracts. Insofar as they instrumentalize law, then, these contracts are not reducible to the treatment they describe; they are conceived as devices that make treatment more effective. In design, they are metaphorically legal, but really efficacious.[60] They bind patients to norms of behavior that would transform them from dysfunctional marginal figures into responsible members of the communities to which they have been liberated from institutional care. But what happens if the law fails to make treatment work—if, instead of reducing patients' resistance to treatment, contracts instead give them leverage to remain ill?

Indeed, in practice, as I saw it in Thrace, therapeutic contracts seemed to have little binding power even within the space of therapy. The dilemmas bred by contractual breaches provided frequent occasions for therapists to work out the nature of their responsibilities toward patients. That these occasions took the form of tedious, repetitive, inconclusive debates that actually amplified and congealed their responsibilities toward patients, rather than resolving them, did not mitigate the high stakes of the debates, which implicated the health and survival of patients, as well as therapists' capacity to help. When therapeutic contracts did not produce treatment outcomes that would redeem and thus dissolve them, they produced dependencies that were nearly impossible to dismantle.[61]

One particular patient at the Association had a knack for playing on the weakness of his therapists as contracting parties. Now twenty-eight years old, Aris had been treated at the Association's child psychiatry institute in Alexandroupolis since the age of twelve. When he reached eighteen, he was transferred to the Association's community mental health center. *He's been using us up since the beginning, one by one,* said the head of his treatment team. Aris was diagnosed with antisocial personality disorder, compounded by hysterical retardation. In staff meetings, he was often described as a "problem patient." He was violent and manipulative. He lied. He did not take his medications properly and was suspected of selling them. He would fail to attend therapy appointments and then turn up at unscheduled times, demanding to be seen. He would plead for money or insist on using the telephone in the front office to call his estranged wife in Bulgaria. If his requests were not granted, he would scream and curse and throw things. He often chose Saturday mornings to make these visits because he knew that the new secretary, whom he could intimidate, would be alone in the office at those times.

For this intolerable behavior, and for his failure to cooperate in therapy, Aris had been dropped as a regular Association patient the year before. Because he continued to live in one of the Association's sheltered residences, however, the staff continued to bear a responsibility for him that could not be divided into discrete financial and therapeutic components. Since his exclusion, Aris had been supposed to check in periodically with Stella and Andreas, his former psychologist and psychiatrist, to coordinate his medications and receive supportive counseling. But within six months, the two therapists had begun devising ways to end this relationship. Andreas had tried once already to terminate therapy, but the following day Aris had shown up at the Association, crying and bleeding from cuts he had made on his arms. Andreas dismissed this behavior as "more drama," and another therapist who was there at the time agreed: *I saw him through my office window, just a minute beforehand. He was acting normally, chatting with some friends on the street.*

Yet the Association could not cut off relations with Aris entirely, because it accepted grants from the state to support him, and it could not evict him from the sheltered residence without undertaking elaborate legal proceedings to transfer responsibility for his case to another state agency. The plan at this point, instead, was to "start over" with a new contract. As Andreas set it forth, the new contract would deploy the Association's leverage on his apartment: *If Aris misses a therapy appointment, we'll cut off his electricity. And the next time, his water, then his rent. I know it sounds terrible, but it's the only way to handle this kind of patient.*

By summertime, the relationship had deteriorated further, and Aris sharpened his tactics. He began threatening secretaries and accountants at the Association over a dispute regarding repairs to his apartment. His therapists admitted that the Association bore responsibility for making the repairs, which they had pledged but failed to do for months. But they insisted that their failure did not excuse Aris's alarming behavior. At a staff meeting, accusations of hypocrisy landed on every therapist who had ever had contact with the patient. Several took his part, arguing that the Association, by sending him mixed messages and neglecting to set consistent limits, had trained him to expect that he could behave badly with impunity. A nurse recalled how the late hero of the Association, a beloved senior psychiatrist who had recently died, used to give patients cash handouts when they ran into trouble. (Later, one of the staff explained to me that this practice was frowned upon—though not prevented in this case, due to the status of the psychiatrist—because, although it appeared philanthropic, it amounted to "buying loyalty" from patients without cultivating their cooperation.) *Since his death, no other therapist has been good enough for Aris*, the nurse said. *That's a real problem. But let's not forget that he's ill. Can we really expect him to hold up his end of the contract?* The social worker replied, *Whether he can respect the contract or not, he understands how it works. He knows he can shame us if we don't hold up our end.*

Each time Aris's case came up in a meeting, Andreas would reiterate the decision made by Dr. Politis, the head of the Association, to cut all ties with this patient. Politis was invoked as the final authority, the only one who could make the ultimate decision. Andreas ventriloquized his commentary on the case: *What more can we do for this patient? We've tried everything and failed. We're human beings. There comes a point when we have to ask ourselves: when can we call it enough?* But the decision itself was only the symbolic register of terminating therapy. Enforcing the decision was the practical task that fell to the junior staff. Responsibility for enforcement circulated relentlessly among them. Some feared Aris's violence; others took courage from it. One psychiatrist asked pointedly of her colleagues: *Are we therapists or not? It's part of our work to terminate therapy when necessary, and we have to be willing to take risks when dealing with volatile patients.* A secretary, who worked in the front office and thus on the frontline of this battle, argued that the "therapists upstairs" had no business passing those risks on to them.

The debate over Aris recurred at staff meetings throughout the summer. Participants occasionally reminded each other, and themselves, that the debate was recurring. But the last chance for Aris to make good on his contract continued to recede into the future.

Toward the end of August, Aris phoned the Association during a staff meeting just as his case was raised for discussion. The new secretary, who took the call in the meeting room, indicated to the staff that he was threatening her: if someone did not come to inspect his apartment the very next day and see to the repairs as promised, he would "make trouble" at the Association. The call set off another bitter argument. Stella protested the criticism launched at her by her colleagues: *Since Aris has missed all of his appointments, we haven't had any chance to tell him about the agreement we came up with at the last staff meeting!* She ultimately agreed to visit Aris at his apartment the following day, both to arrange the repairs and to deliver the final contract—not a verbal agreement this time, but a written document setting out the terms of living in the Association residence. Angered, Stella put the rest of the staff on warning: *The next time we discuss Aris at a staff meeting, I'll bring the district attorney with me, to explain our obligations.* For the first time since the inception of his treatment, those obligations were dislodged from the space of therapy and relocated in the domain of law.

In Aris's case, a breached therapeutic contract announced, but did not achieve, the end of the debt relationship between patient and therapist. It marked the limit of tolerance for the burden placed on therapists by an uncooperative patient, but it did not relieve them of that burden. Oscillating between ethical powers of binding between therapists and patient, on one hand, and legal powers of binding between the Association and the state that funded and sanctioned its services, on the other, the contract in this sense was an apparatus of indecision. An apparatus, insofar as it deployed clinical instruments for evaluation and treatment with a cause-and-effect mechanics of responsibility. Indecision, insofar as it lacked any means to authorize expectations of responsibility: the contract contained no philosophy of the subject, no map of the psyche, no psychomedical expertise that would determine the patient's capacity to uphold his end. It was designed to inculcate that capacity in the patient. What Aris learned from it, instead, was how to leverage his responsibilities to recall therapists to their own.

The legalistic design of therapeutic contracts perhaps implies too strong a distinction between the metaphorical and material efficacy of law. As the legislation of Greek psychiatric reform shows, "real" law, too, works metaphorically, asserting ends as if it could produce them, while actually producing effects that do not correspond to those ends. This was precisely the kind of in/efficacy at work in the case of Aris, whose therapeutic contract set forth expectations of change that it did not bring about. In failing, his contract produced a different effect altogether: namely, the contractual relationship itself—between patient, therapists, and the state—in which entitlements to treatment were leveraged against the mounting debts of care.

Taking Charge

During her admission to the hospital clinic in August, just before she attempted suicide, Fatmé attended group therapy several times, silently. When Niki, the psychologist, finally called on her to talk, she told the other patients about a violent fight with her husband that had driven her to seek refuge here. She began to cry. Niki intervened: *You've had to face really difficult circumstances. You've had problems, worse than many of us. But fate makes us all equal, Fatmé. I believe we're all responsible for how we handle what we're given. You've been sick for twenty years. Haven't you learned from your experiences? Haven't you gotten better at handling your illness and putting yourself back together?*

Fatmé bowed her head and stayed quiet. Niki, who knew her history, listed the achievements by which Fatmé had "risen above" her illness: her two jobs, her healthy children, her cooperation in treatment. But Fatmé resisted this reformulation of her story. *All these things: you say they're achievements, but they're also burdens. I've never been free.* At that moment, a notoriously volatile young patient, diagnosed with schizophrenia and mental retardation, entered the room abruptly, laughing. He demanded a coffee from Niki and smoked two cigarettes simultaneously while the startled group watched and waited. Finally, he turned to Fatmé and shouted an insult about her husband. She stood without a word and left. Niki swiftly called the group to a close, halfway through the scheduled session.

Other patients rose better to the occasion. One session in December was dedicated, in the spirit of the holidays, to the topic of "what we do to have fun." After a lively start, the discussion took a grim turn as, one after another, patients confessed that they really did not have fun anymore. They felt empty. They took drugs or got into fights to spark some excitement, but it was never enough. One patient said the only way truly to have fun was to be free from all social constraints, and that was "impossible for a mental patient." Niki picked her fingernails and stared at the floor. But Lakis, a young villager diagnosed with schizophrenia, corralled the discussion with comic relief. In a dramatic voice, he announced to the group: *Having fun is a struggle, you have to fight for it! What I do is, I make myself go out even when I don't feel like it. Or, other times, when I stay home, I'll get up in front of the mirror and sing and dance, like I'm in a concert.* He stood up, threw his head back and crooned a few bars from a pop song, aiming intense expressions of joy and grief at his air microphone. Other patients began to laugh. A few sang with him.

Lakis sat back down, grinning. *I know I'm ridiculous. But that's the whole point.* An older patient suggested that Lakis must be healthier than he was himself, since he could not even summon the strength to struggle. But Niki had registered the logic of the intervention: *When we're ill, we sometimes take ourselves too seriously, and this keeps us from having any enjoyment in life. Does anyone besides Lakis see the lighter side?* A few patients joined in, suggesting activities like cooking, listening to music, watching the soaps on TV. Others said they were looking forward to taking leave from the clinic to go home for the holidays.

❋ ❋ ❋

In his two-volume textbook on social psychiatry, Sakellaropoulos devotes one page to the philosophy of group therapy, which he notes has not been a priority for psychiatric reform in Greece. Group therapy, on his account, aims at enlisting unconscious conflicts in the formation of a group dynamic. The basic "principles" are the same in group as in individual therapy, but in a group, "the therapist tries to comprehend and mobilize the personal conflicts of each member, so that they can be expressed by way of the group dynamic."[62] In an orthodox analytic group, a reserved and neutral leader guides the "regression" of group members by promoting the free expression of their emotions and fantasies, and focuses interpretation on the group dynamic through the internal relations of transference among group members. According to the text, other kinds of group therapy follow the same procedure, but with greater "flexibility": it is always a matter of attending to the conflicts of group members, but this can involve focusing the group's attention on one patient's conflicts or exploring the shared conflicts of the entire group.

This basic model served Dr. Liakos, a codirector of the hospital clinic, in finally accomplishing his long-standing plan to establish a new group therapy program there. Leadership of the new group was assigned to Manolis and Kalliope, the two most experienced residents, who would transfer it to a new pair of therapists after six months. The new group was for psychotic patients only. It would have a stable and exclusive membership; no new patients or guests would be admitted. They would meet twice weekly at a precise time; tardiness on the part of patients or therapists would not be tolerated, as it would disrupt the evolution of group transference over the course of each session. (This requirement, much discussed in the absence of Dr. Liakos, was novel and rather problematic for a staff accustomed to keeping appointments more loosely.) Periodically, the therapists would meet with Dr. Liakos to discuss what had transpired, as in an orthodox psychoanalytic supervision.

Manolis, for one, appeared to resent the self-reflective tasks that accompanied his leadership of the new group: *Liakos hasn't trained us in analytic theory, and I just don't see the need to "explore my own experience" of the group.* He joked about Liakos's notoriously feeble grasp of patients' cases: *The reason he never remembers what his patients say is that he's paying so much attention to how he feels about it!* Yet he and Kalliope dutifully kept notes of each session and read them aloud, interrupted by Liakos's interpretive commentary, during the seminars he occasionally gave for the staff. During its first few weeks, the new group acquired among the staff the repute of a pretentious experiment with questionable therapeutic value.

But that was the new group. The old group, active at the hospital clinic for more than a decade, was run—like other such groups I had observed at state psychiatric hospitals in Thessaloniki and Chania—independently of psychoanalytic principles. I attended about twenty-five sessions of this group at the Alexandroupolis hospital clinic over the course of a year. It met for an hour twice weekly under the leadership of Niki, the clinic's psychologist, in addition to rotating nurses and psychiatric residents. Patients of any age and diagnosis were welcome. The composition of the group changed each session, as patients were admitted and discharged, well or indisposed, bored or occupied with other things. It met in the morning, so coffee and juice were provided to the patients—some of whom attended for just that reason, as they readily admitted to the group. Attendance was voluntary, in theory, but the nurses encouraged turnout by vigorously collecting patients from their bedrooms at the appointed time. It was not clear that all the patients understood why they were attending the group; some evidently believed they were obligated, in the same way they were obligated to meet with doctors and take medications. They were not supposed to arrive late or to leave the group once seated, lest they disturb the "comfortable and respectful atmosphere," but these rules were not often enforced.

According to Niki, the "philosophy" of the group, which she would announce at the start of each session, was that the patients were "in charge." It was for them to propose and agree on a topic, and all members were encouraged to contribute to the discussion. The staff was supposed not to answer their questions directly, nor judge their comments right or wrong, but rather to help patients engage one another in "constructive communication." Often the patients in attendance expressed distress or confusion at having to choose a topic, and asked the staff to tell them what to discuss. At these moments, the staff would wait for an outgoing patient to take charge, or cobble a topic together from drifting commentary, finding a theme in patients' words after the fact. "Good themes"—a closed set, repeatedly mined—included conditions of life in the clinic, relations between patients, relationships with doctors and family, medications and health problems, the stigma of mental illness, hopes and fears on returning home from the clinic, work, and holidays. The discussion of politics and religion was not permitted; Niki felt these were divisive topics that could disturb the group dynamic. Personal stories were also discouraged. If patients strayed too far into the details of their own cases, Niki steered them back toward the general theme, encouraging them to express an opinion rather than a story: *We're not here to discuss personal issues; we're addressing a topic we can all relate to.* She also set the parameters for patients' comportment in the group. It was inappropriate, for example, to "say everything" to the group, to monopolize the conversation, or to treat others rudely or aggressively. Niki continually had to lay down the law with recalcitrant and disruptive patients who did not understand, or did not heed, these parameters. From a rhetoric of general mutual interest, she summoned a screen of egalitarian support around her exclusive position of authority over the group.

But patients on occasion saw through the screen. One morning, for example, a spirited elderly woman joined the group well into the session. Interrupting another participant, she started immediately in on the troubles she was having with the nurses, which had delayed her that morning. Niki shushed her a few times, quietly asking her to listen to the others. But the patient would not accept a private reprimand: *Aren't we supposed to talk about our problems? Isn't that what we're here for?* The others looked to Niki for a response. She explained: *You know what group is like— we all decide together what topic to discuss, and we try to stick to that topic. We can't all talk at once, we have to wait our turn.* The patient smiled and sat back in her chair. *Oh, so it's like teacher and students, eh?*

And so it was. Group therapy in the hospital clinic functioned less as a space of open expression and listening than as a site for the inculcation of the value of personal responsibility. Niki told me that this kind of group was more "supportive" than "therapeutic," and she did not often discuss what happened in the group with the clinicians treating the patients who attended. But she identified three features of the group sessions that facilitated their recovery. First, group therapy was "cathartic": it provided patients an opportunity to express thoughts, feelings, and difficulties that they could not address with their doctors. Second, it was "educational": patients learned "coping strategies" and "lessons of hope" from one other. Finally, it was "occupational": it fostered social activity that kept patients "integrated" and "functional" despite the "artificial" conditions of life in the clinic. The therapeutic strategy practiced by Niki and her colleagues was to transform the cathartic dimension of the group experience into educational moments: dissatisfaction, fear, pain, and confusion were shaped into motives for taking an active role in one's own recovery.[63] If patients were not getting along with their roommates at the clinic, they would be asked to describe their roommates' positive qualities. If patients disputed the treatment they were receiving, they were encouraged to trust their doctors and be sure to "say everything" in therapy, even those things that scared or shamed them. If patients ran into conflict with their family members, they were advised to think about why the conflict persisted and what they could do to resolve it. If patients protested the filthy conditions of the lounge, they were instructed to clean up after themselves before complaining.

In her discussion of group therapy in a French community mental heath center, Livia Velpry notes that the normative criteria that frame the views patients express, either as valid opinions or as symptoms of illness, are disavowed as norms or principles of group sessions. These criteria operate, instead, as "implicit expectations" fostered through the "ritualized" repetition of questions that elicit conformist statements from patients about their practices, hopes, and values.[64] In the group sessions I attended at the hospital clinic in Alexandroupolis—which, being supportive rather than therapeutic, were not integrated into the treatment of individual patients and did not serve as opportunities for psychological evaluation—the validity of patients' views had more to do with their moral than their mental states. The conformism elicited from patients in this group was to an ethics of personal responsibility.

"How we get well" was the topic of a discussion already underway when I joined a group therapy session at the clinic one morning in May. It was the day after Chrisanthi, a chronic patient who lived in one of the Association's sheltered residences downtown, had attempted suicide by overdosing on heroin. News had spread around the clinic that she was being kept alive on a respirator in the intensive care unit. Frosso, a middle-aged villager diagnosed with severe depression, and a close friend of Chrisanthi, followed the discussion with her eyes but refrained from speaking as, one after another, patients offered bits of potted wisdom for the occasion: *Medications are not enough. You have to want to get well.* The resident in charge of the group observed Frosso's poorly veiled turmoil and called on her to contribute to the conversation.

Frosso sat back in a defensive posture and addressed the group. *I have to admit that I don't have any hope of getting well. I can't say that I want to. And I don't try. I hate to say it, but I feel like Chrisanthi proved me right. I always considered her a strong and capable person, someone I could look to for strength and guidance. Someone who took charge of her life. And look what happened to her.*

At this, another patient intervened. Earlier, this man had introduced himself to the group as an alcoholic and told them that he had voluntarily admitted himself to the clinic for detox and rehabilitation. (One of the nurses told me later that this patient liked to think of himself as a "big man" but, despite his appearance of leadership, he was really an egotist and a troublemaker.) He turned to Frosso, offering himself as an example: *I really do hope to get well, for my sake and for my family. I'm trying. But it depends on my confidence that I really can get well. I noticed that you didn't come to the ice cream party last night in the lounge. I understand why: it's the sort of event you would normally go to with Chrisanthi. You were upset by her accident, and you felt vulnerable and afraid without her. But when you skipped the party, you lost an opportunity to gain strength and confidence from the rest of us. You would have felt better with company, and you would have had fun. You need to take charge of yourself. It's up to you to create your own path away from illness.*

Frosso looked away: *Maybe you're right. But I don't have the will to do it.* The resident diverted attention away from Frosso, asking other patients whether they wanted to get well. Several quickly assented. But Tasos, a young man admitted just a few days earlier during an apparent psychotic break, approached the question askance: *I came here because I think I'm Jesus.* He looked around as some in the group started laughing. *If I get well, if I find my own identity, everyone in the world who depends on Jesus will suffer. I don't want to do that to them.* He started laughing with the others. The resident, attempting to respect the logic of his apparent delusion rather than the group's laughter, asked: *Well, if you're Jesus, shouldn't you want to sacrifice yourself for the others?* Tasos only laughed more. The resident pointed out, *You keep saying that you "think" or "believe" you're Jesus. You don't speak as Jesus, which you would do if you completely lacked insight into your illness.* Tasos admitted that he was probably confused.

At that moment, a frail, elderly patient sitting beside him laughed out loud. Tasos turned to him, teasing: *You believe I'm Jesus, right? Isn't that what you told me yesterday?* The old man, smiling, denied Tasos's claim: *I don't know what you're talking about!* He won hearty congratulations from the resident. Affecting schoolmarmish seriousness, she warned Tasos not to "turn" the old man "the other way": *He's such a good patient! When he's well he goes about his work on the farm and watches his animals; and when he's not well, he realizes he needs help and he comes to us. Such a patient man! When he came to the clinic, he spent the first night in a different ward because we had no bed for him. And yesterday he waited all afternoon for his lab tests. He never once complained. Tasos, you could learn a lot from him about how to cooperate in your treatment.* On behalf of the group, the resident translated Tasos's ironic stance toward his illness into a refusal of his responsibility to get well. She left untranslated the threat such irony posed to the coercive force of group morale.

✳   ✳   ✳

Whether or not patients in Thrace could achieve the ethical capacity for responsibility that psychiatric reform introduced as a condition of their freedom, they often either did not achieve it or did not gain recognition for achieving it. The invitation to responsibility issued to them in this context inaugurated not an ethics, but a moralism—a process not of negotiation, but of divested autonomy and unilateral persuasion. The ideal framework for treatment that Lamberakis proposed, contingent on equality in the therapeutic relationship, was not often reached in practice. "Cooperation" stood, instead, as the norm.

Patients in Thrace did not always respond to the moralism of cooperation by complying with its therapeutic program. The scenes I have presented in this section attest to the quite effective strategies of countermoralism practiced by some patients. One strategy was to expose failures on the part of therapists to live up to their responsibilities to patients: failures to sustain a therapeutic tie with patients, to secure them financial and social support, to respect their autonomous judgment. Patients were sometimes able to leverage these failures to negotiate the terms of their treatment and to pursue other goals.

Another strategy of countermoralism was to contest the coercive valorization of personal autonomy and responsibility by means of which patients were asked to "cooperate." As some occasionally suggested (*so it's like teacher and students, eh?*), contrary to mobilizing their autonomy and responsibility on a foundation of equality between patients and therapists, cooperation instead served to reinforce patients' dependence on therapists' expertise and approval.[65]

Noncooperation produced asymmetrical effects on either side of the therapeutic relationship, corresponding to the asymmetry of its power dynamic. For therapists, broken contracts and derailed group sessions yielded a banal condition of frustration, occasionally enlivened by accusations and deflections of guilt in the inconclusive discussions that recurred at staff meetings. For patients, on the other hand, breakdowns in these techniques—at times passively endured and at times actively produced as disruptions of the normative regime—exposed the unavailability to them of effective ways to improve their health and circumstances. The process of persuasion sustained patients' dependence on therapeutic relationships, yet it often failed to satisfy that dependence with well-being.

THE OTHER ASYLUM

The monastery was rooted there, on the horizon of his illness, long before I met Kleandis. Thalia introduced us about ten days into his admission that winter, predicting that, unlike some other patients, Kleandis would be thrilled to speak with me. I did not take the point until much later, after a series of protracted and grueling sessions, when his uncontrolled verbosity had begun to erode my understanding. Our first conversation started in the early afternoon as most of the staff were leaving for the day; it took several hours to unfold, as Kleandis drew himself out of his nervous and exaggerated courtesy and fixed on our common status as subordinated students. He was animated as he told me about his academic studies, but his tone and gaze fell when he spoke of his illness— of the chronic outbreaks and therapeutic failures that had furnished the structure of his life over the past five years, of the horrors contained in his unofficial medical history. *The monastery is my last hope for recovery,* he told me. *It's the only way I can see to break out of this vicious cycle.*

Perhaps thinking that I would find this idea strange, in the symptomatic sense, Thalia had explained to me that seeking sanctuary in monasteries was once a common practice in the "traditional culture" of rural Greece. But Kleandis spoke to me of a more intellectual interest in churchly life, which had grown from his university studies of Byzantine history and the ancient liturgical languages of Greek and Latin.

It was, in any case, to no ordinary monastery—of which there were plenty in rural Thrace—but to Mount Athos, the great holy mountain of Greece, that Kleandis aspired. At the furthest tip of the last peninsula of Halkidiki, an Aegean beach resort area northeast of Thessaloniki, Mount Athos stood about four hundred kilometers from his own village. The mountaintop holds a gated complex of twenty Byzantine-era monasteries, which Kleandis described to me as an "asylum": a refuge of order and tranquility where he would ritually nurse himself back to health. The Athonites were known for their rigorous observance of Byzantine practices of chanting and meditation. As it was, Kleandis gravitated toward ritual, but he told me there was more to the monastic life than this that attracted him: he longed as well for the inner peace that he thought could be achieved through ascetic purification.[66]

Dr. Lamberakis, who had treated Kleandis in the past, said Kleandis had admitted to him that he washed compulsively in order to "cleanse himself of sin." *These were his own words,* Lamberakis announced at a staff meeting. *The symbolism couldn't be clearer.* Kleandis's confession indicated that his obsessive thoughts bore some sexual content, but Thalia reported that he would not "open up" on the subject. He declined to discuss it with me as well. It was perhaps for this reason that the experience of obsession he expressed to me seemed to lack any subjective quality. He described abstractly the scenes that would force their way before his mind's eye: faces he knew, fragments of memories. *I don't even like watching TV at home, because the images show up later, inside my mind. No, they don't have any special meaning. They come to me randomly [τυχαίως]. They fill my head until it feels like I'm going to burst.*

Though he did not connect it explicitly to his desire for purification, Kleandis remarked on the mandated absence of women from the grounds of the monastic complex at Mount Athos. *Living in an all-male environment wouldn't be much of a change for me, you know. I'm a virgin. I've never had a girlfriend. I've been ill since I was fifteen, and I never became a competent person. That's my illness, in the big picture. That's what keeps me from recovering. I know living at home is a regression to childhood. Some day I'll have to turn this around and grow up, I'll have to get married and have children. But I have no chance of finding a wife as long as I'm living like this.*

On one level, the obstacles Kleandis faced were medical: his hypothyroidism left him overweight and sluggish; his psychiatric medications diminished his "natural" [φυσιολογικό, i.e., sexual] functioning; and he was radically preoccupied by thoughts and behaviors to which he could never expect a woman to adapt. On another level, though, the obstacle was, as he put it, "existential." *I'm alienated from society, and especially from*

the romantic part of life. I come from a traditional village. Women are totally dependent on men where I come from. Men provide their home, their safety, their family.
People get married very young, when both spouses are still pure. And marriage lasts a
lifetime. When he had moved to Thessaloniki to attend university, he said,
he had learned that modern Greek women were more independent; they
earned their own money, made their own decisions, and liked to "try out"
a range of men before settling on a partner later in life. I have nothing to
offer women like that. But living in the city changed me. I don't want a traditional
marriage anymore, like what my parents have.

Kleandis expected that moving to a monastery would allow him to
postpone his confrontation with these "social" problems to the moment
his illness was resolved, which he felt now could only happen outside
the clinic. The monastery thus served him as an alternative asylum to the
psychiatric hospital — not only a refuge, but also a site of isolation and
marginality.[67] The symmetry of these alternatives was plain and clear to
him. After all, he knew the other asylum very well;[68] he had traveled its
institutional conduit, fleeing the stigma that followed him through his
village all the way across the threshold of the state hospital in Thessaloniki. Perhaps this experience colored his imagination of the monastery,
conferring a resemblance between the self-punitive life of ascetic sacrifice and the ferocity of "heavy" medications and electroshock. This resemblance, for him, was elaborated over time: it was only because those
radical psychiatric treatments had failed — had in fact damaged his organism beyond redress — that he turned toward another powerful source
of aid and succor. When psychiatry relinquished it, responsibility for his
recovery fell into his own hands, and he raised them in prayer.

A Clear Dimension of Self-Punishment

In the clinic, the priority in Kleandis's treatment was to mobilize his self-
control against the danger he posed to himself and others in moments
of extremity. Though the legislative discourse on involuntary committal
gives a different impression, the problem of danger among the mentally
ill in Greece is plainly not restricted to psychotics. As Dr. Politis pointed
out to his staff, dangerous mental illness implicates even the most reformable of psychiatric subjects — patients like Kleandis, who are taken
to be logical and reasonable, in touch with reality, available and ame-
nable to psychotherapy. And yet, like psychotics, Kleandis was subject to
motives beyond his control. His pathology was severe enough to debar

his personal responsibility for his behavior and to warrant his delivery instead to the law.

In his textbook, Sakellaropoulos describes "obsessive/compulsive disorder" (ψυχαναναγαστική/καταναναγαστική διαταραχή) as "the most organized and most severe form of neurotic disorder."[69] The DSM-IV classifies OCD as a clinical (Axis I) anxiety disorder.[70] According to the text, the severity of the disorder is indicated by the "marked distress" of the patient, and by his or her social and functional impairment, due to the time-consuming nature both of the behaviors and of the patient's efforts not to "yield" to them. Obsessions are defined here as "persistent ideas, thoughts, impulses, or images" that patients experience as "intrusive and inappropriate," often because they conflict with the self-image and moral code of the sufferer. According to the DSM, obsessions have an "alien" quality—they do not "belong" to the patient. But unlike psychotic delusions, these thoughts are typically felt to originate from within the person's mind, rather than from outside. "Compulsions" represent the person's attempts to "neutralize" these obsessive thoughts with "repetitive behaviors . . . or mental acts" such as washing, checking, counting, or chanting, whose goal is not pleasure or gratification, but rather a reduction of "anxiety or distress" caused by the obsessions. The DSM emphasizes the excessive and irrational nature of these behaviors, insisting that "by definition, [they] are not connected in a realistic way with what they are designed to neutralize or prevent." Indeed, to be diagnosed with OCD, the patient must recognize the "excessive or unreasonable" nature of his or her obsessions and compulsions; unlike psychotic delusions, they are subject to "insight" and "reality testing."

This clinical picture is of a patient who cannot identify with his or her random and alien obsessions. Yet despite this disavowal, compulsions represent a need to take responsibility for these obsessive thoughts, as if in the mode of penance. Sakellaropoulos puts it this way: "All the gestures and practices of the obsessive obtain the meaning of exorcizing harmful thoughts . . . and have a clear dimension of self-punishment."[71] The DSM, too, makes reference to "a pathological sense of responsibility" that typifies OCD.[72]

This detail is offered in the DSM as a descriptive symptom rather than an etiology of the disorder, but its disavowed roots are planted firmly in psychoanalysis. In the case of Kleandis, the biopsychiatric view of OCD as a disease of "unknown cause" repeatedly confronted the psychoanalytic theory of desire as cause, and symptoms as metaphors of desire.

The symptoms he presented to his many therapists over the years had accrued as many interpretations. Prominent among them was a metaphorical reading of his orientation to purity and sin: *the symbolism couldn't be clearer.* In this light, his dependency and rage toward his parents appeared as a drama of Oedipal ambivalence in a grown man who abstained from sex with appropriate partners while pursuing physical intimacy with his mother; a man who despaired of inheriting the farm and the place in the village community held by his weak, elderly father. As another of his therapists said, for this patient there were "questions of incest," in regard to which his obsessions and compulsions appeared as signs of a traumatic calamity unfolding in the intimate space of his family home. The disorder from which Kleandis suffered could thus be understood as the self-punishment of a moralist in his struggle for personal responsibility.[73]

As a clinical disorder with irreducibly symbolic symptoms, OCD attests to the persistent relevance of psychoanalytic interpretation in Greek psychiatry after reform. Yet the case of Kleandis is not just a psychoanalytic story of a patient's guilty struggle to claim responsibility for his health by working his way out of a moral conflict between normative demands and libidinal cathexes. Those dynamics can certainly be discerned in his story; but other dynamics are at work there as well that elude the Freudian terms of psychosexual drama. The disastrous failure of pharmaceutical and psychotherapeutic treatment gave Kleandis's guilty struggle for responsibility a shape around his helplessness to "try harder on his own behalf." His illness thus shared with his treatment the structure of submission to compulsion. More than an internal battle waged by all subjects on the path to maturity, his guilt refracted a distinctively liberal mandate to reform that made an ethical disability out of his clinical pathology.[74]

As a "good subject for psychotherapy," and as a patient who developed and endured his illness as he repeatedly entered and exited clinical supervision, Kleandis had learned to take an avidly interpretive stance toward his disorder. His prolix discourse—itself, in its excess, a symptom— contained elements of the cognitive-behavioral, psychoanalytic, and biopsychiatric treatment he had undertaken over the years. His therapeutic lexicon instrumentalized his proclivity for self-reflection as it substantiated the urgency of his participation in treatment. Yet this fragmentary language, the durable debris of interpretation, did not effect a closure to his cycle of suffering and treatment. His deterioration, as it intensified his dependency on his parents, also tied him to an order of meaning outside the clinic—the order of "traditional" Greek culture, targeted for reform along with psychiatric practice and policy in Thrace: the culture of rural village life, of stigma, gender hierarchy, and the conservative institution of the family. This was the social world of Kleandis's parents, perduring at the edges of the new liberal order in Greece, where treatment appeared as the only path to sanctuary. Despite his estrangement, this was his world, too.

❋ ❋ ❋

Even though he had been interned, under restraint, at a state psychiatric hospital; even though he had taken heavy medications for years; even though he was tormented by his own "random" ideas and behaviors—despite all this, Kleandis told me that he wasn't "crazy" (τρελός). He had not known, in the early years of his illness, whether he might be. He had associated that word with the stigma he tried to evade by seeking treatment in Thessaloniki, so far from home. But when he began therapy in Alexandroupolis, his psychiatrist assured him that OCD was not "madness" (τρέλλα), but rather a "neurotic illness" (νευρωτική νόσος). And since then, he had learned that in fact he was not like the other patients in the clinic, with whom he shared his space, his meals, and often his medications. *Most of them are psychotics. Their illness is a part of them, and they'll never be cured. All the doctors can do for them is help them manage their lives with medication. I think one of the reasons I try to avoid admission here is that I hate to see these people suffer, without being able to connect with them on a human level.*

What then, I asked Kleandis, did *crazy* mean to him, at this point? He said, *Honestly, I can't answer that question—I really don't know what it means. It's more than I can understand.*

His doctor's insistent resolve on his distance from madness corresponds to an institutional novelty yielded by psychiatric reform in Greece. Patients like Kleandis, who carry neurotic diagnoses and thus the hope of therapeutic redress, do not qualify for the limited spaces in halfway houses, sheltered residences, and group homes created since the 1980s. The state policy of deinstitutionalization reserves most of these spaces for psychotic patients discharged from long-term residence in state hospitals. It relies on the families of neurotic outpatients to take responsibility for their accommodation and day-to-day care, on the presumption that they can manage these milder forms of mental illness.[75] The clinical division between psychosis and neurosis in this way folds into the logic of scarce state resources, refusing the option of madness to an increasing number of patients like Kleandis. The institutional fate from which they are spared by this refusal takes with it, for some, a vital refuge.

The last time I saw Kleandis, shortly before my departure from Alexandroupolis, he was on his way into the hospital clinic; I was on my way out. On our previous meeting, he had struggled for hours to express his aspiration to find a research position in the United States—an opportunity for both legitimacy and escape. This entirely implausible plan, contingent on help that I could not give, marked a dead end in our conversation, which for the first time had concluded without resolution or future.

I had not expected to see him at the clinic again. But he told me now that he had finally given up on the monastery. The monks had never responded to his application, and his interest in Mount Athos had waned along with his belief that that other asylum was a real alternative to the clinic. He still yearned to relinquish responsibility to an authority that could elaborate and care for his symptoms, a structure that would determine his moral character along with his cure. But it mattered less to him now whether "the good" to which he submitted was sacred or clinical. In despair, he had shaven off his supplicant's beard, and at the behest of his mother, he turned once again to therapy.

For Kleandis, responsibility took an unanswerable turn away from the decision of the subject. Obsessive-compulsive disorder figured a cycle of self-perception and self-reflection that yielded the desire, but not the capacity, for ethical transformation. Deprived of this capacity by the law-like force of compulsion, Kleandis shifted his sights from responsibility toward submission. But in his case, as in many others, the treatment to which the patient submitted would continuously and ruinously fail—exposing the inadequacy of both medical care and legal protection to foster his well-being.

This impasse between humanitarian psychiatry and intractable pathology determines the ethics of responsibility for mental illness in Greece—for patients, doctors, communities, and the state. Well-being emerges on one side of this impasse; asylum persists on the other. Kleandis lingered at the gates of asylum, bound there by the law of compulsion, holding out for delivery at the hands of another.

Reprise:

Diagnosis

In 1887, the year preceding the "last year of [his] sane life," according to an editor,[1] Friedrich Nietzsche wrote a preface for his second edition of *The Gay Science*, published first in 1882. In those brisk and brash remarks, he hailed the exuberance and gratitude he had acquired in his emergence from the pain of a "severe sickness"—an experience that revealed to him the dependence of modern philosophy on illness:

> The unconscious disguise of physiological needs under the cloaks of the objective, ideal, purely spiritual goes to frightening lengths—and often I have asked myself whether, taking a large view, philosophy has not been merely an interpretation of the body and *a misunderstanding of the body*.
>
> Behind the highest value judgments that have hitherto guided the history of thought, there are concealed misunderstandings of the physical constitution—of individuals or classes or even whole races. All those bold insanities of metaphysics, especially answers to the question about the *value* of existence, may always be considered first of all as the symptoms of certain bodies. And if such world affirmations or world negations *tout court* lack any grain of significance when measured scientifically, they are the more valuable for the historian and psychologist as hints or symptoms of the body, of its success or failure, its plenitude, power, and autocracy in history, or of its frustrations, weariness, impoverishment, its premonitions of the end, its will to the end.

I am still waiting for a philosophical *physician* in the exceptional sense of that word—one who has to pursue the problem of the total health of a people, time, race or of humanity—to muster the courage to push my suspicion to its limits and to risk the proposition: what was at stake in all philosophizing hitherto was not at all "truth" but something else— let us say, health, future, growth, power, life.[2]

Following immediately upon *The Gay Science*, Nietzsche again rendered "the bold insanities" of moralism symptomatically in *The Twilight of the Idols*: "Judgments, value judgments concerning life, for or against, can in the last resort never be true; they possess value only as symptoms, they come into consideration only as symptoms—in themselves such judgments are stupidities."[3] In his earlier work, Nietzsche had already vigorously promoted the method of diagnosis to discern these symptoms. In "The Philosopher as Cultural Physician," he described the task of the new philosopher (also an old and forgotten one) who would conduct "a study of the symptoms of the age."[4] In modernity, he commented elsewhere, "the philosopher has become a being who is harmful to the community. He annihilates happiness, virtue, culture, and finally himself. Formerly, in the role of cultural physician, philosophy had to be in alliance with the cohesive forces"[5]—that is, with the forces of the state as a means to culture. The "philosophical physician" Nietzsche awaited, then, insofar as he diagnosed, would also perform a remedy, working in the service of culture to restore vitality to humanity.

For those who take Nietzsche as a philosophical ancestor, these texts establish diagnosis as an analytic response to the madness of moralism—a response that aims not to achieve health in any straightforward sense, but rather to recuperate madness from moral philosophy: *understanding the body as a creative philosophical activity*. Gilles Deleuze and Félix Guattari, in their antidefinitive questioning of philosophy, observe that "the diagnosis of becomings in every passing present is what Nietzsche assigned to the philosopher as physician, 'physician of civilization,' or inventor of new immanent modes of existence."[6] This formulation relates diagnosis to invention,[7] a creative activity allied not with the will to truth, but rather with the will to power—the "instinct for freedom" that, Nietzsche argues in the *Genealogy of Morals*, has been "pushed back and repressed,"[8] turned back on itself, foundering in that "madness of the will" known as guilt.[9] In diagnosing this madness, the *Genealogy* shows diagnosis to be incommensurable with the scholarly pursuits of those earnest and indecent "men of knowledge" driven, unwittingly, by bad conscience.[10] The alliance of diagnosis with life introduces a disjuncture between Nietzsche's method of diagnosis and those earnest men's pursuit of truth: "No, this bad taste, this will to truth, to 'truth at any price,' this youthful madness in the love of truth, have lost their charm for us . . . We no longer believe that truth remains truth when the veils are withdrawn; we have lived too much to believe this. Today we consider it a matter of decency not to wish to see everything naked, or to be present at everything, or to understand and 'know' everything."[11]

Nietzsche phrases this deprecation of the will to truth, of the scholarly ambition to unveil, as disgust—not just an assault to his sense of decency but something more embodied: a digestive problem, a "bad taste" in his mouth, "nausea."[12] Diagnosis thus risks contagion between those such as himself, who suffer and grow sensitive to this illness of the soul, thereby gaining the competency to diagnose it, and, on the other hand, those who remain ignorant—who believe they understand the value of life and health but are in fact deluded, mad. This delusion is also a form of suffering, but it remains masked in scholarship. In diagnosing this madness, Nietzsche counterposes to it another: a rapturous but knowing philosophical activity that bolsters the vitality of bodies along with culture, creating a new context for life.

Deleuze gleans from Nietzsche this curative and creative "symptomatological method" running through so many of his own works,[13] from *Nietzsche and Philosophy* to *Coldness and Cruelty* to *Anti-Oedipus*, culminating in *Essays Critical and Clinical*. There, he elaborates the encounter between literature and clinical psychiatry written into life by artists and philosophers who, suffering madness, become, themselves, the most thorough and creative symptomatologists—better, Deleuze insists, than clinicians at diagnosing symptoms, "because the work of art gives them new means."[14] Those "new means" are creative precisely insofar as they emerge from madness:

> We do not write with our neuroses. Neuroses or psychoses are not passages of life, but states into which we fall when the process is interrupted, blocked, or plugged up. Illness is not a process but a stopping of the process, as in "the Nietzsche case." Moreover, the writer as such is not a patient but rather a physician, the physician of himself and of the world. The world is a set of symptoms, whose illness merges with man. Literature then appears as an enterprise of health: not that the

writer would necessarily be in good health . . . but he possess an irresistible and delicate health that stems from what he has seen and heard of things too big for him, too strong for him, suffocating things whose passage exhausts him, while nonetheless giving him the becomings that a dominant and substantial health would render impossible. The writer returns from what he has seen and heard with bloodshot eyes and pierced eardrums. What health would be sufficient to liberate life wherever it is imprisoned by man and within man, by and within organisms and genera? It is like Spinoza's delicate health, while it lasted, bearing witness until the end to a new vision whose passage it remained open to.[15]

For Deleuze, the crucial distinction for creativity, in writing as in philosophy, is not between health and madness, but between "good health"—that is, a "dominant and substantial health" in harmony with the present—and the "irresistible and delicate health" of the writer-physician whose illness has opened the possibility of a future vitality. This delicacy is not madness but its residue, left by the writer's emergence from the depths of that "fallen state."

Michel Foucault takes the particular character of those depths as a symptom of the modern age in his heady conclusion to *Madness and Civilization*.[16] The mutually limiting relation between madness and the work of art that he sees in the age of reason—in the work of Sade, Goya, Swift, Rousseau—was, he says, a relation of "exchange" wherein truth made itself visible in madness in the form of a question about the origins of language and artistic inspiration. Against this historical "accommodation" between madness and reason, Foucault poses the modern arrangement where, he contends, madness no longer questions, challenges, or limits truth. Its classical exchange with the work of art is succeeded by silence: "Madness is the absolute break with the work of art: it forms the constitutive moment of abolition . . . the contour against the void."[17] For this new age, Foucault takes Nietzsche—with Artaud, Van Gogh, Nerval—as a decisive figure: "Nietzsche's last cry, proclaiming himself both Christ and Dionysus, is not on the border of reason and unreason . . . it is the very annihilation of the work of art, the point where it becomes impossible and where it must fall silent; the hammer has just fallen from the philosopher's hands."[18]

Foucault's diagnosis of the modern age, his analysis of the means it invents for being and knowing itself, turns on the symptom of Nietzsche's madness. Here, diagnosis appears as a genealogical method—a "curative science" that, Foucault writes, "has more in common with medicine than with philosophy," if philosophy is the metaphysical moralism that Nietzsche derided with such delight. The "effective history" yielded by genealogy, for Foucault, takes the body as its primary material:[19]

> The genealogist needs history to dispel the chimeras of the origin, somewhat in the manner of the pious philosopher who needs a doctor to exorcise the shadow of his soul. He must be able to recognize the events of history, its jolts, its surprises, its unsteady victories and unpalatable defeats—the basis of all beginnings, atavisms, and heredities. Similarly, he must be able to diagnose the illnesses of the body, its conditions of weakness and strength, its breakdowns and resistances, to be in a position to judge philosophical discourse. . . . Genealogy, as an analysis of descent, is thus situated within the articulation of the body and history. Its task is to expose a body totally imprinted by history and the process of history's destruction of that body.[20]

This passage argues for the nonmetaphorical currency of the body in philosophical diagnosis. For Foucault, the persistence, flexibility, and mutability of this body as the material on which history is inscribed make it possible for the philosopher to read historical change genealogically. And just as history, as the narration of "ideal continuity," is relinquished in genealogy,[21] so metaphysical moralism is relinquished in diagnosis. Philosophy emerges instead as the thought of individuals, produced in and through bodies. There is an identification here between the body of genealogy and Nietzsche's own sick body—for what was his illness, if not the "destruction" of his "body" by "history"? This experience of bodily devastation drove him to "question further, more deeply, severely, harshly, evilly and quietly," since "the trust in life [wa]s gone: life itself ha[d] become a *problem*."[22] The life and philosophy of the body put each other at stake, and at risk.

For Nietzsche and these heirs, then, diagnosis is not a medical metaphor for philosophical activity or social analysis. Rather, if philosophy is a strategy of the body in its life, growth, and health, then a diagnosis of its symptomatic philosophy—its moralism—is an argument for the body, rendering critical judgment of the extent and direction of its vitality in view of the self-evident benefit of life and health. This body is not a metaphorical tool, but a material site of the will to power, sensible to the "historical sense" of genealogy, and generative of a philosophy that vitalizes and cures.

If the language of a sick body expresses moral judgments about the value of life, as Nietzsche suggests, then what method of interpretation can expose the sickness, the madness, of which this degradation of language is a symptom? In an epigrammatic essay on the "techniques of interpretation" of Nietzsche, Marx, and Freud, Foucault observes the historical development of systems of interpretation to address a persistent, twofold suspicion of language: first, that "language does not mean exactly what it says," but indirectly expresses a deeper and hidden meaning; and second, that things other than language—sounds, gestures, material itself—can speak.[23] Illness is an experience that shapes both these suspicions and the interpretative techniques that concretize and qualify them. The suspiciousness of language and the distinctively modern "malevolence" of the sign lie at the heart of diagnosis.[24]

Foucault finds modern interpretation circular, collapsing into the absence of a primary uninterpreted object: the material to be interpreted is never composed of "the thing itself" but of signs, which already constitute interpretations of other signs. Interpretation, he submits, is by its nature an incomplete act, an infinite task that threatens a vital danger: "What is in question in the point of rupture of interpretation, in this convergence of interpretation on a point that renders it impossible, could well be something like the experience of madness."[25] This structural madness of interpretation, this "fascination" and "struggle," is a potentiality that Foucault sees realized in Nietzsche.[26]

In diagnosing Nietzsche as a madman, here, Foucault makes a methodological point about modern hermeneutics. Is this a shift in register between clinical diagnosis and the philosophical variety that is Nietzsche's legacy, or an assertion that their distinction is untenable—even impossible? By what, save the madness of interpretation itself, could a psychological diagnosis of Nietzsche be authorized for philosophy? The literality of the body or the mind that is diagnosed by its philosophy cannot be settled, within this genealogy of thought, without broaching Nietzsche's own madness.[27] After all, he declared, "We philosophers are not free to divide body from soul as the people do."[28] If madness is a sickness, an experience of pain from which the philosopher emerges refreshed and bursting with profound levity, it is not only an object of interpretation but also a likeness: a shade of interpretation when pushed to the shallow depths of an empty origin.

Is this madness of interpretation so very different from the madness of moralism—the absurd negativity Nietzsche finds in philosophy that ventures value judgments about existence? I perceive the moralism of responsibility in Greek psychiatry as just such a philosophy. Though this book does not escape the field of power and desire in which that philosophy is grounded, I hope the diagnosis it offers might shift the context of interpretation away from psychiatry's truth claims and toward the moral responsibilities it produces. The risk is that this diagnosis may come to exhibit symptoms of another moralism, in the service of another truth game.

Postlude:

A Peaceful Place

Greek psychiatric reform began in Thrace, where patients and therapists formed Greece's first regional community-based mental health care network. Today, they continue to labor, more and less collaboratively, at the therapeutic and cross-cultural frontiers of Greek psychiatry. These frontiers coincide with the national border between Greece and Turkey. In the first decade of the new century, under securitarian conditions marked by the politicization of Islam and a surge in migration from the east, European control of this border is orchestrating another psychiatric innovation.

The case of Mohamet—whose attributed name was but a cipher for his ambiguous status as a patient, immigrant, refugee, criminal—traces the institutional configuration of that innovation. The elusive identity of this patient, who did not speak, matched the provisionality of his proliferating diagnoses: schizophrenic catatonia, post-traumatic stress disorder, malingering. He presented to psychiatrists a sheer surface for the madly contradictory inscription of state power, humanitarian ethics, cultural diagnostics, and the ill will of language that were coalescing in the clinics of Thrace around the moralism of responsibility. Originating in an obscure social order beyond the border, and disappearing into a domestic asylum forgotten to reform, Mohamet's case disclosed a biopolitical novelty in the guise of a reversion: the ghost of carceral psychiatry resurfacing on the terrain of immigration, eradicating one more fissure in the body politic where souls lost to society might find shelter.

❀ ❀ ❀

It was nearing winter when Mohamet was transferred to the old hospital in Alexandroupolis from an immigration detention center in the nearby town of Venna. He had been apprehended by border guards with some other young men while trying to cross the Turkish border on foot. According to Dr. Filalithi, who spoke with a nurse at the detention center's dispensary, Mohamet had been behaving bizarrely for more than a week. He had seemed fine when he first arrived at the center, but then he stopped talking—even to his friends. He refused food and water. He defecated in his clothing. He did not move, nor sleep. No one was able to break through to him, and he soon became gravely ill.

Filalithi was holding her weekly seminar on the evening Mohamet was admitted to the hospital clinic, so she presented the case briefly to the residents and staff in attendance. She suggested that, with my interest in culture, I might learn a lot from this case. I was permitted to shadow Kalliope, the resident assigned to Mohamet, as she tended to him that night. First, he had to be collected from the lab in the main building of the hospital, where his blood had been drawn and screened. The results cleared him of organic illness.

We found Mohamet in the lab's anteroom, seated awkwardly on a cot, staring into space. He was emaciated and no more than twenty years old. The police officer at his side told us that Mohamet had not moved or spoken during the medical procedures. Kalliope tried to engage his attention—speaking to him and then yelling, laughing, hopping through his sightline, clapping, manipulating his limbs—but she got no response. The officer, kindly in his way, told us he had succeeded in giving Mohamet some water from a paper cup—an indication, Kalliope said, that the patient had "some degree of orientation to reality." But that was the extent of their progress. The officer lifted Mohamet to his feet and escorted him, shuffling and stumbling, with us to the clinic. He was installed in its single private room, handcuffed to his bed, and left to rest in police custody.

Mohamet's dark complexion and eastern provenance led several of the doctors hovering around him that evening to guess that he was "Arab"; some judged him to be Iraqi, others Palestinian, others Persian. He seemed to recognize the words *Palestine* and *Kurdistan* when Dr. Lamberakis pronounced them loudly, as if Mohamet were deaf. When Aspa, a Pontian medical student, spoke the Turkish word for *sit*, Mohamet sat down. This compounded the diagnostic puzzle, for he was clearly not

Turkish—but would an Arab understand Turkish? One of the nurses observed, *You can tell he's Muslim because he's afraid of women. He won't look at us, he completely avoids physical contact.*

Kalliope consulted Lamberakis and Filalithi about Mohamet's diagnosis. They could not attribute his symptoms to simple catatonia, because he was able to execute certain movements: he would sit or walk when they encouraged him, and jerk his hand back when they reached for him; his limbs would fall back into position rather than hang in paralysis when the doctors raised them manually. He repeatedly touched his nose and chin, like a tic. He uttered sounds, though no one at the clinic could tell if these were words. Lamberakis speculated that he might be presenting negative symptoms of schizophrenia: flat affect, avolition. *But if so,* he said, *it's the most extreme case we've ever seen.* And since communication was impossible, there was no way to determine the extent of positive symptoms of schizophrenia, such as cognitive disorder and disorganized speech.

Other therapists floated other diagnostic possibilities. Mohamet might be suffering from cognitive delay consequent to some trauma, or even from post-traumatic stress disorder. Perhaps he had fled a war; perhaps he had experienced or witnessed some unspeakable horror. The doctors ordered a high dose of Aloperidin (US Haldol), an antipsychotic medication, in hopes that it might stimulate a response that would clarify the nature of his illness.

The presence of the police guard evinced another theory. Kalliope told me later that night that a number of illegal immigrants transferred to the hospital from the detention center during the last year had escaped once their guards released them to medical authorities: *The police won't let him go because they think he might be faking, and he'd run away the minute he's left alone.* Mohamet's guard stayed with him all night. He reported the next day that Mohamet had not slept much: *Maybe the restraints bothered him?* Twelve hours after his first dose of antipsychotic medication, Mohamet was still not speaking or making eye contact.

Later that morning, when I stopped by to visit, the police officer informed me that Mohamet had just tried to escape. His handcuffs had been removed so that a nurse could give him a second injection, and he immediately sprang to the window and jumped out. The officer gave chase and caught Mohamet, who was slow, weak, and disoriented. He was hastily restored to his room and his handcuffs.

The escape attempt tended to corroborate—though inconclusively—

the suspicion that Mohamet was feigning his illness. Another guard was dispatched to relieve the first one, and the police chief called Dr. Fila-lithi to debate the future of Mohamet's custody. Filalithi told me later that the chief had insisted on upholding the new immigration laws: *The hospital is obliged to contain* [να κλείνει] *the patient in a secure room. But we have only one room like that in the whole hospital, and it's located in the orthopedics ward.* Dr. Lamberakis, who collaborated on the case, said he feared that Mohamet would not get adequate medical attention in this locked room, which was on the other side of the hospital from the psychiatry clinic; and that isolation might exacerbate his catatonic condition, which still could not be diagnosed.

The debate continued for days. Mohamet was transferred to the locked room in orthopedics, and his psychiatrists agonized over his abandon-ment. They conferred with the doctor at the detention center, who said he was unable to ensure that Mohamet would be administered psychoactive medications on a regular basis if he were sent back to the center. After ex-tended discussion, and consultation with the two clinic directors, Lam-berakis and Filalithi came to the conclusion that Mohamet would receive better psychiatric care at the state hospital in Thessaloniki, which had a large locked ward. *Over there,* Filalithi said, *he can be "secured" without being restrained. He'll have the company of other patients, and constant medical super-vision. He might open up and begin to talk if he feels safe.* A custodial institu-tion — backbone of the bad old days of psychiatric care — began to seem a humane alternative.

Four days after his initial admission, Mohamet was transferred to Thessaloniki, accompanied by a team of armed guards. His file went with him, and the hospital clinic never heard from him again. Lamberakis, who was teaching a class of undergraduate medical students that week, talked to them about the case. It was an example, he told them, of how psychiatric care can also be political: *In my view, psychiatrists should not concern themselves with the political aspects of a case. We're supposed to work only for the good of the patient.* He confessed utter confusion as to the clinical nature of Mohamet's illness. *We might have been able to figure it out, if we'd had enough time to do a thorough evaluation. These new immigration laws are paranoid and inhumane. I feel terrible not being able to care properly for my patient.* Refused privacy, forcibly restrained and medicated, and ultimately transported by armed escort to a remote custodial hospital, Mohamet received treat-ment antithetical to the standards of humane and effective care that de-termined psychiatric ethics in this setting, under normal circumstances.

A year later, I began to perceive what kind of circumstances they were. Just before leaving Alexandroupolis, I happened into contact with Petros, a young doctor who had recently been appointed to the same immigration detention center where Mohamet had landed the winter before. I secured an invitation to visit. Petros was a local, born in Komotini and educated at the medical school in Alexandroupolis. As a student, he had participated in a special nine-month psychiatry program, treating patients discharged from state psychiatric hospitals who were now living in the community. He had worked with several psychiatrists from the hospital clinic, including Dr. Filalithi, and told me that he maintained a deep respect and affection for them. *But I decided against psychiatry as a specialty. It requires special gifts that I don't have — not just with language but with people. I think I'm better suited to scientific work, like surgery.*

Like many recent graduates of medical school in Greece, Petros was stalled indefinitely in waiting for a residency post to open up. I had heard by then many theories as to why the upper ranks of the profession were so full, and why the state was so slow to fund new positions in order to accommodate the number of medical school graduates and meet the needs of the growing patient population. Psychiatry, being in low demand, offered fewer obstacles in this regard than other branches of medicine. The surgical specialty Petros had chosen was more competitive; he expected to wait another two or three years before beginning his training. In the meantime, he made a living working overnight shifts in various wards at the General Hospital of Xanthi, and running the dispensary at the detention center.

Petros explained that the latter post, which entailed four or five clinical sessions per week, had been created when the detention center was opened several years before as part of the same EU program that supplied an international team of specially trained border guards — the precursors of Frontex. When the previous doctor had left the center to start a private practice, many candidates sought the position. *That was until they found out what kind of people they would have as patients,* Petros said. He was hired partly through the efforts of the nurse who worked there, Ioanna, who was a family friend. *But mainly I think it was because I showed enthusiasm for this kind of work. I'm committed to providing these people good medical care for as long as they're detained. Whatever people say, they have a right to that care.*

The previous doctor, too, had had an enthusiastic disposition, according to Ioanna. The pair of them were the first clinicians to approach the new institution, with wide eyes. It was they who demanded that hot water be installed in the facility; who brought extra blankets and clothing with them for the inmates; who ordered new mattresses to replace the plastic mats on which the inmates had slept in the early days. *We improved the conditions bit by bit as we went along,* she told me. *That's the kind of work this place demands.*

The detention center was housed in an old train depot, long since closed to railway traffic but still visible to passing trains through the overgrown brush. It was a plain cement structure, configured like a warehouse with an open plan, high ceilings, and picture windows. That summer, the aging cement was crumbling at the joints. The roof was falling in and the windows were boarded up, leaving only small slats at the top to let in the daylight. The complex was surrounded by barbed wire, and the gate tended by armed border guards who amiably waved us through. I was not permitted into the main building, but Petros described it to me. He said the space had been divided with makeshift partitions into seven large but severely overcrowded rooms, each kept locked. An effort was made to lodge relatives and traveling companions in the same rooms, but otherwise the inmates were not grouped by age, sex, language, or national origin. They were not permitted to circulate except when they were let in small groups into the dusty courtyard for a short period of recreation each day. At this time, the facility housed about 150 inmates, but the previous winter the number had been closer to 800, and conditions had been very desperate.

It's no wonder the dispensary is so popular with the inmates! Petros said. Groups of up to a dozen patients would be selected by the guards for each clinical session, according to the urgency of their complaints and the amount of time they had already waited to see the doctor. The dispensary occupied a tiny, poorly ventilated annex at the back of the main building. It comprised a consultation office with a waiting area, and a pantry where a small stock of medications was kept—mostly analgesics and antibiotics ordered from the pharmacy at the General Hospital of Komotini, a ten-minute drive away. The entire group of patients would be locked into the waiting area by the guards, and there they waited, as a group, for each patient to be seen—up to four hours, on some days— before being escorted back to the main building. Most presented minor injuries or ailments that could be treated at the center with a routine course of medication. Medical emergencies that exceeded the scope of the dispensary were handled at the hospital in Komotini. But *some of the inmates use the dispensary as recreation*, Petros told me. *I can sympathize. But I really resent it when I'm struggling to figure out what's wrong with them, and they're giving me vague complaints that never get resolved.*

Inmates could expect to lodge at the center for two to three months, at which point they would be released with official papers granting them one month either to vacate the country—forcibly, if necessary—or to petition the state for residency. Ioanna said, *It's obvious that most of the inmates don't know this information. They know nothing about their legal status or what's going to happen to them.* No translators were employed to communicate their rights and options to them. Many would have no legal redress, in any case. Ignorance and speculation further constricted the horizon of their hope. Despair and anxiety set in. Fights broke out among them. They had trouble sleeping. They began to manifest signs of psychological disturbance.

As we saw patients at the dispensary that day, Petros and Ioanna observed these signs of disturbance, diagnosing them generically, attributing them to the traumatic circumstances the inmates had fled in their homelands, or to the conditions of their containment here. But this was not a psychiatry clinic. Petros could not offer therapy, and he would not dispense psychoactive medications—not even the sedatives that many inmates requested for temporary relief. *I'm afraid they'll get addicted*, he said. *And then, once they've left the center and have no access to medical care, they'll be facing withdrawal, which is agonizing. Or they'll find drugs on the street, and this is the start of a criminal life.*

Petros had first become concerned about addiction when one of the inmates attempted suicide. *He got his hands on a sharp piece of metal that he probably picked up in the recreation yard. He slashed his wrists in the middle of the night and bled for hours before he was found.* He was taken to the emergency room at the hospital in Komotini and held there for several days of observation. Petros thought this inmate, whom he had seen a few times at the dispensary, had been addicted to drugs: *The suicide attempt was probably triggered by withdrawal psychosis.*

The inmates were examined that day with the aid of two young translators, enlisted on the spot from the group waiting at the dispensary. Both were Balinese, and they spoke to each other in their native language. One knew Arabic as well, and the other English. Often both were needed to render communication between patient and doctor. Petros spoke a haphazard, highly formal English with the translator, so—reversing the customary direction of my ethnographic encounters—I aided in English-

Greek translation. Petros seemed to delight in the linguistic chaos, though he commented from time to time, *I think something's being lost in translation!*

Most of the patients were middle-aged and alone at the center. In addition to the translators, we saw an Iraqi man with abrasions and an infected bite he had gotten from another inmate in a fight. An Iraqi woman with a rash. A Bangladeshi man with a shoulder injury. A Burmese man with nausea and headaches. A young Somali woman with abdominal pain. A Palestinian man who spoke to us in French about numbness in his leg that persisted, five days after his surgery at the hospital in Komotini for an infected gunshot wound.

The last patients were two young Liberian men who had been apprehended separately and became friends at the detention center. Both had come to Greece from Liberia by ship. One was picked up in the Mediterranean by a Greek fisherman sidelining as a trafficker, and was not caught by the police until he disembarked in Thessaloniki. He was suffering from severe headaches: *I haven't slept in days,* he said, in English. *I'm haunted by memories of the war. I saw my three brothers murdered before my eyes. My parents just disappeared one day.* His companion complained of relentless aches and pains throughout his body. He, too, was unable to sleep; he could not stop thinking about what had happened in the war. *Bloody images come to me all of a sudden. I jolt awake and I can't get back to sleep.* Though Petros administered painkillers to the men, he refused them sedatives. Their symptoms of psychological disturbance did not rise to the level of urgency required for him to make a psychiatric referral and transfer them to clinical custody.

In fact, Ioanna told me, the only psychiatric referral to be made by the detention center that year was for Mohamet, the mystery patient. He had been transferred to the hospital in Alexandroupolis because, at the time, the hospital in Komotini had no psychiatrist on staff. This had happened before Petros began working at the center, but Ioanna remembered Mohamet well. *I never found out what happened to him, but I'm sure he didn't come back here. He was a very desperate case. But we see that happen to a lot of the inmates: they're fine when they arrive, but they deteriorate, and we lose them.* In this space of deferred asylum, medical care was complicated by the difficulty of communicating with aliens, and absolutely confounded by the impossibility of relieving the pathogenic conditions of their containment. Mental illness was created here, not treated.

At the dispensary that day, the second of the two Liberian men told us he had been apprehended on a train just west of Alexandroupolis. He had come up the Aegean Sea by ship, as part of the United Nations evacuation fleet from Liberia during the worst phase of violence. He jumped ship when they docked at the port of Alexandroupolis and hopped a train to Thessaloniki. *I've been here for fifteen days and I have no idea when they'll let me go*, he said. Petros told him, in English, that he would likely be held for two months and then released, on condition that he leave the country. The man shook his head, looked at his friend. *Leave where? I want to stay in Greece. I didn't see much of it, but I saw the sea, and I saw farms through the windows of the train. I could live here. It's such a peaceful place.*

NOTES

INTRODUCTION

1. Throughout this text, I use different formal modes to represent different contexts and functions of speech. As I elaborate in part 1 (page 66), speech that I reproduce verbatim appears in direct quotation. I use italics to paraphrase or recollect speech, reconstructed from detailed notes, and indirect discourse to paraphrase or recollect speech in my own interpretive voice. Finally, I employ free-indirect discourse to present communication whose function exceeds the speakers' and my own interpretive voices.

2. I spent several months working in Thrace during 2001 and 2004, and conducted continuous research there from September 2002 through September 2003. Prior to this project, I worked in other clinical settings in Greece, including state psychiatric hospitals in Thessaloniki (June–August 2000) and Chania, Crete (December 1999).

3. "Turk," "Pomak," and "Gypsy" were fraught and contested identifications in Thrace, whose meanings and effects I explore in part 2. I use the term *Gypsy* (γύφτος/-ισσα) especially advisedly: like many designators of minority identity, this term has pejorative and positive connotations, depending on its use. In using the term myself, I aim to flag an abject social status, rather than to obscure it with a more neutral term. The Gypsies of Thrace—a Turkish-speaking Muslim community comprising about 7 percent of the regional population and about 20 percent of the regional Muslim population at the time of my research—entertained ambiguous associations with both the Turks of Greece and the Roma of Eastern Europe. These associations had strong but very different political resonances in Greek political discourse. On the Roma side, the precarious citizenship of Gypsies in Thrace evokes the classification of Gypsies as a criminal population, seen explicitly in the Berlusconi administration's census and fingerprinting scheme introduced in Italy in 2008—echoing similar policies in Bulgaria, Romania, and Serbia. See Alexandrakis's (2003) ethnography of a Roma community on the margins of Athens.

4. By the early 1990s, the total population of Thrace numbered around 362,000.

Of this total population, about a third (120,000) self-reported as Turkish-speaking Muslims, broken down into three categories: about 65,000 Turks, 31,000 Pomaks, and 24,000 Gypsies. Oran notes that the Turko-Muslim third of the total population of Thrace has a much higher birthrate than the Greek population—2.8 as compared with 0.7 (Oran 2003: 107). See also Alexandris (2003) and Voutira (2003) for population statistics on Thrace.

5. See Fassin and d'Halluin (2005, 2007) and Ticktin (2005) for discussions of this overdetermined nexus of suspicion toward immigrants developing among the legal, medical, and policing organs of the state at the borders of Europe.

6. See Blue 1991 for a discussion of this "folk genetics" as well as the stigma borne by the first generation of deinstitutionalized outpatients in Greece.

7. I am excluding from this description the activities of the Community Mental Health Center run by the hospital clinic staff on separate premises in downtown Alexandroupolis. It was at this center that clinic psychiatrists conducted long-term therapy with their more stable patients. Since these patients constituted a much smaller and almost completely separate group from those admitted to the hospital clinic, I have treated the clinic as a discrete therapeutic context. I did not conduct substantial research at the center, where I attended some staff meetings but few treatment sessions.

8. I have rendered thus the question Michalis asked: "Που να'πευθύνομαι για να ξέρω τί έγινε, ποιός έχει ευθύνη"; I heard the first predicate construction as a contraction, in which the vowel in the prefix was swallowed, rendering the verb semantically indeterminate. I have assumed Michalis meant "να απευθύνομαι" (To whom can I address myself . . . ?). But he might have meant "να υπευθύνομαι"—with muddled syntax, something like, "How can I take upon myself the responsibility . . . ?" The phrase might also be neologistic, based in a distortion of the root ευθύνη (responsibility), which he reiterates at the end of the question. A final consideration is that Michalis was speaking modern Greek, which bears syntactical differences from Pontic Greek, his native tongue.

9. Papas is a famous Greek actress and singer, known especially for her role in Zorba the Greek (1964). In 2002 she was awarded the Woman of Europe medallion by the European Union for "integrating the EU" through her international training centers for actors. At that time—about four years after Michalis's psychotic break, and a year before this encounter—her biography and commentary on Europe were popular topics in the Greek press.

10. Noting that "the pestering question of identity" has long been debated epistemologically—that is, in terms of who can "claim knowledge"—Neni Panourgiá remarks of neo-Hellenism in the nineteenth century: "Greek intellectuals understood only too well that in order for them to be considered European they first had to prove that they were as 'Greek' as the rest of Europe. . . . What needed to be proven, in the first place, was their modernity, and the only way of proving that was through the proof of their ancient pedigree" (2004: 174). James D. Faubion

(1993) examines Europeanization as an ambition internalized by these intellectuals, who legitimated the Greek nation-state with historical, folkloric, and philological knowledge, as well as with the great classical tradition of poetry. Stathis Gourgouris (1996) argues against viewing Europeanization as an explicit or unitary project of Hellenism in the Greek Enlightenment, except in retrospect. See also Jusdanis 1991 and Herzfeld 1987a.

11. See Paul Rabinow's treatment of the topos of *anthropos* in modern knowledge (2003).

12. References to this recursion could number in the thousands, with no small debt to Freud, Nietzsche, and Hegel. I have immediately in mind certain contemporary works in social theory and anthropology, including Judith Butler's treatment of agency in the feminist legacy of Antigone (2002); Neni Panourgiá's journey through the ongoing production of the Oedipus myth (2008, 2009); and anthropologists of the psyche who have played such an important role in refiguring *anthropos* through radical cultural difference, from James George Frazer (1922) and Ruth Benedict (1934) to Georges Devereux (1951, 1953, 1963) and Gananath Obeyesekere (1990).

13. In this book, I usually render ψυχή with the term *psyche*, its direct cognate in English. While "soul" is the conventional translation in philosophical works, *psyche* better conveys the dual medical and moral usages of ψυχή in the psychiatric settings where I worked. There, the word νοῦς most often signified "mind," the seat of cognition and antithesis of σῶμα (body); while πνεῦμα alternately denoted "spirit" (as in *spiritual*) or the root "ment-" (as in *mentality* and *mental health*).

14. Simon 1980: 55–56; Claus 1981: 2, quoting Rohde 1966; Holmes 2010: 6.

15. Claus 1981: 2. Simon describes the Platonic ψυχή as "the self that . . . thinks, decides, initiates, and is conscious of what it does" (1980: 161). See Brooke Holmes's (2010) account of the body's centrality to this conception of the psyche. Holmes shows how the body (σῶμα) became visible in philosophical, medical, and dramatic works of the fifth and fourth centuries BCE by way of changing interpretations of bodily symptoms. She charts a "fragmentation of agency" among gods and demons (14), bodily processes, and physicians' interventions, which positioned the body as a new problem for empirical knowledge and ethical attention in this period. Against conventional dualistic accounts that trace personhood and ethical subjectivity in the classical world to the emergence of ψυχή, Holmes finds a different ethical horizon and locus of personhood in analogies and interactions between σῶμα and ψυχή (36–37), especially the "haunting" of ψυχή by the "daemonic energies"—the impersonal, unconscious, unruly workings—of σῶμα (4).

16. As, for example, Saba Mahmood does for the concept of habitus in Greek and Arab-Islamic traditions of ethical formation and pedagogy. Mahmood traces the transmission of this concept from Aristotle through medieval Islamic scholars such as Abu Hamid al-Ghazali and Ibn Khaldun to community ethicists in contemporary urban Egypt, in whose practices of piety "this Aristotelian legacy continues to live" (Mahmood 2005: 137).

17. In this venture, I am indebted to Simon (1980), who presents a thorough and imaginative genealogy of the modern psyche, exploring the ancient Greek ancestry of dramatic, philosophical, and medical orientations to mental illness in the West.

18. On this interior domain, see Holmes's (2010) discussion of the body's "cavity," and its signification by symptoms, in classical thought.

19. As Andrew Lakoff (2005) shows in his account of postreform psychiatry in contemporary Argentina, even in clinics where psychoanalysis has retained a strong presence, its theorization of subjectivity is increasingly viewed as the vestige of an obsolete progressivism, and its diagnostic and therapeutic techniques as potentially "irresponsible" in light of advances in scientific (i.e., pharmaceutical and "evidence-based") treatment.

20. Foucault 1990a, 1990b, 1988a.

21. Foucault 1988a; 1990b: 28, 30. See Rabinow 1997; Campbell and Shaw 2009.

22. For one, James D. Faubion (2001a) examines the practices of "self-reading" and "self-writing" that compose the creative "scriptural" or "hermeneutic" ethics of his principal subject, an American millennialist prophet (150). For another, Anand Pandian (2008 and 2009) explores the ethical work on self and others undertaken by members of a rural south Indian "criminal tribe" at the crossroads of postcolonial development projects and Tamil moral traditions. Pandian presents *cultivation* as a repertoire of agrarian practices and a constellation of virtues (civility, propriety, restraint, toil, sympathy)—a particular, studied array of desires, habits, metaphors, and bodily techniques—that together form the present ethical horizon symbolized as "development."

Prominent among these recent ethnographies, and most directly relevant to my own engagement with ethics, is Mahmood's (2005) work on the women's mosque movement in contemporary Egypt. Mahmood takes the virtue of piety—in line with variously construed Islamic doctrine—to be both expressed and produced by an array of ethical practices, especially bodily movements and dispositions. Following Foucault, she pays careful historical, theological, and ethnographic attention to the "way of life" to which these practices are "germane," rather than exclusively to the ratiocinative forms of "moral deliberation" granted primacy in Kantian ethics. Such moral deliberation appears, in her account, as a capacity contingent on the disposition formed first through such habituated practices (27). Mahmood grounds her analysis of these practices in a critique of liberal conceptions of freedom, to which she sees pious Muslim women posing a radical challenge. It is their conscious "subordination" to the "transcendent will" of God that leads Mahmood to problematize liberal and feminist presumptions of a desire for freedom at the heart of human agency (3–4, 10). In her view, the agency of women's ethics of piety in Egypt can be found in the "capacities and skills" that piety requires, the "product" of "discursive traditions" rather than of the "consciousness of subjects" who practice those traditions (29, 32). Thus the submission to duty by women participants in the mosque movement, and the "precise embodied form" taken by their "obedience to a moral code" in their daily lives (27), are the decisions not of subjects, but of discourses in which these women become subjects.

To the extent that psychiatric patients, too, are enrolled in an ethical project by some agency other than their own autonomous rational will, and are transformed in the process into subjects of a moral discourse, their submission to treatment bears a strong affinity to the subordination of pious women to the will of God in Mahmood's account. In both cases, the constitutive task of ethical subjectivity is to assume subjective responsibility for an extrinsic duty. This task is what Mahmood, with Judith Butler, cites as Foucault's *paradox of subjectivation* (Mahmood 2005: 17, 20n35; Butler 1993: 15): "The very processes and conditions that secure a subject's subordination are also the means by which she becomes a self-conscious identity and agent" (17). Mahmood's departure from Butler is to consider, as ethical, practices that do not subvert the norms that give rise to them in this way—that find a telos other than "liberation" in the terms of progressive liberal politics (14). This departure dislodges ethics from the mutual entailment of freedom and agency—a set of values to which, as Mahmood points out, liberalism and feminism make exclusive political claims, against other "value systems" such as Islamism. Yet the ethics in which psychiatric patients are engaged by reform insistently repose that entailment. Freedom in this context both requires and produces agentive responsibility: it is a legal condition of the decision to undertake treatment (consistent with the "procedural" account of freedom, as Mahmood construes liberal theory, 10–12), but also the normative goal of that treatment (consistent with the "substantive" account of freedom): a liberation from mental illness and institutional life. Psychiatric reform thus poses freedom as a special problem for the ethics of responsibility that cannot be reduced to cultural or political conflicts over values.

23. This is to adapt Paul Rabinow's hypothesis that ethics may be considered a new diacritic of "the human," the object and subject of contemporary anthropology (2001).

24. Durkheim 1997.

25. On this distinction, see Rabinow's (1997) introduction to Foucault's collected work on ethics.

26. This task takes the form of subjectivation, in Foucault's terms, but diverges in an important way. The "paradox of subjectivation," as Judith Butler calls it (1993: 15), is "that the subject who would resist (regulatory norms which she/he opposes) is itself enabled, if not produced, by such norms." The reform of psychiatric patients, however, obligates them to make an ethical good—a telos—out of their subordination to regulatory norms that they do not necessarily oppose, and indeed to which they may aspire. A compelling and not wholly incommensurable theorization of this paradox is developed in the work of Jacques Lacan. In his reading of Freud, the status of the unconscious is not "ontic" but "ethical" (Lacan 1978: 32–33): it is an alien will that emerges within the subject, binding him to the symbolic order in which, alone, he may be recognized as a subject—which is to

say, with Kant, as the author of his will. The Real, as the alien and arbitrary cause of desire, must ultimately be assumed by the subject in a moment of responsibility for him to "become," in the sense of Freud's famous phrase: "where It was, there shall I become." Lacanian psychoanalysis aims at this achievement, effecting a reconfiguration of the subject's relationship to desire so that he can act as its responsible cause. To make this ethical leap, the subject has to sacrifice the good, that series of desirable objects that have substituted for the real satisfaction of desire in an imaginary structure of fantasy that binds him to the symbolic order. Lacanian psychoanalysis pushes subjects to act ethically in this sense—that is, "in conformity with [their] desire" (1992: 311) thus construed, rather than in the "service of goods" that describe the framework of "traditional ethics" (1992: 314–15). The confrontation in the subject's unconscious between impulses to pursue its desire and the internalized moral imperative to repress those impulses is revealed in neurotic symptoms despite or to spite the subject's conscious intentions. These symptoms express the ambivalent alienation of the subject from the symbolic order, which, as a condition of his intelligibility, cannot be resolved by psychoanalysis; but the subject's struggle has a trajectory that it can discern and adjust. Psychoanalytic ethics are thus allied not with socially prescribed norms—the "morality of the master" (1992: 315)—but with the patient's desire revealed through this procedure, regardless of its permissibility in the sociomoral order (see also Certeau 1986: 56).

I see "care of the self," that variegated suite of ethical practices explored by Foucault, as consistent with Lacanian psychoanalytic ethics, even if the latter describe a deontology (in which the subject's duty or obligation is bound to his desire, as against normative social goods), rather than immanent, voluntarist yet nondecisionist practices of the sort Foucault examines. Lacan, offering psychoanalysis as an empirical practice rather than an axiomatic moral system, suggests it is an "open question" whether psychoanalysis has an ethics, which he defines as the judgment of actions that themselves "contain" judgment (1992: 311). If psychoanalysis does have an ethics, it is because the practice restores focus to the "meaning of an action," revealing the desire that "inhabits" the action (1992: 312, 313) in a "catharsis" of self-knowledge that permits the patient to assume authorship of his own desire. If psychoanalytic ethics conceive responsibility as precisely this authorship of desire—discharged therapeutically but discovered hermeneutically—then responsibility transpires within the field of truth, enrolled in its laborious progression from concealment to revelation. This procedure, with its commitment to "deep" and "hidden" meaning (1992: 312), exemplifies the "hermeneutics of suspicion" to which Foucault turns a critical eye (Foucault 1998; Dreyfus and Rabinow 1983). As far as the patient's work on the self is concerned, however, I see Foucault's and Lacan's formulations of ethics converging on the same paradox of subjectivation.

27. Foucault 1990b: 287; Faubion 2001b: 96. Also see Foucault 1988a.

28. My approach to this kind of ethical "disability" owes much to Stefania Pan-

dolfo's work (2006, 2007). Pandolfo explores the restitution of provisional, discontinuous, singular forms of ethical subjectivity in the aftermath of a loss of self in Moroccan communities where the moral authority of law, history, and culture has been drastically disrupted. She asks what forms of life can be lived, and what forms of ethics can be chosen, under such conditions of radical unfreedom. In "Bghit nghanni hnaya" (2006), she tells the story of Roqiya, a young psychiatric patient whose rejection by her community, and whose abolition in madness, attest to the impossibility of "inhabiting the present" in contemporary Morocco. On Pandolfo's telling, however, this story also expresses the possibility for a self, dispossessed of its "right to the city," to reground itself as a "counter-subject." Pandolfo sees countersubjectivity articulated through the very absence of belonging wrought by ruptures in symbolic transmission—of culture and history, and of the legitimacy they confer—in the traumas of war, colonization, and postcolonial modernization.

In "The Burning" (2007), Pandolfo turns from the scene of madness to that of suicide, and the imbrication there of psychical, existential, and sociopolitical grounds of ethics in contemporary Morocco. The act named by the paper's title—the hazardous attempt to cross the Mediterranean and migrate illegally to Europe—divulges an eschatological horizon for ethical subjectivity under conditions of dispossession that form a male, urban complement to those in which Roqiya went mad. From a debate between two young men about the theological status of the burning, Pandolfo discerns in its risk the possibility of ethical subjectivity in a departure toward the "ethical community to come," a "practice of freedom" in the shadow of death (337). Against the virtue of "patience" (339) required by the "voluntary servitude" (338) accepted by those who stay in Morocco, the burning instead proffers a "notion of individual agency and responsibility" in the struggle for change, to be achieved either in exile or in "active rebellion" (340). That this struggle may end in the agent's death confers on the act, for those who desire it, the mien of martyrdom (332, 340). The young men's debate recurs to Al-Ghazzali's ethics of jihad as a work on the self, a refinement of character by freeing oneself from this-worldly attachments. Pandolfo argues that, in this mode, jihad names an eschatological ethics of a self born in the "experience of finitude," where the next world occupies the horizon of this one (345). Its trajectory of self-creation through an encounter with alterity, to which many are impelled by despair, is intertwined with the path of illegal migration from Morocco: "In both cases, the long-term horizon is made possible by the opening of a gap, a departure from one's 'self' and one's attachments" (347). Pandolfo perceives the theological premises of this ethics as fragmentary and debatable; they do not partake of a secure symbolic authority, nor do they constitute the grounds of an unproblematic belonging to a religious community. Submission to God's will is a deeply confounding enterprise in this context, and ethical subjectivation through divine law thus appears in other terms, as a "solitary and eclectic" (346) practice of self-authorization grounded only in the subject's own responsibility.

For Pandolfo, this solitary struggle for life attests to the robust reflexivity of the subjects who undertake it; though it carries the threat of extinction, the eschatology of the burning is not a true closure of subjectivity. But acute despair threatens such a closure and may end in the utter abjection of madness or the unsanctified death of suicide. Pandolfo follows this despair to another existential space beyond the theologically grounded ethical de/subjectivation in an encounter with finitude—to the space of the uncanny, on the verge of which these youth of urban Morocco are stranded. The appeal of the burning that draws them in this place is not a desire but a compulsion, an "addiction" that "befalls" them in the way that death might (353), luring them into the "end of time" (354). Ethics can dwell in eschatology, but not in the uncanny. To the extent that the burning permits an ethics to be chosen, then, Pandolfo understands it as an ethics of self-fortification for this confrontation with obliteration—an "art of danger," of "cultivating the volition and skills of a healer, who develops the interior strength to encounter the demonic without being seized" (352). In her participation in this debate over the burning, as in her listening to Roqiya's song, Pandolfo sees a possibility for ethics in the space of radical alterity, beyond all normative criteria of subjectivity. But she broaches this possibility as an open question to be answered according to the singular coordinates of the lives at stake. For some—those who reach the uncanny space of compulsion—the answer may be "no."

29. See Faubion 2001b: 97.

30. Rose 1999: 154. See also Beck 1992; and Lupton 1999.

31. Foucault 1991; Rose 1989, 1999.

32. Castel 1981; Cohen 1985; Ierodiakonou 1983a, b, c; Ierodiakonou with Iakovidis and Bikos 1983; Rose 1989, 1998, 1999.

33. In her second book on the trials of culture in postcolonial Australia, Elizabeth Povinelli (2002) develops a pertinent analysis of nondiscursive experience through which bodies and affects are implicated in reasoned ethical discourse in its appeal to freedom. The opening scene of the text registers the "panic" of a native woman provoked by the deliberations of her community over authorizing a mining venture that might alleviate some of its poverty, while at the same time threatening its traditional claim to the land. Povinelli reads this woman's panic as the "corporeal index" of a competition between her affective and rational "levels of obligation" (2–3). Similarly, she attributes to the "shifting grounds" of public debate over intolerance toward "repugnant" traditional cultural practices a rising "nausea" among native and settler Australians (28), enjoined in asymmetrical but equally disjunctive ways to enact their commitments to a "national meta-ethics" of multiculturalism (17). Povinellli takes such affective experiences as signs of a "superanimation" of liberalism—feelings that supply a reason beyond reason to account for the moral obligations that incite those metaethics (16). In her view, they symptomatically express an "impasse of discursive and moral orders" (3) in liberalism—a "non-passage" from moral sensibility to reasoned, enlightened discourse

in the operations of obligation (14), itself regulated by the law of recognition that evaluates traditional culture in Australia and determines its present compensation for the damage wrought by colonialism. Her critical analysis of liberalism in this context therefore turns, ethnographically, to diverse scenes of the peculiarly affective moralism of Australian multiculturalism: its demand that citizens commit themselves liberally to the national community by way of their feelings about how others should feel about traditional culture, even as they appeal to the abstract, discursive, rational structure of law to mediate those feelings (27).

34. Lakoff (2005) discusses in depth this failure to "stabilize" psychiatric nosology (2, 38). See also Young 1995; and Luhrmann 2000.

35. In Vita, João Biehl (2005) considers the possibility of a mad ethics. He presents Vita, a custodial (or, arguably, rehabilitative) institution in Porto Allegre, Brazil, as a residual space generated by social and economic liberalization in Brazil, occupied by increasing numbers of marginal or "useless" citizens abandoned by their families and communities, the state, and perhaps themselves: the addicted, the severely disabled, the mentally ill, or those dying from untreated diseases. The institution of Vita emerges, in this work, in counterpoint to the story of Catarina, a resident struggling not to slip into its space of social death. In her case, Biehl says, "medical science has become a tool of common sense, foreclosing various possibilities of empathy and experience. . . . Both the empirical reality through which living became practically impossible for Catarina and the possibility of critique have been sealed up" (258). In relief to this sealed-up and intractable reality, Biehl traces the emergence of Catarina's voice—the advent of an "I"—through her writing, "bordering on poetry," of a set of dictionaries: a massive trove of words concatenated in metonymic chains that name the nodal points of her memory, including the events that led to her abandonment in Vita. In Biehl's view, Catarina's writing "grounds an ethics" that guides her memory (24): like the small objects carried around by other residents of the institution (211), her words materialize her tie to her family, to a past and a life before and outside Vita—a route back to the social and political order of recognition, not through a moralism of "good or evil directed at her" (278), but through her attachment to the positivity of the tie. For Biehl, this nonmoralistic attachment constitutes an ethics, at least in the specific case of Catarina. Yet it seems that the attachments fostered by other residents of Vita may not—perhaps, I speculate, because they are frozen in dead objects, which mount only a mute protest against abandonment, rather than opening onto the world through language. While I am persuaded by this gradation of ethical capacities among dehumanized (or, as Biehl cautiously puts it, "ex-human") subjects, I would not want presumptively to bind "mad ethics" exclusively to discursive forms of expression; I also imagine nondiscursive symptoms of mental illness as candidates for ethical practice.

36. See Foucault's discussion of ethics in relation to the will to truth in Nietzsche (Foucault 1998b, 1997b).

37. Ellen Corin discusses "figures of the negative" in her own clinical practice (for instance, the appearance of transformative "void spaces" that are absences, more than silences, in analytic sessions) and in the philosophy of language and symbolization, from Hegelian negation to Derridean *différance*. The work of the negative, as she takes it, is to "rupture" and "destructure" representation, to "unveil the opaque, inaudible, and unknowable inherent in every narrative" (2007: 304–5). While this work of the void is dangerous, she suggests that it may, for some, free a space for a kind of creativity—though she insists that negativity is not, itself, equivalent to creativity. Pandolfo renders a Moroccan figure of the negative that resonates profoundly with those described by Corin: the figure of *fitna*, "a polysemic concept at the limit of representation and thought, mark of an intractable difference, fracture, rift, schism, disjunction, or separation—separation from oneself—the figure of an exile that is constitutive of the position of the subject, as both a possibility and a loss" (1997: 5).

38. This attempt, on the level of methodology, is my response to the debate between Jacques Derrida (1978) and Michel Foucault (1998a) on madness as a limit that either constitutes or is foreclosed by reason—argued in terms of the status of madness vis-à-vis the dream as cause for intellectual doubt in Cartesian rationalism. This debate can be construed as a conflict between the normativity of reasoning about madness and the negativity of madness as unreason. In my view, negativity does not disappear at the moment when madness is reduced to mental illness in the normative discourse of modern psychiatry, as Foucault construes the "division" that silenced madness in the nineteenth century (1988b: ix). The practice of reason yet sustains a relationship with negativity: the unknown, the destructive, the alter of reason. But madness need not be treated as negativity *as such* to register the ravages it wreaks on reasoned attempts to reduce it. (For Foucault, even the "dark freedom," the corrosive void, the "possibility of abolishing both man and world" that he sees represented in Goya's *Madhouse*, however exquisite an iconography of negativity, was but a positive historical form of it [1988b: 279].) The question that this conflict between normativity and negativity makes possible, in the analytic space between Derrida and Foucault—a question posed by philosophy to a nominalist anthropology—is: what difference to madness is made by its present normative constraints? The questions of method that I raise in this book concerning the diagnosis of madness in the contemporary clinic are ancillary to this more fundamental problem. In my view, a strictly nominalist analysis that would eschew the philosophical formulation of madness as pure negativity, and insist on its normativity as the sole legitimate site of analysis, compounds the moralism of clinical judgment with a moralism of critique.

39. Simon contends that for Plato, "sicknesses of the psyche are equated with vice," noting this passage from *The Sophist*: "Cowardice, intemperance, and injustice . . . all alike are forms of disease in the psyche" (quoted in Simon 1980: 168).

1. Madianos 1994; Blue 1991: 335, quoting Mavreas 1987.

2. See Madianos 1994 for an authoritative account of Greek psychiatric reform from within the academy. Blue 1991 records a condensed version of this narrative, which the author gathered from senior psychiatrists at four major hospitals in Greece in the late 1980s. I heard it from clinicians at Alexandroupolis as well as the B' University Clinic at Stavroupolis Psychiatric Hospital in Thessaloniki, one of the major clinical engines of reform, where I worked in the summer of 2000.

3. Sakellaropoulos 1995.

4. Ibid., 51–52.

5. Ibid., 50.

6. Blue 1991: 339.

7. Ibid., 332–33.

8. Ierodiakonou 1983a, 1983b, 1983c; Ierodiakonou with Iakovidis and Bikos 1983; Paraschos 1983.

9. Michalis Madianos emerged as a key figure in psychiatric reform as it evolved through the 1980s. He has since published the definitive work on the history of psychiatric reform in Greece (see Madianos 1994).

10. The five points of comparison between European systems of psychiatric care were: (1) the existence of special legislation regarding the mentally ill; (2) the geographical sectorization of psychiatric services; (3) the operation of advisory councils and scientific coordinating committees; (4) the existence of a national institute for research on mental health; and (5) the implementation of a system for evaluating the efficiency of the services offered. These infrastructural criteria were added to other bases of comparison, such as the per capita saturation of services, psychiatrists, medical staff, beds, and various kinds of institutions and services. Other European nations had better ratios. A regional breakdown within Greece according to these measures illustrated the centralized nature of the system (Stefanis and Madianos 1980: 242).

11. Ibid., 241.

12. Ibid., 246. See also Paraschos 1983 for a proposal, ultimately abandoned, to build small regional hospitals.

13. This separation was enacted formally in 1981. See Blue 1991: 338; Stylianidis and Papadakos 2000: 348.

14. Stefanis and Madianos 1980: 248.

15. Ibid., 249.

16. Upon the activation of the Maastricht Treaty in 1993, the EEC (European Economic Community) took the new name and new form of the EU (European Union).

17. See Luhrmann 2000; Lakoff 2005.

18. Campbell and Shaw 2009; Castel, Castel, and Lovell 1982; Lester 2009; Rose 1998, 1999.

19. According to Castel, the construction of this sectorial *dispositif* in France required that psychiatry, always perched awkwardly between magic and science, justify its "originality" and its necessity as a medical specialty. This involved, on the one hand, a differentiation from neurology on the basis of its object, conceived as a "relational" rather than an "organic" disorder; and on the other, an obedience to "scientific principles," notably in the use of psychoactive medications available from the 1950s onward and the later emphasis on genetic research. After 1968, sectorial psychiatry acquired political legitimacy from its unstable alliance with psychoanalysis, which purported to "incarnate the truth of the political critique of psychiatry" (1981: 25), and which provided a "fixed model" for approaching the "problematic of the subject" (12). Castel reads the "political neutrality" of psychoanalysis, derived from its autonomy from the state, as a kind of quietism, since the "struggle for liberation is carried out in 'the other scene,'" rather than in the socioeconomic field (26).

20. Castel 1991: 281.

21. Ibid., 291.

22. Castel 1981: 153, 1991: 295.

23. Castel 1991: 281–82.

24. Castel 1981: 126, 128.

25. Ibid., 127.

26. Ibid., 139–40.

27. Ibid., 137.

28. Castel 1991: 281.

29. There was not, for example, a single Alcoholics Anonymous chapter in the entire district of Thrace in 2003, despite disproportionately high rates of alcoholism in the region.

30. Rose 1998: 196 (quoting Baistow 1994), 12, 153.

31. Blue 1991: 339; Stylianidis and Papadakos 2000: 348; COM 2: 20.

32. Ierodiakonou 1983b. In Greece, the medical degree results from a six-year undergraduate program, followed by one year of rural service and specialized residencies of various lengths and compositions.

33. Quoted in Sakellaropoulos 1995: 57.

34. COM 2: 7.

35. According to Blue (1991: 2–16), a group of young doctors assigned to Leros for their rural medical service in 1981 were so horrified by the inhumane conditions they encountered there that they brought their findings to the press and lobbied the Ministry of Health to halt new admissions to the hospital until reforms were undertaken. The European press picked up the story, and soon Leros became a political quagmire in Greece and an international scandal. It was the only psychiatric hospi-

tal singled out for special improvement programs in EEC measure 815/84 (see note below).

I discovered, soon after I met him, that a psychiatric resident at the hospital in Alexandroupolis had completed part of his residency at Leros. He told me that, despite the desperate state of most of the patients who lived there, it was a desirable place to go for residency: due to special funding from the European Union, it had the best equipment and the highest salaries of any psychiatric setting in Greece. After the scandal, he said, certain reforms were undertaken at Leros, and now some one hundred patients were cared for "very well." They were housed in new semi-independent houses throughout the island and participated in occupational therapy and other activities. But this is a front, he told me. The other four hundred to five hundred patients still live at the main hospital. Conditions have definitely changed there since 1990, but these people still don't receive anything like adequate care. They live an institutional life, like in the bad old days. What upset me most were the children in the back ward: deformed, sick, mentally retarded, mostly abandoned by parents who couldn't care for them. And what could the psychiatrists do about it? It broke my heart.

36. The other portion of this fund was reserved for the development of vocational training in urban areas not already covered by the European regional development fund (OJ 1). The proportion of total funding diverted to each program shifted in the course of implementation, depending on the specific projects proposed each year. In March 1989, funding for psychiatric reform projects was suspended, and thus vocational training projects started to be proportionately "overfunded" (OJ 5: 11).

The ECU (European Currency Unit), based on the combinatory weighted values of the national currencies of EEC member states, was an artificial accounting unit used in the European Monetary System created in 1979. The ECU was replaced at a 1:1 ratio by the Euro, a real currency, in January 1999. See McCormick 1999: 75; Gandolfo 1987: 380–93, 404–11.

37. Monies were to be disbursed in the form of 60 percent advances when projects commenced, with the balance to be paid within a year of their completion. This procedure explains the frequent accounting of figures in commission documents as percentages of percentages, and references to the "cancellation" of funds already disbursed (OJ 1).

38. OJ 5: 12.

39. OJ 2.

40. Ibid. The funding for this committee's "technical assistance, assessment, and monitoring of projects" would be derived from the existing reform package. This meant 100 percent of its funding, an amount not to exceed 2 percent of the total award of 120 million ECU (OJ 2; OJ 4).

41. COM 1: 3.

42. OJ 5.

43. COM 2: 23.

44. OJ 5: 9, 11; COM 2: 23.

45. OJ 5: 3.

46. OJ 5: 4.

47. Stylianidis and Papadakos 2000: 348–49.

48. Included in the original measure 815/84 was funding for five small projects at Leros, including group homes, rehabilitation facilities and programs, and staffing investments. Hardly any of these projects was completed by 1989. The auditors observed that an attempt at "restructuring" had been made, but "from the point of view of the treatment of patients, the situation ha[d] remained unchanged" (OJ 5: 5). The new plan, called Leros I, was to be implemented in 1991–92, but delays continued. The plan was revised once again, renamed Leros II, and finally completed in 1993–94.

49. COM 2: 24.

50. COM 2.

51. These residences, in decreasing order of the intensity of needs among the patients who live in them, include permanent group homes (οικοτροφεία), short-term halfway houses (ξενώνες), and sheltered apartments (προστατευμένα διαμερίσματα).

52. COM 2: 6.

53. OJ 5: 12. Stylianidis and Papadakos (2000: 349) break down that average admission length by type of care center: 159 days for psychiatric hospitals, 97 days for private clinics, and 15 days for inpatient units in general hospitals.

54. For more detailed discussions of Psychargos, see Karastergiou et al. 2005; Madianos and Christodoulou 2007; Tountas, Karnaki, and Pavi 2002; WHO 2001: 33–34.

55. Stylianidis and Papadakos 2000: 351.

56. Sakellaropoulos 1995: 58.

57. Ibid.

58. Blue 1991: 319–20.

59. Stylianidis and Papadakos 2000: 349.

60. Madianos 1994: 275.

61. Blue 1991: 319, 326 (quoting Athanasiou 1989).

62. See note (70), below.

63. Stylianidis and Papadakos 2000: 349.

64. Ibid., 354.

65. Ierodiakonou 1983b.

66. See also Blue 1991: 350, 371.

67. Ierodiakonou 1983a, 1983b, 1983c; Ierodiakonou with Iakovidis and Bikos 1983.

68. See Paraschos 1985.

69. Association for Social Psychiatry and Mental Health 2002b: 8.

70. The IKA (Social Insurance Institute), a massive semiprivate insurance agency in Greece, also employs its own physicians. The agency's centers are dispersed throughout the country; in some areas, they are the only accessible source of healthcare. See part 2 for a discussion of IKA's role in psychiatric care provision in Thrace.

71. Paraschos 1985.

72. See Paraschos 1985; Sakellaropoulos 1995a.

73. Stylianidis and Papadakos 2000: 353.

74. Lakoff (2005: 8, 47, 65) documents a similar development in the mental health movement in Argentina, which embraced both social and pharmaceutical psychiatry as "humanizing" modes of care.

75. Association for Social Psychiatry and Mental Health 2002b: 2–3.

76. Ibid., 7–8.

PART 1. FALSE FACE

1. See the 2002 *Webster's Third New International Dictionary*, s.v. "diagnosis"; "dia-"; and "know." Compare Bambinioti 2002: 478.

2. Geertz 1983: 24–25. The essay, "Blurred Genres," was first published in 1980 (*The American Scholar* 49 [2]: 165–79).

3. Foucault 1997b: 295.

4. Ibid.

5. This is perhaps why Crapanzano, though he offers a critique of semantico-referential metapragmatics, cannot propose a fully *pragmatic* metapragmatics for Western social science: such a knowledge cannot be intelligibly valorized in that truth game.

6. Foucault 1997b: 296.

7. Foucault 1982: 346.

8. Bourdieu 1991: 19.

9. Ibid., 33.

10. Ibid., 80, 66.

11. Ibid., 67.

12. Ibid., 105. Only the observer of the game, who steps out of play and construes its logic, can "totally brea[k] the spell, the *illusio*, renouncing all stakes, that is, all the gambles on the future" (82). Bourdieu's attribution of *illusio* to the logic (*ratio*) of game-playing shows that practice, too, is a truth game, but only for the observer seeking "objective" knowledge. See Rabinow 1996 (esp. 7–13) for a critique of Bourdieu's concept of *illusio* and of the corresponding method he proposes for objective scientific practice.

13. Bourdieu 1991: 71–72, 73.

14. Ibid., 67.

15. Ibid., 85, 86. Judith Farquhar (1994) finds coherence in practice by a different route. Encountering "apparent contradictions" between explanations of symptoms and treatments in traditional Chinese medicine (1), and failing to elicit a theoretical resolution to these contradictions from practitioners themselves, she comes to understand the valorization of practical logic over theoretical abstractions in this particular truth game. She thus refuses Bourdieu the privilege of *always* allocating the universal value of truth to the objectivity of the system rather than to the efficacy of the practice.

16. Bourdieu 1991: 130, 133, 136.

17. See "Common Sense as a Cultural System" in Geertz 1983.

18. Ibid., 56, 59.

19. Ibid., 82.

20. Ibid., 102.

21. Lévi-Strauss 1963: 167–85.

22. See part 3 for a discussion of Basaglia's influence on Greek psychiatric reform. See Giordano (2011) for a comprehensive account of his legacy in Italy, and a discussion of the resonance between his work and that of Frantz Fanon in a contemporary Italian ethnopsychiatric clinic.

23. Neither Basaglia nor Laing, however, identified himself with the antipsychiatry movement. See note 31 below.

24. Goffman 1961a.

25. See Rabinow 1983 on the method of "bracketing truth" in anthropology. While he argues that this practice, grounded in cultural relativism, promotes ethical nihilism, I am pointing instead to the way that this relativism manages, despite itself, to promote culturally specific values.

26. See, for example, Estroff 1981; Good 1992; and Luhrmann 2000.

27. See Lakoff 2005.

28. Lewis 2006; Petryna, Lakoff, and Kleinman 2006.

29. Lakoff (2005) documents this remarkable practice under the rubric of "diagnostic truing."

30. While I focus here on language and diagnosis in community-based care, Livia Velpry makes a similar point about language and psychotherapy in France: "It is important how what the patient says organizes and structures the therapeutic framework: the patient's words are clinical material that providers use during treatment. It is apparent that by changing the regime from imposition to collaboration, and thus modifying the patient's position in his or her relationships with care providers, the status of discourse and the definition and limits of therapy are altered." Velpry 2008: 251.

31. Rather than a discrete and monolithic movement, antipsychiatry is perhaps best understood as a retrospective label for a disparate array of critical theories and experimental practices emerging across Europe and the United States between the 1950s and 1970s. See Foucault 2006; Scheper-Hughes and Lovell 1987; and

Giordano (2011) for accounts of this array. In his course summary for the Collège de France, Foucault dates the "age of antipsychiatry" to the "suspicion, and soon after the certainty, that Charcot actually produced the hysterical fit he described" (2006: 341). Distinguishing antipsychiatry from the "movement for 'depsychiatrization'" (342) inaugurated by critics of Jean-Martin Charcot, Foucault argues that "what is at stake in antipsychiatry . . . is not at all the truth value of psychiatry in terms of knowledge (of diagnostic accuracy or therapeutic effectiveness). The struggle with, in, and against the institution is at the heart of antipsychiatry" (344).

32. Clare 2003; Breggin 2008; Good 1992; Hacking 1999; Healey 1997, 2002; Lakoff 2005; Lewis 2006.

33. Crapanzano 1992: 12.

34. Crapanzano ventures the psychological metaphor of repression here in the same mode of playful speculation with which he places in parentheses the question: "(Is it possible that what we call 'unconscious' is that which is masked in any communicative exchange and *placed*, for whatever reasons, somewhere, in the psyche?)" (1992: 24).

35. Byron Good argues in a similar direction, showing that ethnographers have conventionally relied on an empiricist notion of language in regard to "belief," taking the "sincere assertions" of native theorists as the accurate representation of behavioral rationales that, themselves, remain fundamentally discrepant from social scientific (i.e., "true") knowledge (Good 1994 [esp. chap. 1]).

36. Crapanzano 1998: 739–41, esp. 741n11.

37. Austin 1965.

38. Szasz 1974: 138.

39. Ibid., 210–11.

40. Ibid., 215.

41. This communication, though mobilized around psychiatric expertise, is not an array of what Hubert Dreyfus and Paul Rabinow, in their critique of Foucault's archaeology, call "serious speech acts"—claims whose truth is constituted by the rules of a game of expert knowledge "autonomous" from the "everyday" or "pragmatic" context in which the claims are spoken (Dreyfus and Rabinow 1983: 48, 54). Psychiatric expertise here is not a discrete discursive arena in which the seriousness of a diagnostic claim can be analyzed independently of its use. The truth of diagnostic words is, instead, put to pragmatic use by patients and therapists when they bind one another to their responsibilities through moralism.

42. Crapanzano 1992 (esp. chap. 6), 1998.

43. Pandolfo 1997, 2006.

44. Ewing 2006b: 90.

45. Foucault argues that "relations of power," meaning "relationship[s] in which one person tries to control the conduct of the other," are possible only when the subjects of the relation are free—however relative, limited, and contingent that

freedom may be. These relations, operating within the field of ethics only on the "ontological condition" of freedom, are thus not determined or determinative but "mobile, reversible, and unstable" (1997b: 284, 292).

46. Nietzsche 1947: 281.

47. Ibid., 282.

48. This approach is inspired by Stefania Pandolfo, who, in her rendering of poetic, philosophical, sacred, and everyday speech in the Dra' Valley of southern Morocco, attends "to the concrete way things are said, to a reflection on the specific vocabularies, rhetorical figures, and conceptual configurations" (1997: 5).

49. Ibid., 4, 6, 312n7; Deleuze 1989: 223–24.

50. Rose 1998: 177.

51. Ibid., 178, 174, 178.

52. Ibid., 178, 186.

53. Crapanzano 1992: 24.

54. Goffman 1961a; Young 1995.

55. Kleinman 1995.

56. Cohen 1998: 301.

57. American Psychiatric Association 2000.

58. Berlant 2000: 1, 6.

59. Szasz 1979: 124.

60. Szasz 1974: 227.

61. Lacan developed a theory of desire as the truth of the subject and charted Freud's invention of the psychoanalytic procedure to discover this truth through a strategic reduction of symptoms to signifiers. For Freud, Lacan says, the dread "other" situated in this field of truth is not the *deceiving* God of the Cartesian nightmare but a "*deceived* Other" (1978: 37)—the analyst himself, whom the patient fears misleading, and who can indeed be misled. The patient's unconscious desire to deceive the analyst is "that truth which makes it perfectly possible, contrary to the supposed paradox, to declare, *I am lying*" (37–38). This deception does not undermine analysis, because the patient's speech is granted symbolic value in its signification of motive rather than its semantic reference.

62. Lacan makes this assertion in a discussion of deception, which characterizes the "reality of the hysteric" that impelled Freud's invention of the analytic procedure (1978: 32–3).

63. Certeau 1986: 55–56.

64. As I noted earlier, the "illusion" of the game for Bourdieu is the repression of its objective truth, and the "self-deception" of its players about that repressed truth is a condition of the game's social function. The overt deception of others can only be a tactic in such a game, never a threat to the pragmatic illusion that makes it work. Thomas Szasz offers a similarly functionalist view of deception, through a different classification. He argues that lying constitutes a distinct strategy or mode of play rather than a mere tactic in a game of communication: where honest game-

playing aims at mastering a task or skill, dishonest game-playing aims at controlling the opponent (1974: 226). For the hysteric, who nurtures the ambivalent hope that her lies will be both "unmasked" and accepted as true (224), lying is a means of managing risk by "controlling the response of the other player[s]," because the hysteric is better able to predict their responses to lies than to truth. This is especially so in cases where the hysteric and her advocates have entered a chronic situation of collusion, where all players tacitly acknowledge and tolerate lying because it serves a stabilizing function in their relationships. In such games, which therapists can also play, dishonest communication is a negotiation of power: for one player to accept the other's lies is an acknowledgment of their mutual dependence, as well as their mutual attachment to the game (227).

Because dishonesty may promote greater relational stability and attachment than honesty, Szasz considers lying a "reasonable" and often a *winning* strategy for patients. He valorizes H. S. Sullivan's (1966) portrait of hysteria as "inexplicit malingering," enacted by the patient to "satisfy unacceptable impulses in a personally satisfactory way which exempts him from social blame" (Szasz 1974: 220). On this view, the suffering of the hysteric is actually a masked "stratagem." Less inclined than Sullivan to see hysterical symptoms as "unconscious" or "unwitting" (218), however, Szasz considers them "moral choices" that take dishonest communication as their medium (222). While he thus charges patients with personal responsibility for these choices, he is not inclined to moralize about them; rather, he issues a therapeutic mandate to maximize choices, including dishonesty, that are available to patients in determining their own behavioral strategies (259).

65. Bourdieu 1991: 107.

66. McKinney (2007: 286–87) observes a different norm of credulity among therapists treating victims of trauma—especially the trauma of war and of state or insurgent violence, about which patients' accounts may be instrumentalized in legal testimony for asylum claims. McKinney shows a norm of not doubting the truth (the "accuracy") of a patient's account—as distinct from its reality *for the patient*—emerging from therapists' attainment to the status of "ethical witness" to the patient's trauma. This status is premised, moralistically, on the innocence of the patient, which excludes the possibility of fantasy or a pathological process at work in the patient's account of trauma.

67. American Psychiatric Association 2000: 298–302.

68. Ibid., 299.

69. Velpry 2008: 247.

70. Ibid., 246. She notes that therapists consider "covertly delusional" those patients "who appear 'normal' and well-functioning in superficial conversations, but who are revealed to have delusional thinking in more profound exchanges." The covertness or overtness of a patient's thinking seems to have little bearing on the criteria therapists use to determine it as "valid" or "delusional."

71. Ibid., 241.

72. Ibid., 243.

73. *Retsina* is a type of wine made with pine resin. It is considered an ancient and traditional Greek drink, widely and often cheaply available, including at street-corner kiosks and hospital cafeterias.

74. Sakellaropoulos 1995: 411.

75. Greater clarity cannot be introduced into my analysis of the critical diagnostic terms at stake here—*intention, motive, consciousness, desire, illness, pathology*—than inhered in their usage. Their opacity, contingent redundancy, and situational inaptness are features of this usage that cannot be overcome. Instead, my analysis takes the shape of their broad field of reference, and identifies moments when meanings and distinctions can be pinpointed in the context of usage. Thus, with experience in these psychiatric settings, I came to understand that patients with personality disorders were disliked and treated with less respect than patients presenting clinical disorders. This implicit understanding made sense of a more explicit diagnostic division between clinical and personality disorders that appeared to carry a moral distinction between intentions and motives—which in turn appeared to rest on a context-specific conception of consciousness. This is not to conclude that "the unconscious" as such has a specific definition for clinicians in Thrace that refers to that set of distinctions. The "economical" logic of this truth game does not exercise such control over the field of semantic reference.

76. American Psychiatric Association 2000: 685.

77. Ibid., 308–9.

78. Ibid., 685–86. Obsessive-compulsive personality disorder should not be confused with obsessive-compulsive disorder, classified as a more severe clinical (Axis I) anxiety disorder.

79. Feighner et al. 1972: 60.

80. See Rhodes 2004 for an incisive discussion of the nexus between antisociality and criminality, as between the medical and penal systems, in the United States.

81. American Psychiatric Association 2000: 513, 705, 739.

82. Ibid., 702–3; Cleckley 1941: 208.

83. American Psychiatric Association 2000: 705–6.

84. Ibid., 513–15.

85. This ambivalence about patients with personality disorders is not unique to the clinics of Thrace. Tanya Luhrmann (2000), for example, describes the feelings of guilt experienced by a cohort of U.S. psychiatric residents in their work with patients diagnosed with personality disorders (112–18). These residents often blamed the patients for their own suffering—in stark contrast to patients with clinical disorders who, as one therapist put it, "'[come] by their diagnosis honestly'" (115; emphasis added). Luhrmann notes that these residents learned to diagnose personality disorders not through the "disease model" of mental illness, but through the "interaction model" of psychodynamic therapy, by analyzing their

countertransference with patients (112). Rebecca Lester (2009), also working in an American clinical setting, likewise observes the recourse made by therapists to the dynamics of transference and countertransference in their "borderline talk," when deciding on treatment for "difficult" patients whom they suspected were manipulating them with self-destructive behaviors that came to seem "incurable" in the rationality of managed care (33). At the hospital clinic in Alexandroupolis, however, residents and clinicians rarely referred to transference and countertransference when discussing their personal reactions to "difficult" patients. Rather than naturalizing their suspicion or hostility toward these patients as products of challenging clinical encounters, they often phrased these reactions in terms of cultural difference (see part 2).

86. See João Biehl's (2005) discussion of Geertz (1983) on "common sense," and his use of this concept to analyze the contingent structure of expectations and foreclosures that make it seem reasonable to forget a "mad" or "useless" person, and neglect to sustain her life.

87. See Winnicott 1971, 1992.

88. See Sakellaropoulos's article, "Psychoanalytic Psychotherapy and Public Health Care" (1989), reprinted in Sakellaropoulos 1995: 693–708.

89. Sakellaropoulos 1995: 696.

90. Ibid., 698.

91. Ibid., 700–701.

92. See Lacan 1992: 31.

93. See Gal 1991; Herzfeld 1991.

94. Foucault 2003: 10.

95. Spivak 1999: 384; see also Spivak 1994.

INTERLUDE: THE JEWEL OF GREECE

1. Taussig 1999: 51.

PART 2. STRANGERS

1. Campbell 1964; du Boulay 1974, 1976; Friedl 1962; Gilmore 1987a; Herzfeld 1987b; Péristiany 1966.

2. Gilmore 1987b: 11. See Herzfeld 1985 for a distinct view on Greek masculinity.

3. Gilmore 1987a: 94–96.

4. In "Lies, Mockery, and Family Integrity," Juliet du Boulay renders a taxonomy of lies and their motives—from "family defense" to "self-interest" to "mischief" to "slander"—that fall within "self-limiting" cultural parameters in central Greece. She notes that, since these legitimate forms of lying are subject to normative sanc-

tions oriented to the "sacred world" symbolized by the household, they do not disrupt social "equilibrium" but, on the contrary, serve to mediate between "love and trust within the house" and "hostility" outside it (du Boulay 1976: 400, 393).

5. In Tuhami: Portrait of a Moroccan (1980), for example, Crapanzano portrays Moroccan culture as one that is especially hostile to realism in language. He describes the "mode of social organization" in traditional Morocco that involves the continual negotiation of reciprocity and mutual advantage between dyads in a large network of social relationships (78). Truth becomes a contextual matter of what people engaged in dialogue want from each other and what kinds of relationships they create when they talk. Although to outsiders this kind of negotiation appears incoherent, contradictory, or dishonest (80), Crapanzano argues that it represents a coherent attitude toward truth: a relativist, pragmatic, and rhetorical orientation that is based in the locally circumscribed, mutually dependent, and constantly changing nature of dialogic social relationships. Among traditional Moroccans, according to Crapanzano, the Western psychological notion of an internalized conscience, or superego, is not the site of morality; personal guilt does not play a role in controlling individual behavior. Instead, the "social honor" of the individual (79) constitutes an exterior, public "locus of propriety" (78), and it is the threat of public exposure—shame—that functions as the moral regulator of society, obliging people to fulfill their promises and discharge their debts (78). Language, in this pragmatic orientation to honor and shame, does not simply or primarily represent what is "real." To characterize the distance between speech and reality in this context as hypocrisy, then, stems from a confusion of cultural categories: "hypocrisy" imputes a psychological interior where there is only a public face.

6. Herzfeld 2005: 6, 3.

7. See Demetriou 2004 for a discussion of Pomak and its shifting relation to Turk in Greek and Turkish nationalist discourses on the Muslim minority of Thrace, as well as emergent multiculturalist discourses. See also Hart 1999 for a parallel discussion of Albanian and Greek communal demarcations in regard to the politics of blood, culture, Islam, and Christianity in the borderland between Greece and Albania; Karakasidou 1997 on problems of integration and identification faced by refugees from Asia Minor in Greek Macedonia; and Voutira 2003 on the resonance or repetition of those problems faced by Pontian immigrants in Greek Thrace.

8. Herzfeld (1987a): 189.

9. Ibid., 85, 75.

10. Ibid., 64.

11. Panourgiá 1995: 8.

12. See Hirschon 1993 for an account of the gendered division of "open" and "closed" bodies and spaces in "traditional" Greek culture, which strongly resonates with Evyenia's description.

13. See Arvaniti et al. 2009 for a study, conducted by members of the psychiatric

staff at the hospital clinic in Alexandroupolis, on the persistent problem of stigma toward the mentally ill, even among health workers and medical students at the General Regional University Hospital of Alexandroupolis.

14. See, for example, Ierodiakonou 1983a, 1983c; and Ierodiakonou with Iakovidis and Bikos 1983. A more recent study on psychological problems presented by Christian and Muslim patients at a primary healthcare clinic in Iasmos, Thrace, conducted in 2000 by psychiatric personnel from the General Hospital of Alexandroupolis, ventures this familiar explanation for the high rate of somatoform symptoms in this patient population: "Patients in Iasmos consult their GP almost exclusively for somatic reasons, even though a substantial portion of them suffer from mental health problems. Somatization may partly explain why psychological problems as reasons for consultation were so rare. The higher mean score among Moslems on the *somatic complaints* subscale . . . may be explained by the fact that the more traditional, poorly educated groups tend to focus their attention and worries on bodily signs indicative of a medical condition. Poor knowledge of psychological terminology may lead to a somatic, metaphoric way of experiencing, or at least describing, psychological distress" (Androutsopoulou et al. 2002: 292).

15. Ierodiakonou 1983a, 1983c; Ierodiakonou with Iakovidis and Bikos 1983. See the prelude for a discussion of his research and interventions in Thrace during the 1970s and 1980s. I met and interviewed Charalambos Ierodiakonou at AXEPA, the psychiatry ward in the General Hospital of Thessaloniki, in June 2000.

16. Ierodiakonou 1983c: 547.

17. Ibid., 546–47.

18. Ibid., 549.

19. Ibid., 548.

20. Ierodiakonou 1983a: 231; Ierodiakonou with Iakovidis and Bikos 1983: 521.

21. Ierodiakonou with Iakovidis and Bikos 1983: 521.

22. See Basaglia 1987: 283.

23. The word she used, κρίση, denotes a range of medical problems, including epileptic seizures and manic outbursts.

24. This term is a shortened form of *Pomak Mahometan*, a term used less frequently than simply *Pomak* to designate a reputedly Slavic ethnolinguistic group with ancestral ties to Bulgaria and political ties to Turkey, comprising about 30 percent of the Turkish-speaking Muslim population of Thrace.

25. See Mezzich et al. 1996 and Gaines 1992 for comprehensive collections on contemporary transcultural psychiatry and its influence on psychiatric practice internationally.

26. Livaditis 2003: 14–15.

27. Ibid., 582.

28. Ibid., 14.

29. These indices reappear in a study, coauthored by Miltos Livaditis, on Chris-

tian and Muslim patients seeking primary healthcare at a rural clinic in Iasmos, Thrace (about seventy kilometers from Alexandroupolis): "The area is characterized by a high degree of traditionality, i.e., strong family and community bonds, well defined, long-standing social roles and responsibilities, gender-based discrimination with restricted autonomy for women" (Androutsopoulou et al. 2002: 286).

30. American Psychiatric Association 2000: 897–903. See Charles C. Hughes's critique of the classificatory and terminological assumptions undergirding "culture-bound syndrome" in the (then forthcoming) DSM-IV, and the positioning of its Appendix I as an "afterthought" (Mezzich et al. 1996: 289–307).

31. American Psychiatric Association 2000: 487; emphasis added.

32. Blue 1991; Danforth 1989; Dunk 1989; Lock 1989, 1990.

33. See Kleinman and Kleinman 1985.

34. Kleinman 1988: 14.

35. Kleinman 1995: 9, 10–11.

36. See Csordas 1994.

37. Scheper-Hughes 1992: 185–86.

38. Ibid., 196; Lock 1993: 142.

39. Lock 1989; Dunk 1989.

40. Livaditis 2003: 451–52.

41. Ibid., 444–64.

42. Livaditis 2003 cites a longitudinal study in Aegean outpatient clinics that showed a decrease in the rate of hysteria from 6 percent of cases in 1948–50 to 3 percent in 1969–71 (449).

43. Ibid. Though Livaditis does not cite him directly, this comparison is central to Arthur Kleinman's early work (see Kleinman and Kleinman 1985).

44. Kleinman comes to a similar, and similarly guarded, conclusion (1988: 48). Corin 2007 cites the finding of the International Pilot Study of Schizophrenia, "that the course and outcome of schizophrenia are more benign in that part of the world [India] than in Western societies"—as a point of departure for analyzing the role of Hindu "myth models" in articulating schizophrenic "limit-experiences" among patients in Chennai (289, 289, 300).

45. As, for example, Loring Danforth (1989) discusses the worship of Saint Constantine and the dancing-firewalking rituals of the Anastenaria in Macedonia; and as C. Nadia Seremetakis (1991, 1993) treats the mediation of pain and grief in mourning rituals practiced by Inner Maniats.

46. See João Biehl's (2005) discussion of the pharmaceuticalization of psychiatric care after deinstitutionalization in Brazil, which has in many cases taken shape in the drastic overmedication of patients as a form of chemical dependency.

47. The Muslim market here is called the "bazaar" (το παζάρι), to distinguish it from its Greek counterpart, the "folk market" (η λαϊκή [αγορά]).

48. Livaditis and Vorvolakos (2001) confirm this view: "Although Gypsies share

some cultural features with other Muslims in the area, especially in regard to language and religion, in other aspects of culture, as well as in ethnic origin, they present substantial cultural differences."

49. I discovered the reach of this imagined transnational community immediately on starting work at the Association. At our first meeting, Pandelis, a psychiatrist there, spoke to me of his Gypsy patients in Sapes, where he had been working for more than a year. *I really admire their value of loyalty,* he said. *You can see the same thing in* Snatch. (*Snatch* is a feature film released in 2000, starring Brad Pitt as a Gypsy boxer in Great Britain.)

50. Livaditis and Vorvolakos (2001) consider unemployment a characteristic feature of the Gypsy way of life: "A major obstacle faced by the Gypsies is that of unemployment, which functions as if it were natural, and contributes to their economic deprivation."

51. Livaditis 2003: 594.

52. Livaditis and Vorvolakos 2001.

53. In English, *psychopath*, the closest term morphologically to the Greek ψυχοπαθής, evokes a florid, violent psychosis that has little clinically to do with the syndrome in question. A better but still misleading English translation for the Greek ψυχοπαθητικός is "psychopathic."

54. In some diagnostic systems, antisocial personality disorder appears as "psychopathy" or "sociopathy," with slightly different clinical emphases. M. J. Rutherford, J. S. Cacciola, and A. I. Alterman (1999: 849, 851) point out that, while the sociopathy/psychopathy diagnosis, which is more common in European psychiatric practice, places more emphasis on character traits, the antisocial personality diagnosis in the DSM enumerates behaviors, thus bearing a wider scope of potential application but narrower psychomoral implications. See Gondles 1999 for a brief history of shifts in the usage of these diagnostic labels in U.S. psychiatry and popular culture.

55. Sakellaropoulos 1995: 239.

56. Ibid., 240.

57. It is worth noting local deviations from the gendered parameters of the antisocial diagnosis in Thrace. In the United States and Europe, diagnostic metrics for antisocial personality disorder were initially formulated through studies of male patient populations (Rutherford, Cacciol, and Alterman 1999: 850), while those for borderline personality disorder, associated with more "passive" or "self-destructive" traits and behaviors, focused on female patients. See Rhodes 2004; Lester 2009; and Nuckolls 1992 for discussions of the gendered behavioral symptoms of antisocial, histrionic, and borderline personality disorder in the United States. The antisocial type of the disorder appears more common among men than women in the American population: the DSM notes a prevalence of 3 percent in men versus 1 percent in women in the community sample studied by its working group

and a survey of psychiatric literature. Rates are much higher and more gender-skewed for specific patient populations, especially among substance abusers and prisoners (704). But the presentation of Gypsy patients in Thrace rarely fit this alignment of antisociality with gender. As therapists described it, antisociality was a more general cultural trait among Gypsies—one that described a destructive disposition toward oneself and others. Thus, while most Gypsies hospitalized for suicide attempts were women, many of these same patients were equally violent toward others, especially family members. In my experience, when a specific type of personality disorder was diagnosed in a Gypsy patient, it was more often "antisocial" than any other, regardless of the patient's gender.

58. Sakellaropoulos 1995: 241, 240.

59. Sakellaropoulos 1995: 240, 241.

60. Livaditis 2003: 594–95.

61. See Pandolfo 2008; Giordano 2008, 2011; and Fassin and Rechtman 2005 on the ways in which transcultural psychiatry and ethnopsychiatry may resurrect the cultural essentialisms of colonial rule—essentialisms that contain or forestall the political voice of ethnic and migrant patients in their demands for state recognition (in Morocco, Italy, and France, respectively).

62. See Lauren Berlant's discussion of the "culture" invoked in public health discourse on obesity among people of color in the United States—a notion of "endemic environment" in which people are imagined "already saturated by death and available for mourning, compelled by appetites rather than by strategies of sovereign agency toward class mobility" (Berlant 2007: 774).

63. Sakellaropoulos 1995: 242.

64. Ibid., 239.

65. Similarly, in an article on community-based therapy practiced in public schools by politicized therapists in postdictatorship Brazil, Dominique Behague (2008) notes the radical discrepancy of scale between social and individual psychological treatment, and the insufficiency of clinical models to redress social "inequities" and "conflicts" that dispose public school children to behavioral and emotional distress (216).

66. Blue 1991: 174–75.

67. Brown 1995: 53.

68. Ibid., 66. In a later work, Wendy Brown observes the tragic impossibility of surrendering the ideals that found political claims of injury in modern liberalism. Turning to Freud, she allegorizes the formation of political subjectivity in a libidinal framework of masochistic desire: a complex oscillation between the disavowal and the satisfaction of this desire stabilizes the subject's attachment to the political order that punishes it. From this process of subject formation, she suggests, emerges a "political personality" wrought in paranoid paralysis—a powerlessness to dislodge the masochistic structure of desire (Brown 2001: 58).

69. My analysis of this dependency takes a different direction from the critique

of medicalization proposed by anthropologists of "social suffering," who seek to address suffering without personalizing it in the psychological individual, nor pathologizing it in the constructions of biomedical rationality (as, for example, Kleinman [1995: 38, 177] sees the social effects of political violence treated as posttraumatic stress disorder). This critique preserves the distinction between political and medical etiologies so as not to reduce suffering to the institutional discourses of the state (as Veena Das [1995] shows in her work on the Bhopal disaster and other events of social trauma in India; see also Kleinman 1997: 318–19). This antinomy, however, establishes the condition for obfuscating equivalences: mental illness may appear primarily as an index of political crisis, while political crisis takes the social form of mental illness. These equivalences account, in my view, for a tendency in this literature to diagnose medicalization itself as a symptom of structural inequalities and social dysfunction in modern states, rather than viewing mental illness (such as antisocial personality disorder among Gypsy outpatients in Thrace) as a failure of the distinction between political and medical causes and effects.

70. Rebecca Lester similarly notes the peculiarly circular and expansive way in which a generic, ungrounded concept of culture operates in cross-cultural approaches to eating disorders: "Culture becomes something of a catchall term for anything not strictly psychological or biological, and . . . a way of displacing concerns that might otherwise require a more profound examination of the cultural bases of the diagnostic criteria themselves" (Lester 2004: 609).

71. Herzfeld 1992: 122.

72. Ibid., 77, 81.

73. Ibid., 73.

74. See Sarinay 2000 for a vehement argument, from a "Turkish point of view," on the Pontus issue and its "revision" in Greek historical scholarship. This revisionist history, according to Sarinay, excludes the Greek nationalist strategy of resettling Pontii from throughout the Ottoman lands to the small region along the eastern Black Sea to establish a "native" claim to the territory for the emergent Greek nation-state.

75. See Karpozilos 1991 on Pontian culture and language in the Greek minority under Soviet rule.

76. The treaty, which designates as "Christian" and "Moslem" the minority groups to be exchanged or exempted, is reprinted as the appendix in Hirschon 2003: 281–87. See Oran 2003 for a more detailed picture of the ethno-religio-linguistic landscape of Thrace at the time of the treaty.

77. Eftihia Voutira, citing a report from the Ministry of Macedonia and Thrace, estimates 140,000 Soviet Greeks emigrating to Greece by 1995, when state policy shifted from "welcoming" to "containing" Pontian immigration from the FSU (Voutira 2006: 396, 398). The total number of Pontian immigrants to Greece from the FSU was estimated at 160,000 by 2005 (Voutira 2006: 398; Edgar et al. 2005: 111), about one-fifth of whom settled in Thrace (Edgar et al. 2005: 111).

78. See Voutira 2003, 2006 on the Greek state's approach to Pontian immigrants in the 1920s and 1990s. See also Vergeti 1991 for a detailed demography of Pontian immigrants to Greece throughout the twentieth century. While the greatest surges in migration occurred during the 1920s (amounting to about four hundred thousand Pontian Greeks from Asia Minor) and the late 1980s to the mid-1990s, Vergeti notes smaller waves in the mid-1930s and mid-1960s.

79. Pontian immigration thus illuminates what Étienne Balibar calls the "polysemic nature" of borders: that is, "the simple fact that they do not have the same meaning for everyone," but are "designed . . . not merely to give individuals from different social classes different experiences of the law . . . but actively to differentiate between individuals in terms of social class" (Balibar 2002: 81–82). In this sense, the community of Pontian immigrants in Greece is ambivalent, intimate, uncanny—but not "clandestine," in the way Michèle Sinapi (2008) and Pierre Legendre (2007) discuss "known communities" of undocumented immigrants in Europe.

80. I have in mind Freud's famous case study on paranoia: an analysis of German Senate president Daniel Paul Schreber, based on Schreber's own memoir of his "nervous illness" published in 1903. In the study, Freud argues that paranoia can be traced to the subject's fixation at an early stage in libidinal development: the stage of homosexual desire, repressed under the force of social and familial prohibition. Barred from an external object of desire, the libido attaches instead to the subject's own ego, generating a narcissistic structure that may develop into megalomania. For Freud, then, paranoia is typified by the subject's withdrawal of attachments from the outside world. Delusions of persecution represent the subject's attempt to recover an attachment to others, often through a regressive libidinal surge toward a new object (1963: 138); but this new object that "instigates" the attachment—a substitute for a parent or a sibling—becomes, instead, a persecutor and an enemy. The subject's love, experienced first internally, is repressed and then projected onto the substitute and inverted: my love for the other becomes the other's hatred for me, which then justifies my fear of him. Because the subject's repression of forbidden love is unconscious, he experiences that love-turned-hate as extrinsic, and feels no conscious responsibility for his persecution.

81. My approach is inspired by Vincent Crapanzano's reading of Schreber (Crapanzano 1998), where he develops the notion of "interlocutory collapse" in Schreber's authorship of his own paranoia while refusing the diagnostic, symptomatic, and allegorical readings of Schreber proffered, respectively, by Sigmund Freud, Elias Canetti, and Eric Santner.

82. Balibar 2002: 92.

83. Balibar defines "active citizenship" as a form of citizenship "characterized by the full exercise of political rights" (Balibar 2004: 59).

84. See Voutira 1991 on these distinct moments and trajectories of Pontian displacement.

85. See Agtzidis 1991; Kokkinos 1991a; and Xanthopoulou-Kyriakou 1991 on the fate of the Pontian diaspora in Ottoman territories, pre-Soviet Russia, and the Soviet Union. See Bryer 1991 for a history of Pontian Greeks before their displacement from the Pontus region during the Ottoman and Soviet periods.

86. The Greek name is Εθνικό Ίδρυμα Υποδοχής και Αποκατάστασης Αποδήμων και Παλιννοστούντων Ομογενών Ελλήνων. See Kokkinos 1991b and ΕΙΥΑΑΠΟΕ 2001 for overviews and reviews of programs during the institute's decade of operation.

87. In his case study of Schreber, anticipating the accusation that he has borrowed his theorization of paranoia from Schreber himself, Freud writes: "Since I neither fear the criticism of others nor shrink from criticizing myself, I have no motive for avoiding the mention of a similarity which may possibly damage our libido theory in the estimation of many of our readers. Schreber's 'rays of God,' which are made up of a condensation of the sun's rays, of nerve fibers, and of spermatozoa, are in reality nothing else than a concrete representation and external projection of libidinal cathexes; and they thus lend his delusions a striking similarity with our theory. His belief that the world must come to an end because his ego was attracting all the rays to itself, his anxious concern at a later period, during the process of reconstruction, lest God should sever his ray-connection with him, — these and many other details of Schreber's delusional formation sound almost like endopsychic perceptions of the processes whose existence I have assumed in these pages as the basis of our explanation of paranoia. I can nevertheless call a friend and fellow-specialist to witness that I had developed my theory of paranoia before I became acquainted with the content of Schreber's book. It remains for the future to decide whether there is more delusion in my theory than I should like to admit, or whether there is more truth in Schreber's delusion than other people are as yet prepared to believe" (1963: 154). The "paranoid" tenor of Freud's preemptive self-defense, along with his insistence on the convergence of his and Schreber's independent theories, corroborate the conclusion that Freud phrases as a playful provocation in the last line of this passage: namely, that a deep intimacy unites psychoanalytic theorization with the psychical process of paranoia.

88. Balibar 2002: 84.

INTERLUDE: THE PERSIANS

1. Aeschlyus 1956: 84, line 1033.
2. Ibid., 77, line 807.
3. Ibid., 74, lines 742–43.
4. Ibid., 65, lines 495–96.

1. A 1992 study at the state psychiatric hospital in Thessaloniki, in line with international research, found Anafranil exceptionally and discretely effective for OCD: "Anafranil seems to have an anti-obsessional effect *per se* and its influence on OCD has no relation with depression" (Dimitriou et al. 1992: 7).

2. Ibid., 4.

3. A fifteen-year retrospective study, published in 1980 just as reform was initiated, examines the prescription of neuroleptics to hospitalized schizophrenics, starting from the observation that chronic schizophrenia does not respond well to medications of any kind: "The drugs cannot prevent or disrupt the unrelenting downward-spiralling process of chronic schizophrenia." Psychiatrists in hospital settings were therefore challenged to "help [patients] come out of their social withdrawal, flatness of affect and poverty of feelings, and assume a more appropriate emotional and mental functioning within their human environment" by methods other than just medication (Paraschos et al. 1980: 381). Over the fifteen years of the study, the authors observe a steady rise in dosage—beyond the level of "general acceptance" (385)—of the two main families of antipsychotic medications, which they attribute not to a biochemical tolerance among patients but to a growing tolerance on the part of therapists to the risks of prescribing higher doses.

A 1983 study focuses on a "hard-core group" of chronic psychotic patients "judged never likely to be discharged" and "usually characterized as violent, disorganized, mentally deficient, and socially isolated." Such patients, treated only by medication and "custodial care," constituted 60 to 70 percent of the state hospital population in Greece in the early 1980s (Manos et al. 1983: 457). The authors of the study created a "therapeutic milieu" in a men's ward at the state hospital in Thessaloniki, with the goal of rendering their permanent conditions more "humane" and "active," elevating human contact and communication through "group therapy, occupational therapy, [and] recreational therapy" (458). According to the study, these patients showed vast improvement in functioning within three months. They returned to poor functioning when these therapists were reassigned to another clinic.

In 1986–87, another group of researchers from the Thessaloniki state hospital instituted an aftercare program for discharged chronic psychotic patients (Lavrendiadis et al. 1987). This "returning patients' clinic," which convened every other week at the clinic from which the patients had been released, assured better contact between outpatients and staff, and thus better continuity of care. According to the authors, the program successfully prevented many relapses and readmissions and would serve as a good model for other aftercare projects to be initiated at community mental health centers and general hospitals in Greece.

4. In one prominent study, Nikos Manos and his colleagues observe, "Thus the state hospital has never been phased out and remains a vital link in the chain of mental health services" (1983: 457). See also Castel, Castel, and Lovell (1979: 298) on the "myth of deinstitutionalization" in American psychiatry.

5. Though they account for it somewhat differently, João Biehl (2005: 144, 179), in Brazil, and Andrew Lakoff (2005, esp. chap. 4), in Argentina, cite the same historical shift from psychosis to neurosis (or from schizophrenia to mood disorders) in psychiatric epidemiology and diagnostic trends since the 1990s.

6. By 2003, two small centers for the treatment of substance abuse, KETHEA (Κέντρο Θεραπείας Εξαρτημένων Ατόμων/Therapeutic Center for Addicted Persons) and OKANA (Οργανισμός κατά των Ναρκωτικών/Organization against Narcotics), had been founded in Alexandroupolis, but both were private. While they took some patients on referral from state services, they were under no obligation to treat such patients, and treatment depended on complex negotiations for coverage with IKA (Social Insurance Institute), OGA (Agricultural Workers' Insurance Organization), and/or welfare. The state psychiatric hospital in Thessaloniki thus remained the closest public facility for detox and recovery.

7. Foucault 1988b.

8. Foucault: 1978: 73.

9. Foucault 1991: 102–3.

10. Foucault 1997e: 59.

11. Foucault 1997a: 73.

12. Ibid., 76.

13. Ibid., 77.

14. Despite Foucault's injunction to analyze the "triangle" of sovereignty, discipline, and governmentality together rather than as discrete, successive regimes (1991: 102), heirs of his research project, particularly those invested in the paradigm of the psyche, have not always risen to the challenge. Robert Castel, as noted in the prelude, is extravagantly epochal in his pronouncements on psychiatric power. Nikolas Rose, on the other hand, by way of a gentle critique of Deleuze's "metaphorical" remarks on "societies of control" (Deleuze 1990; Rose 1999: 233), is careful to characterize these rationalities of power genealogically, as complementary and coexistent "styles of thinking" (246) that arise out of "contingent conditions" (275)—rather than historically, as successive unities, or sociologically, as functionalist logics of power. We can thus expect to find these styles overlapping in "problem spaces" (275) such as psychiatric reform, producing various effects there according to the contingent contours of the situation.

And indeed this is what Rose draws from his reading of Stan Cohen's work on "decarceration" (Cohen 1985; Rose 1999: 237), a term that, in the psychiatric context, corresponds roughly to deinstitutionalization and the diffusion of community-based care. With Deleuze (1990: 2, 4) and Cohen (1985), as against the liberatory ideology that gave rise to it, Rose suggests that the decarceration of psychiatric patients yielded *not* a reduction of psychiatric power but a shift and even an expansion of control, as psychiatric encounters proliferated in number and kind across newly dispersed networks of care. In a Foucauldian vocabulary, this proliferation of "contacts" corresponds to a transformation of discipline (with occasional sovereign relations of domination) into governmentality. Yet *governmentality* is not the only modality of power in the "psy" field under the new regime of control. Rose observes that the process of decarceration retains incarceration as a "strategy of exclusion" (240) in which *discipline* and *sovereignty* continue to operate, while the neoliberal modes of consumption, responsibility, and community that characterize *control* predominate as "strategies of inclusion" in the mainstream.

What is excluded, in this new mode of incarceration, is what Castel named the problem of danger. To tie Rose consistently to the nomenclature of the distinction he borrows from Castel: "Danger" is a threat posed to the community by individual subjects, in a governmental regime of discipline; "risk" is a threat both faced and posed by a population under specifiable social, economic, political, and biological conditions in a governmental regime of control. (Rose cites Feeley and Simon 1994 on the "actuarial regime" by which, the authors argue, such conditions are regulated in "the new penology," as opposed to the prior disciplinary regime by which criminal individuals were excluded and interned; 236.) When Rose speaks, then, of a "new territory of exclusion" (262) to which "risky" persons are consigned in neoliberal governmentality, he is no longer concerned with risk, but with danger, which reasserts a disciplinary logic at the extreme point beyond all control.

Such *residually* dangerous individuals compose a "minority" whose "risk" (i.e., danger), according to Rose, is more or less "permanent." (Though he does not say so, Rose must take the position that this "minority" group is not a "population" in the biostatistical sense, since it is precisely the resistance of the individuals in question to normalization as a population that consigns them to the residual space of exclusion.) Under the rubric of the "penal-welfare complex" (270), he compiles a list of marginal types composing the "social problem group" (254) that populates this space of permanent danger. Deinstitutionalized psychiatric patients are lumped in here with the poor, the homeless, and the criminal (260, 270)—those "unable or unwilling to enterprise their lives or manage their own risk, incapable of exercising responsible self-government" (259), a "semi-permanent quasi-criminal population, seen as impervious to the demands of the new morality" (271). Rose likewise reduces the tasks faced by the mental health professionals in charge of decarceration to the problem of evaluating danger, of determining which patients can and which cannot be managed in the new risk environment of dispersed outpatient care (260–61): "The demand that psychiatry should be concerned with the assessment and administration of risky individuals, rather than with diagnosis, treatment and cure, does not mark a new moment in its political vocation. Nonetheless, its role is revised in the new configuration of control. What is called for is the management of a permanently risky minority on the territory of the community" (262). Thus in Rose's account does treatment recede from the horizon of knowledge and ethics in the "psy" field. Likewise, the only patients who continue to be excluded and interned in custodial institutions are those considered "too risky" for outpatient management: "Confinement becomes little more than a way of securing the most risky until their riskiness can be fully assessed and controlled" (1999: 261). This "too risky" class of psychiatric patients falls into the same "permanently risky" group as recidivist criminals—people whose danger to the community can only be controlled by permanent incarceration.

On the other hand, if the danger this group poses is only "semi-permanent" (271), as Rose also contends, it is because the mentally ill are reformable in the same way that poor and criminal elements of the non–mentally ill population are imagined to be. His attention to this question is largely focused on neoconservative welfare reform in the United Kingdom and the United States, and its attendant neoliberal discourse of "responsibilization" among the poor, pitched against their purported "culture of dependency" (256). These people are such apt targets of "moral reformation" (266) in this discourse, Rose argues, that poverty is often preemptively equated with moral irresponsibility—as if poverty were the penalty for not trying hard or earnestly enough to "achieve full membership in the moral community" through work (267).

Rose offers a clue to how we might resolve the ambiguity of danger's im/permanence in the new territory of exclusion when he describes the kind of subjectivity at stake in policies of "moral reformation" in the new risk-management environment: "This is not a psychological subjectivity with social determinants, as in welfare regimes. It is an ethical subjectivity, and a cultural subjectivity" (265). Even though the subjectivity targeted by reform is not, then, "psychological," it is available to "ethical reconstruction" (263) via a range of "psychological techniques" designed to transform dependency into autonomy (268)—techniques not derived from psychiatry and medicine but "recycled" from the now discrete and largely private-sector field of psychology (269).

Rose is able to call the subjectivity that is subject to transformation here "ethical," rather than "psychological," because he does not attend to the severely mentally ill as targets of reform, but instead takes the normalized psyche as given. Take, for example, the "workfare ethos" of neoconservative welfare reform, which Rose says offers a "new ethical gloss" on the puritan work ethic: "Paid work engenders pride and self-respect, or self-esteem, and ties the individual into respectability, identity and community" (266). While this same goal forms an explicit rationale in occupational therapy for schizophrenics, the rationale in that context is therapeutic and, strictly speaking, has nothing to do with the logic of control by which these patients might be integrated as producers and consumers into the neoliberal market economy.

While his approach to power is more empirically supple, Rose thus joins Castel in restricting his analysis of the contemporary psyche to the expansion of "psychological culture" outside the clinic and the proliferation of "psy" technologies in the private self-management of normal subjects. When he includes the severely mentally ill in the category of "risky minorities" consigned to permanent exclusion and incarceration, he cannot countenance their treatment and their engagement in ethical reform, which actually transpire in the clinical space. When, on the other hand, Rose includes the mentally ill in the category of recalcitrant but reformable groups, thus commensurating psychiatric reform to welfare reform, he neglects the special problems that severe pathology poses to ethical reform.

15. Basaglia 1987: 273.

16. Ibid., 274–77.

17. Ibid., 284.

18. Ibid., 287.

19. Ibid., 290–91.

20. Article 16.1, UN Resolution 46/119, "Principles for the Protection of Persons with Mental Illness and the Improvement of Mental Health Care" (1991).

21. Matsa 1989: 66–67.

22. Ibid., 68.

23. Ibid., 69.

24. This discussion excludes another critical disjuncture: the determination of criminal responsibility in forensic psychiatry and the penal code.

25. See Article 95 of Statute 2071, discussed below.

26. Two more recent bodies of legislation on mental health care in Greece have been passed since 1992: Statute 2519/97 ("Development and Modernization of the National Health System, Organization of Health Services, Drug Regulations and Other Provisions") and the Mental Health Act of 1999, Statute 2716/99 ("Development and Modernization of the Mental Health Services and Other Provisions"). Statute 2519/97 established an independent division in the Ministry of Health and Welfare for the protection of patients' rights, a monitoring committee for the protection of patients' rights, and a communication office for the public in every Greek hospital, including psychiatric hospitals. It also provided for the formation of a three-member committee for the protection of citizens' rights. Statute 2716/99, a more expansive body of legislation that outlined the Psychargos plan for psychiatric reform, approved by the European Union in 1998, minimally elaborated those provisions of the 1997 statute, extending the purview of the monitoring committee for the protection of patients' rights to private clinics as well as public hospitals (see Papadimas 1999: 6). Yet the 1997 and 1999 laws did not enact changes to the 1992 legislation regarding involuntary confinement, according to a report to the European Commission by the Greek Ministry of Health in 1999: "We consider that the provisions of the articles of Act 2071 of 1992 regarding the procedure of admission, the legal means, the interruption or termination of involuntary hospitalization, secure the patient's rights and himself/herself. This is the reason why, although Act

2716 of 1999 on the development and modernization of mental health services was enacted, none of these provisions was modified, and only the provision of article 16 was added to the new law for further protection, in terms of involuntary hospitalization at a private mental clinic" (Papadimas 1999: 8).

27. Tziaferi 1989: 62–63.

28. Papasteriou 1989: 58.

29. Fotiadis 1989: 75.

30. Article 94 of the Greek statute describes the conditions for *voluntary* inpatient treatment—an innovation in the law introduced in 1978 (Statute 5345) in anticipation of the growth of a responsible patient population capable of self-scrutiny and self-referral. According to Article 94, patients must be able to judge in the interest of their health in order to admit themselves voluntarily, and the medical director of the relevant service must agree to the need for treatment. Voluntary inpatients, unlike involuntary patients, retain the exercise of all their personal rights and freedoms. Treatment can be terminated at their own request or at that of the psychiatrist in charge of their case.

31. In the same interview, Lamberakis described the formal procedures of involuntary committal according to the letter of the law. He also indicated the conditions under which clinicians, patient advocates, and judicial officials could make their way, "in practice," around those formal procedures. He continued:

And of course, in practice, a lot has to happen [for a person to be admitted by reason of danger]. Prior to the judge's decision, the district attorney will have ordered an emergency admission [έκτακτα] to the hospital—it's urgent because the person is dangerous and has to be admitted today, and nothing else can be done. And then afterward, the district attorney sends the matter to the judge, who decides whether to ratify that decision as "good." This happens quite frequently. But according to the law, the patient has the right to get a lawyer—before the admission, but he can also do it afterward—to go to the courthouse and contest the district attorney's emergency order. Now, the district attorney is not going to want to have his decision overturned. So this has made district attorneys hesitant to grant these orders too easily.

A relative of a patient can go to the district attorney to tell him there's a problem. But the district attorney here in Alexandroupolis won't grant an order easily if the patient isn't a chronic patient. Or she'll order an examination first, which the district attorney has the right to do. If the patient won't come by himself, the police escort him to the psychiatrist to be examined—otherwise how would the exam happen? But even to grant an order of examination, the district attorney thinks carefully about it—only in cases where, for example, *we* tell the district attorney that, yes, what the relatives are saying is true, there really is a problem and you have to order an examination. Or if the patient is chronically ill, and constantly in and out of the hospital, and it's known that he's in treatment and is relapsing, and that when he relapses he gets violent. . . . In those cases, it's easier to get an order for examination. But always, to hold the patient after the examination, there must always be a psychiatric opinion either that the patient is dangerous to himself or others, or the second reason, that if he isn't treated his health will get worse. . . .

The actual order says that the police are to bring the patient to be examined by a psychiatrist, and that he can leave afterward if the district attorney doesn't order an admission. If we determine that the case is urgent, we tell the district attorney to grant the order. But if we say that the exam is inconclusive, and we should wait and see, or that there's no need for admission, the patient can leave. The law says that the relatives have the right to request an order . . . but the district attorney can order it without their request if, let's say, some neighbors come to him to report a problem, and there's some danger. But we always try to have the relatives involved.

32. Sakellaropoulos 1995: 65.

33. Ibid.

34. Ploumpidis 1995; Stylianidis and Ploumpidis 1989: 643.

35. Stylianidis and Ploumpidis 1989: 645.

36. See also Stylianidis and Papadakos 2000: 348; Blue 1991: 333.

37. Stylianidis and Ploumpidis 1989: 646.

38. These review procedures are specified in Articles 97 and 99.

39. Papagiorgiou 1989: 80, 82–83.

40. Basaglia attributes this space of "practical action," which he considers an ambiguous good, to the essential contradiction between psychiatry's medical and penal functions (1987: 277, 289).

41. Stylianidis and Ploumpidis 1989: 648.

42. Ibid., 649.

43. Mitrosili 1996: 12.

44. Δυστυχώς δεν θα έχουμε καν μετάβαση από το σύστημα «εν αμφιβολία υπερ της ασφάλειας» στο σύστημα «εν αμφιβολία υπερ της ελευθερίας» (Orphanoudakis 1989: 106).

45. Sakellaropoulos 1995: 65.

46. Castel 1981: 126.

47. See Davis (n.d.) for a thorough discussion of therapeutic contracts and their imbrication with Greek law and debt.

48. See Young 1995, especially chapter 6, on the multiple functions of the contract in an inpatient treatment unit for veterans diagnosed with post-traumatic stress disorder in the United States. See also Castel 1981 on the diffusion of the therapeutic contract in a range of new psychiatric management techniques. He associates the contract, like "differential treatment" generally, with the classic conception of mental illness as a relational rather than an organic disorder, and a classic psychiatry oriented to face-to-face encounters rather than to the technocratic compilation of population profiles. He observes a contract "similar to that

of psychotherapy" emerging in behavior-modification therapy, where the parties agree to a "corrective program" without, however, any reflection or work on the dynamic nature of the relation between therapist and client (110).

49. See Perrin and Newnes 2002.

50. Allan Young (1995) shows that contracts could be employed by therapists to eject a patient from treatment for technical infractions, when a consensus had been reached that the patient was uncooperative or untreatable in a more general sense.

51. See Levendusky et al. 1983.

52. See Stacey 1997 on the neoliberal initiative for patients' "responsibility to health" in Great Britain.

53. Cohen 1999, 2001, 2005.

54. Cohen 1999: 146–47. See also Scheper-Hughes 2005 on the international sale of kidneys. She shows how a "patient-centered ethic" of organ transplantation (where the "patient" in question is the recipient), whose keystone is the patient's "right to purchase" organs, counts on vast geographic and economic distance between recipients and donors, as well as on the invisibility of the latter in public bioethics discourse. She notes the harmonization of this patient-centered ethic with "neoliberal readjustments of societies worldwide to meet the demands of economic globalization": "The uninhibited circulation of bought and sold kidneys exemplifies a neoliberal political discourse based on juridical concepts of the autonomous individual subject, equality (at least, equality of opportunity), radical freedom, accumulation, and universalism" (145, 149, 148).

55. This is to put aside for a moment the many treatment decisions made for patients *involuntarily*—another site of vigorous debate.

56. See Mahmood 2005: 10–12 for a critique of such procedural reasoning in liberal thought.

57. Cohen 1999: 148, 146.

58. Ibid., 148.

59. Ibid., 161–62.

60. Bill Maurer's work on Islamic banking (2005) can perhaps aid in resolving this enigma of efficacy. Maurer explores a variety of Islamic financial contracts whose warrants are arguably subtended by an alternative law to that of mainstream international finance: namely, the law of Islam. He observes that the "reality" of these contracts is constantly questioned, even by the bankers who engage in them: they are said to have no genuine basis in Islamic law; or, on the other hand, they are derided for being not "alternative" at all, but rather mere semblances of mainstream financial contracts, whose guise of Islamic values disguises their implication in straightforward capitalist accumulation. Yet Maurer shows that these recurrent questions about the reality of Islamic contracts do not impinge on their operation (74); they are secondary considerations to the efficacy and use of these contracts, to how they work to make transactions possible. He notes that their efficacy bears a very peculiar relationship to law: their "continuing circulation, and the

obviation of possible falsity that permits it, is made effective through and also, at times, against law" (59). Maurer points to something else at work in their efficacy, "another kind of truth" than their correspondence to reality (62), which he calls "value storage": the "moral precepts and commitments, as well as 'memories' of a time before"—before the emergence of neoliberal global capital, perhaps, or a time when Islam furnished a viable system of value—that attended the conception of the alternative and that underwrite its ongoing operations (61–62).

61. See Don Handelman's (1976) parallel discussion of "transactions" between welfare officials and clients (particularly non-European immigrant clients) in Israel. While the interactions he examines transpire outside the rubric of formal or informal contracts, Handelman astutely specifies the multiple determinants of expectations on both sides of such relationships, and the increasing number of those determinants over time. He shows a mutual dependency growing between officials and clients, one fostered by open-ended negotiations over the exchange of welfare benefits (on the part of officials) for promises to be "rehabilitated" (on the part of clients). Through an extended case study, he traces the increasing purview of the welfare office and other state agencies over the life of one client and his family, extending from employment and housing to medical care, disability income, police interventions, loan deferments, and pension eligibility. In this case, welfare officers were unable to disentangle their negotiations with the client over his employment—their "official" role—from the other responsibilities to him and his family members in which they became implicated through those negotiations. Handelman sees this "social relationship" as "an emergent property" of contacts between officials and clients, "regardless of the more formal or clearly specified attributes of status [i.e., client-patron] which they present to one another" (228, 224).

62. Sakellaropoulos 1995: 684.

63. This process very closely resembles the transformation of patients' complaints into symptoms into grounds for cooperation in treatment, noted by Erving Goffman in the essay, "The Moral Career of the Mental Patient" (1961a: 127–69) and Velpry 2008.

64. Velpry 2008: 248–49.

65. Allan Young (1995: chaps. 6–7) likewise shows the emergence of resistance to moral coercion in group therapy. This same group dynamic, however, draws some patients into the role of therapists, to the point of pressuring "resistant" patients to participate in the collective construction of correct accounts of their traumatic experience.

66. Some research at the intersection of psychology and anthropology has attempted to distinguish ritual, especially in a religious context, from pathologically compulsive behavior, while insisting on their "phenomenological" or "morphological" resemblance (see, respectively, Fiske and Haslam 1997: 211; Dulaney and Fiske 1994: 251). In this vein, OCD is presented as a "pathological manifestation" of

a "normal" human disposition to ritual (Fiske and Haslam 1997: 212; see also Dulaney and Fiske 1994; Smay 2001), thereby presuming a continuum of pathological-to-normal behavior without accounting for discontinuities between individual and culture. Rather than venturing such a normative statement on similarities and distinctions between normal cultural ritual and pathological individual compulsion, I am instead attempting to voice the perspective on their relationship that Kleandis himself intimated. He seemed to see in ritual, as a rigid external structure, a plausible alternative to his pathological compulsions. By displacing these compulsions to a sacred context, he might use ritual to refigure and thereby cure them, while dislodging them from the exclusive orbit of his own responsibility.

67. See A. Jamie Saris's (2008) reflections on marginality and asylum in the case of Tomas O'Connor, which mirrors that of Kleandis in striking ways. Saris shows O'Connor—a "mental patient," a "town character," and an "unrespectable"—tracing, in his daily peregrinations through his village and outskirts in rural Ireland, the multiple configurations of asylum that have determined his social existence. Asylum takes many forms here: not only the hospital where he was interned for much of his life before psychiatric reform in Ireland, but also the local medieval fortress, a symbol of communal protection transformed into the day hospital that he visits each day and that sustains his presence in the village as a poetic critic of institutional authority, as of the British colonial project whose peculiar reverberations he embodies; and finally, perhaps, his wandering itself, a continuous motion that generates his personhood while grounding him in the material coordinates of daily life.

68. This phrase, like the title of this section, alludes to Lawrence Cohen's (2001) inspired scene- and code-shifting analysis of recognition and exchange in organ transplantation in India.

69. Sakellaropoulos 1995: 213. Sakellaropoulos in fact pronounces a grim prognosis for the disorder, which he says is best treated with the drug Anafranil. For the OCD patient, he writes, even psychoanalysis represents an arduous and minimally effective approach: in the best cases, the "rigidity of the superego" can be softened, enabling the ego to incorporate rather than reject the wishes or impulses in question (218).

70. American Psychiatric Association 2000: 456–63. According to the manual, obsessions and compulsions can be distinguished through differential diagnosis from psychosis; from "culturally-prescribed ritual behavior"; from the brooding characteristic of depression, which is not ego-dystonic; from "normal" anxiety, which attaches to "real-life" problems; and from tics, which are functional, non-rhythmic motor movements unrelated to thought content (459). Obsessive-compulsive disorder can also be distinguished from obsessive-compulsive personality disorder, which does not entail true obsessions or compulsions. Instead, this personality presents a "pervasive pattern of pre-occupation" with control that be-

gins early in life and that accrues a painstaking, perfectionist, rule-bound, rigid, and self-critical character that it shares with the clinical disorder (725–29; see also Sakellaropoulos 1995: 230–31).

71. Sakellaropoulos 1995: 215.

72. American Psychiatric Association 2000: 458.

73. In this, Kleandis evokes the classic "obsessional neurotic" defined in Freud's famous case study of the Rat Man. In this work, Freud traces obsessional fears to "former wish[es] . . . now repressed," their unacceptable hostility toward the object subdued by the energetic force of love and censored by moral conscience (Freud 1955: 180). The symptomatic "self-reproaches" of the obsessional neurotic thus do not emerge into consciousness directly, but are "distorted" and "transformed" into obsessional fears incompatible with the ego (227). On Freud's account, these fears produce, out of love, an affect of guilt, which compels the patient to neutralize his fears. But this corrective act—the compulsion—manages to express the hostility contained in the original repressed wish. Thus the reasoned discourse with which an obsessional neurotic persuades himself out of the obsession and into the compulsive act is, rather, a "delirium": while opposing the obsession, the compulsion also accepts and reproduces its premises (222). Freud insists that this ambivalence, which accounts for the stubbornness of obsessions in the face of reason and the paralysis of the patient in the face of his fears, operates as the motive rather than the consequence of obsessional neurosis (199).

The motive force of ambivalence in obsessional neurosis appears in Freud's text as a specific application of the general psychoanalytic principle that, as he told the Rat Man directly, "patients deriv[e] a certain satisfaction from their sufferings, so that in reality they all resis[t] their own recovery to some extent" (183–84). In assigning responsibility to the patient for his own neurosis, this study of obsession risks a moralism for which Freud has been routinely and roundly criticized. For Freud, the conflict between the subject's unconscious wishes and conscious moral code marks his "maturation" and achievement of moral responsibility—or, as the Rat Man translated this process, a victory of the conscious "moral self" over the "evil self of the unconscious" (177). Guilt, as the conscious product of this conflict, inaugurates a dynamic between self-reproach and self-reform, yielding a painful ethical campaign in the adult to claim an ultimately unclaimable responsibility. The obsessional neurotic is one whose excessive guilt preserves a strong enough division between these battling selves that his or her personality verges on disintegration. At stake in this struggle is violence toward oneself and others—precisely the danger posed by Kleandis, and named as the criterion for his involuntary committal.

74. In her essay "Epidemics of the Will," Eve Sedgwick tracks the emergence of the addict as a social and subjective identity, from the opium-eater of the late nineteenth century to the exercise freak of the new millennium. She perceives these disparate figures within the same "paradigm of addiction"—a pathology of the will

that takes, as its converse, not the *merely* free will but the "*healthy* free will" (1992: 584). The force of addiction in this paradigm does not belong to any substance in particular, but rather to "the structure of a will that is insufficiently free," and whose willful assertion itself becomes, therefore, addictive (584). In Sedgwick's genealogy of the metaphysics of will, the alignment of health with the "sufficient freedom" of the will is what yields the distinctive "ethical value" at stake in addiction: "The object of addiction is the exercise of those very qualities whose lack is supposed to define addiction as such: bodily autonomy, self-control, will-power. The object of addiction has become, precisely, enjoyment of 'the ability to choose freely, and freely to choose health'" (583). For Sedgwick, psychoanalysis is too embedded in the "modern heroics of volition/compulsion" to provide an analytic space for addiction beyond absolutist and moralistic metaphysics (591). She turns instead to what she considers a dormant and unmoralized genealogy of habit, retaining a focus on the reflexivity of nonrational practices that could help to illuminate the ethical murk of obsessive-compulsive disorder. Habit, she suggests, "demarcates the space of perceptual and proprioceptive reversal and revelation . . . at which introspection itself can never arrive" (592). Mariana Valverde (1998) takes up Sedgwick's challenge to pursue theories and practices of habit, as against the metaphysical antinomy of compulsion and freedom, in her history of alcoholism in Europe and North America.

See also Lauren Berlant's essay on "practical sovereignty" for an alternative recasting of habit and addiction. Berlant addresses critically our "attachment to a fantasy that in the truly lived life emotions are always heightened and expressed in modes of effective agency that ought justly to be and are ultimately consequential or performatively sovereign. In this habit of representing the intentional subject, a manifest lack of self-cultivating attention can easily become recast as irresponsibility, shallowness, resistance, refusal, or incapacity; and habit itself can begin to look deeply overmeaningful, such that addiction, reaction-formation, conventional gesture-clusters, or just being different can be read as heroic placeholders for resistance to something, affirmation of something, or a transformative desire" (2007: 757–58). Instead of such forms of "effective agency," Berlant explores, in the case of obesity, "affective forms of engagement with the environment of slow death," such as "impassivity and other relations of alienation, coolness, detachment, or distraction"—forms of "relief" rather than desire, which do not aim at self-improvement or "life-building," but rather at "self-continuity" or "life-making" (757–58, 779). In this light, compulsions such as Kleandis's might appear to be life-making and self-continuing but decidedly *not* ethical practices.

75. See Biehl (2005: 22, and part 4), on the family as "the medical agent of the state" in its expanding responsibility for patients at the intersection of community-based and neoliberal structures of psychiatric care—the site at which deinstitutionalized psychiatry is reinstitutionalized (125) in the absence of the family counseling and resocialization so prominent in reform rhetoric (176). Biehl notes the desire

among some residents of Vita to seek permanent refuge within the institution as an alternative to family care (or neglect or abuse). As one resident told him: "'I am weak. I like being dependent here. My thinking is always in here. Here, I feel safe. . . . I hope I can stay here the rest of my life'" (59).

REPRISE: DIAGNOSIS

1. See Michael Tanner's introduction to *"The Twilight of the Idols" and "The Antichrist"* (Nietzsche 1968: 7).

2. Nietzsche 1974: 34–5.

3. Nietzsche 1968: 39.

4. Nietzsche 1979a: 75.

5. Nietzsche 1979b: 121.

6. Deleuze and Guattari 1994: 113.

7. Paul Rabinow, likewise, charts the inventiveness of diagnosis through the work of modern social theorists from Max Weber to Peter Sloterdijk. He sees diagnosis allied with a nominalist critique of the self-evident—a generative critique that, insofar as it facilitates analysis in new and different directions, might be considered not only "critical" and "affirmative" (i.e., not denunciatory) but also, as with Hans Blumenberg (though not Freud), "curative" (2003: 29, 30).

8. Nietzsche 1967: 87.

9. Ibid., 93.

10. Nietzsche 1974: 38, 1967: 15.

11. Ibid. 38.

12. Ibid., 33.

13. Deleuze nominates "symptomatologist" for one of the three vocations of philosophers as practitioners of the "active science" Nietzsche seeks. (The other two philosophical vocations are "typologist" and "genealogist.") The symptomatologist, he says, "interprets phenomena, treating them as symptoms whose sense must be sought in the forces that produce them" (Deleuze 1983: 75).

14. "Perhaps also because they care less about causes." Deleuze 1967: 13, quoted in Daniel W. Smith's introduction to the 1997 English edition of *Essays Critical and Clinical* (Deleuze 1997: xvii). See Smith's thorough discussion of the symptomatological method in Deleuze's corpus.

15. Deleuze 1997: 3.

16. Foucault 1988b: 285–89.

17. Ibid., 287.

18. Ibid.

19. Foucault 1998b: 382.

20. Ibid., 373, 376.

21. Ibid., 380.

22. Nietzsche 1974: 36.

23. Foucault 1998c: 269–70.

24. Ibid., 277.

25. Ibid., 275.

26. Ibid., 275, 278.

27. Rabinow notes that Nietzsche, like Weber, paid a "price in psychic suffering" for the oppositional moralist's "privilege" of diagnosing the modern world (1988: 358).

28. Nietzsche 1974: 35.

BIBLIOGRAPHY

Aeschylus. 1956. "The Persians." ca. 472 BCE. Trans. S. G. Benardete. *Aeschylus II: The Complete Greek Tragedies*, ed. David Grene and Richard Lattimore, 43–86. Chicago: University of Chicago Press.

Agtzidis, Vlasis. 1991. "The Persecution of Pontic Greeks in the Soviet Union." *Journal of Refugee Studies* 4 (4): 372–81.

Alexandrakis, Othon. 2003. "Between Life and Death: Violence and Greek Roma Health and Identity." Master's thesis, University of Western Ontario.

Alexandris, Alexis. 2003. "Religion or Ethnicity: The Identity Issue of the Minorities in Greece and Turkey." *Crossing the Aegean: An Appraisal of the 1923 Compulsory Population Exchange between Greece and Turkey*, ed. Renée Hirschon, 117–32. New York: Berghahn Books.

American Psychiatric Association. 2000. *Diagnostic and Statistical Manual of Mental Disorders*. 4th edn. Washington: American Psychiatric Association.

Androutsopoulou, C., et al. 2002. "Psychological Problems in Christian and Moslem Primary Care Patients in Greece." *International Journal of Psychiatry in Medicine* 32 (3): 285–94.

Arvaniti, Aikaterini, et al. 2009. "Health Service Staff's Attitudes toward Patients with Mental Illness." *Social Psychiatry and Psychiatric Epidemiology* 44 (8): 658–65.

Asad, Talal. 2003. *Formations of the Secular: Christianity, Islam, Modernity*. Stanford: Stanford University Press.

Association for Social Psychiatry and Mental Health. 2001. *Association for Social Psychiatry and Mental Health, 1981–2001*. Amfissa: Association for Social Psychiatry and Mental Health (Εταιρία Κοινωνικής Ψυχιατρικής και Ψυχικής Υγείας) (in Greek).

———. 2002a. *One Step toward Full Citizenship*. European Commission, Department of Employment and Social Affairs. Alexandroupolis: Association for Social Psychiatry and Mental Health (in Greek).

———. 2002b. *Proceedings of the Seminar Series on Mental Health*. Alexandroupolis: Association for Social Psychiatry and Mental Health (in Greek).

Athanasiou, Athena. 1989. "'Hotels' and 'Camps': Private Psychiatric Clinics." *Marie Claire*, December, 283–98.

Austin, J. L. 1965. *How to Do Things with Words: The William James Lectures Delivered at Harvard University*. 1955. Oxford: Oxford University Press.

Baistow, Karen. 1994. "Liberation and Regulation? Some Paradoxes of Empowerment." *Critical Social Policy* 14 (42): 34–46.

Balibar, Étienne. 2002. *Politics and the Other Scene*. 1997. Trans. Christine Jones, James Swenson, and Chris Turner. London: Verso.

———. 2004. *We, the People of Europe? Reflections on Transnational Citizenship*. 2001. Trans. James Swenson. Princeton: Princeton University Press.

Bambinioti, Yiorgiou D., ed. 2002. *Dictionary of the Modern Greek Language*. Athens: Center of Lexicology (in Greek).

Basaglia, Franco. 1987. "Problems of Law and Psychiatry: The Italian Experience." 1979. *Psychiatry Inside Out: Selected Writings of Franco Basaglia*, ed. Nancy Scheper-Hughes and Anne M. Lovell, trans. Lovell and Teresa Shtob, 271–97. New York: Columbia University Press.

Beck, Ulrich. 1992. *Risk Society: Towards a New Modernity*. London: Sage.

Behague, Dominique Pareja. 2008. "Psychiatry and Military Conscription in Brazil: The Search for Opportunity and Institutionalized Therapy." *Culture, Medicine, and Psychiatry* 32: 194–218.

Benedict, Ruth. 1934. *Patterns of Culture*. New York: Houghton Mifflin.

Berlant, Lauren. 2000. "Intimacy: A Special Issue." *Intimacy*, ed. Berlant, 1–8. Chicago: University of Chicago Press.

———. 2007. "Slow Death (Sovereignty, Lateral Agency)." *Critical Inquiry* 33 (4): 754–80.

Biehl, João. 2005. *Vita: Life in a Zone of a Social Abandonment*. Berkeley: University of California Press.

Blue, Amy Victoria. 1991. "Culture, *Nevra*, and Institution: The Making of Greek Professional Ethnopsychiatry." PhD diss., Case Western Reserve University.

———. 1993. "Greek Psychiatry's Transition from the Hospital to the Community." *Medical Anthropology Quarterly* 7 (3): 301–18.

Bourdieu, Pierre. 1991. *The Logic of Practice*. 1980. Trans. Richard Nice. Stanford: Stanford University Press.

Breggin, Peter R. 2008. *Brain Disabling Treatments in Psychiatry: Drugs, Electroshock, and the Psychopharmaceutical Complex*. 1997. 2nd edn. New York: Springer.

Breuer, Joseph, and Sigmund Freud. 2000. *Studies on Hysteria*. 1895. Trans. James Strachey. New York: Basic Books.

Brown, Wendy. 1995. *States of Injury: Power and Freedom in Late Modernity*. Princeton: Princeton University Press.

———. 2001. *Politics Out of History*. Princeton: Princeton University Press.

Bryer, Anthony. 1991. "The Pontic Greeks before the Diaspora." *Journal of Refugee Studies* 4 (4): 315–34.

Butler, Judith. 1993. *Bodies That Matter: On the Discursive Limits of "Sex."* New York: Routledge.

———. 2002. *Antigone's Claim: Kinship between Life and Death.* New York: Columbia University Press.

Campbell, John K. 1964. *Honour, Family, and Patronage.* Oxford: Oxford University Press.

Campbell, Nancy D., and Susan J. Shaw. 2009. "Incitements to Discourse: Illicit Drugs, Harm Reduction, and the Production of Ethnographic Subjects." *Cultural Anthropology* 23 (4): 688–717.

Castel, Robert. 1981. *La gestion des risques: De l'anti-psychiatrie à l'après-psychanalyse.* Paris: Éditions de Minuit.

———. 1991. "From Dangerousness to Risk." *The Foucault Effect: Studies in Governmentality,* ed. Graham Burchell, Colin Gordon, and Peter Miller, 281–98. Chicago: University of Chicago Press.

Castel, Robert, Françoise Castel, and Anne Lovell. 1982. *The Psychiatric Society.* 1979. Trans. Arthur Goldhammer. New York: Columbia University Press.

Certeau, Michel de. 1986. *Heterologies: Discourse on the Other.* Trans. Brian Massumi. Minneapolis: University of Minnesota Press.

Clare, Anthony. 2003. *Psychiatry in Dissent: Controversial Issues in Thought and Practice.* 1979. New York: Routledge.

Claus, David B. 1981. *Toward the Soul.* New Haven: Yale University Press.

Cleckley, Hervey M. 1941. *The Mask of Sanity: An Attempt to Clarify Some Issues about the So-Called Psychopathic Personality.* St. Louis: C. V. Mosby.

Cohen, Lawrence. 1998. *No Aging in India: Alzheimer's, the Bad Family, and Other Modern Things.* Berkeley: University of California Press.

———. 1999. "Where It Hurts: Indian Material for an Ethics of Organ Transplantation." *Daedalus* 128 (4): 135–65.

———. 2001. "The Other Kidney: Biopolitics Beyond Recognition." *Body and Society* 7 (2–3): 9–29.

———. 2005. "Operability, Bioavailability, and Exception." *Global Assemblages: Technology, Politics, and Ethics as Anthropological Problems,* ed. Aihwa Ong and Stephen J. Collier, 79–90. Malden, Mass.: Basil Blackwell.

Cohen, Stan. 1985. *Visions of Social Control.* Cambridge: Polity Press.

Corin, Ellen. 2007. "The 'Other' of Culture in Psychosis: The Ex-centricity of the Subject." *Subjectivity: Ethnographic Investigations,* ed. João Biehl, Byron Good, and Arthur Kleinman, 273–314. Berkeley: University of California Press.

Crapanzano, Vincent. 1980. *Tuhami: Portrait of a Moroccan.* Chicago: University of Chicago Press.

———. 1992. *Hermes' Dilemma and Hamlet's Desire: On the Epistemology of Interpretation.* Cambridge: Harvard University Press.

———. 1998. "'Lacking Now Is Only the Leading Idea, That Is—We, the Rays,

Have No Thoughts': Interlocutory Collapse in Daniel Paul Schreber's *Memoirs of My Nervous Illness.*" *Critical Inquiry* 24 (3): 737–67.

Csordas, Thomas, ed. 1994. *Embodiment and Experience: The Existential Ground of Culture and Self.* Cambridge: Cambridge University Press.

Danforth, Loring. 1989. *Firewalking and Religious Healing: The Anastenaria of Greece and the American Firewalking Movement.* Princeton: Princeton University Press.

Das, Veena. 1995. *Critical Events: An Anthropological Perspective on Contemporary India.* Delhi: Oxford University Press.

Davis, Elizabeth Anne. n.d. "'It wasn't written for me': Law, Debt, and Therapeutic Contracts in Greek Psychiatry." Article manuscript under review.

Deleuze, Gilles. 1967. "Mystique et masochisme." Interview with Madeleine Chapsal. *La quinzaine littéraire* 25: 12–13.

———. 1983. *Nietzsche and Philosophy.* 1962. Trans. H. Tomlinson. New York: Columbia University Press.

———. 1989. *Cinema 2: The Time Image.* Trans. H. Tomlinson and R. Galeta. Minneapolis: University of Minnesota Press.

———. 1989. *"Masochism: Coldness and Cruelty" by Gilles Deleuze and "Venus in Furs" by Leopold von Sacher-Masoch.* 1967. Trans. Jean McNeil and Aude Wilm. New York: Urzone.

———. 1992. "Postscript on the Societies of Control." *October* 59: 3–7.

———. 1997. *Essays Critical and Clinical.* 1993. Trans. Daniel W. Smith and Micahel A. Greco. Minneapolis: University of Minnesota Press.

Deleuze, Gilles, and Félix Guattari. 1994. *What Is Philosophy?* 1991. Trans. Janis Tomlinson and Graham Burchell. New York: Columbia University Press.

Demetriou, Olga. 2004. "Prioritizing 'Ethnicities': The Uncertainty of Pomakness in the Urban Greek Rhodoppe." *Ethnic and Racial Studies* 27 (1): 95–119.

Derrida, Jacques. 1978. "Cogito and the History of Madness." 1963. *Writing and Difference*, trans. Alan Bass, 31–63. Chicago: University of Chicago Press.

Devereux, Georges. 1951. "The Oedipal Situation and Its Consequences in the Epics of Ancient India." *Samiksa* 5: 5–13.

———. 1953. "Why Oedipus Killed Laius." *International Journal of Psychoanalysis* 34: 132–41.

———. 1963. "Sociopolitical Functions of the Oedipus Myth in Early Greece." *Psychoanalytic Quarterly* 32: 205–14.

Dimitriou, E. et al. 1992. "Obsessive-Compulsive Disorder: Therapeutic Aspects." Paper presented at the ninth conference of the SEES-NP, 21–24 September.

———. 1993. "Obsessive-Compulsive Disorder and Alcohol Abuse." *European Journal of Psychiatry* 7 (4): 244–48.

Dreyfus, Hubert L., and Paul Rabinow, eds. 1983. *Michel Foucault: Beyond Structuralism and Hermeneutics.* 2nd edn. Chicago: University of Chicago Press.

du Boulay, Juliet. 1974. *Portrait of a Greek Mountain Village.* Oxford: Clarendon.

————. 1976. "Lies, Mockery, and Family Integrity." *Mediterranean Family Structures*, ed. John G. Peristiany, 389–406. New York: Cambridge University Press.

Dulaney, Siri, and Alan Page Fiske. 1994. "Cultural Rituals and Obsessive-Compulsive Disorder: Is There a Common Psychological Mechanism?" *Ethos* 22 (3): 243–83.

Dunk, Pamela. 1989. "Greek Women and Broken Nerves in Montreal." *Medical Anthropology* 11 (1): 29–45.

Durkheim, Émile. 1997. *The Division of Labor in Society*. 1893. Trans. W. D. Halls. New York: Free Press.

Edgar, Bill, Joe Doherty, and Hank Meert. 2004. *Immigration and Homelessness in Europe*. Bristol: Policy Press.

ΕΙΥΑΑΠΟΕ (Εθνικό Ίδρυμα Υποδοχής και Αποκατάστασης Αποδημών και Παλιννοστούντων Ομογενών Ελλήνων / National Institute for the Reception and Resettlement of Repatriated Ancestral Greeks). 1995. *Report on the Proceedings of ΕΙΥΑΑΠΟΕ, 1991–1995*. Athens: ΕΙΥΑΑΠΟΕ (in Greek).

————. 2001. *Report on the Proceedings of ΕΙΥΑΑΠΟΕ, 1991–2001*. Athens: ΕΙΥΑΑΠΟΕ (in Greek).

Eliade, Mircea. 1998. *Myth and Reality*. 1963. Prospect Heights, Ill.: Waveland Press.

Estroff, Sue E. 1981. *Making It Crazy: An Ethnography of Psychiatric Clients in an American Community*. Berkeley: University of California Press.

Ewing, Katherine Pratt. 1997. *Arguing Sainthood: Modernity, Psychoanalysis, and Islam*. Durham: Duke University Press.

————. 2006a. "Between Cinema and Social Work: Diasporic Turkish Women and the (Dis)Pleasures of Hybridity." *Cultural Anthropology* 21 (2): 265–94.

————. 2006b. "Revealing and Concealing: Interpersonal Dynamics and the Negotiation of Identity in the Interview." *Ethos* 34 (1): 89–122.

Ewing, Katherine Pratt, and Marguerite Hoyler. 2008. "Being Muslim and American: South Asian Muslim Youth and the War on Terror." *Being and Belonging: Muslims in the U.S. since 9/11*, ed. Ewing, 80–104. New York: Russell Sage Foundation.

Farquhar, Judith. 1994. *Knowing Practice: The Clinical Encounter of Chinese Medicine*. Boulder, Colo.: Westview Press.

Fassin, Didier, and Estelle d'Halluin. 2005. "The Truth from the Body: Medical Certificates as Ultimate Evidence for Asylum Seekers." *American Anthropologist* 107 (4): 597–608.

————. 2007. "Critical Evidence: The Politics of Trauma in French Asylum Policies." *Ethos* 35 (3): 300–329.

Fassin, Didier, and Richard Rechtman. 2005. "An Anthropological Hybrid: The Pragmatic Arrangement of Universalism and Culturalism in French Mental Health." *Transcultural Psychiatry* 42 (3): 347–66.

Faubion, James D. 1993. *Modern Greek Lessons: A Primer in Historical Constructivism.* Princeton: Princeton University Press.

———. 2001a. *The Shadows and Lights of Waco: Millennialism Today.* Princeton: Princeton University Press.

———. 2001b. "Toward an Anthropology of Ethics: Foucault and the Pedagogies of Autopoiesis." *Representations* 74: 83–104.

Feeley, Malcolm, and Jonathan Simon. 1994. "Actuarial Justice: Power/Knowledge in Contemporary Criminal Justice." *The Futures of Criminology,* ed. David Nelken, 173–201. London: Sage.

Feighner, John P., et al. 1972. "Diagnostic Criteria for Use in Psychiatric Research." *Archives of General Psychiatry* 26: 57–63.

Fiske, Alan Page, and Nick Haslam. 1997. "Is Obsessive-Compulsive Disorder a Pathology of the Human Disposition to Perform Socially Meaningful Rituals? Evidence of Similar Content." *Journal of Nervous and Mental Disease* 185 (4): 211–22.

Fotiadis, Haritonas. 1989. "Nos-ology and Nos-ignorance." *Proceedings of the Pan-Hellenic Conference on the Synchronization of Greek Legislation on Matters Concerning the Mentally Ill,* ed. Ministry of Health, Welfare, and Social Security (Greece), 74–79. Stavroupolis Psychiatric Hospital of Thessaloniki, 8–9 June 1989 (in Greek).

Foucault, Michel. 1972. *The Archaeology of Knowledge and The Discourse on Language.* Trans. A. M. Sheridan Smith. New York: Pantheon.

———. 1978. *Mental Illness and Psychology.* 1954. Trans. Alan Sheridan. Berkeley: University of California Press.

———. 1983. "Afterword: The Subject and Power." *Michel Foucault: Beyond Structuralism and Hermeneutics,* 2nd edn., ed. Hubert L. Dreyfus and Paul Rabinow, 208–26. Chicago: University of Chicago Press.

———. 1988a. *The History of Sexuality,* vol. 3, *The Care of the Self.* 1984. Trans. Robert Hurley. New York: Vintage.

———. 1988b. *Madness and Civilization: A History of Insanity in the Age of Reason.* 1961. Trans. Richard Howard. New York: Vintage.

———. 1990a. *The History of Sexuality,* vol. 1, *An Introduction.* 1976. Trans. Robert Hurley. New York: Vintage.

———. 1990b. *The History of Sexuality,* vol. 2, *The Use of Pleasure.* 1984. Trans. Robert Hurley. New York: Vintage.

———. 1991. "Governmentality." 1978. *The Foucault Effect: Studies in Governmentality,* ed. Graham Burchell et al., 87–104. Chicago: University of Chicago Press.

———. 1997a. "The Birth of Biopolitics." *Ethics, Subjectivity and Truth,* ed. Paul Rabinow, trans. Robert Hurley et al., 73–79. Vol. 1 of *The Essential Works of Foucault (1954–1984).* New York: New Press.

———. 1997b. "The Ethics of the Concern for Self as a Practice of Freedom." 1984. *Ethics, Subjectivity and Truth,* ed. Paul Rabinow, trans. Robert Hurley et al.,

281–301. Vol. 1 of *The Essential Works of Michel Foucault (1954–84)*. New York: New Press.

———. 1997c. "On the Genealogy of Ethics: An Overview of Work in Progress." 1983. *Ethics, Subjectivity and Truth*, ed. Paul Rabinow, trans. Robert Hurley at al., 253–80. Vol. 1 of *The Essential Works of Michel Foucault (1954–84)*. New York: New Press.

———. 1997d. "Security, Territory, and Population." *Ethics, Subjectivity and Truth*, ed. Paul Rabinow, trans. Robert Hurley et al., 67–72. Vol. 1 of *The Essential Works of Foucault (1954–1984)*. New York: New Press.

———. 1997e. "Society Must Be Defended." *Ethics, Subjectivity and Truth*, ed. Paul Rabinow, trans. Robert Hurley et al., 59–65. Vol. 1 of *The Essential Works of Foucault (1954–1984)*. New York: New Press.

———. 1998a. "My Body, This Paper, This Fire." 1972. *Aesthetics, Method, and Epistemology*, ed. James D. Faubion, trans. Robert Hurley et al., 393–417. Vol. 2 of *The Essential Works of Foucault (1954–84)*. New York: New Press.

———. 1998b. "Nietzsche, Genealogy, History." 1971. *Aesthetics, Method, and Epistemology*, ed. James D. Faubion, trans. Robert Hurley et al., 369–91. Vol. 2 of *The Essential Works of Michel Foucault (1954–84)*. New York: New Press.

———. 1998c. "Nietzsche, Marx, Freud." 1967. *Aesthetics, Method, and Epistemology*, ed. James D. Faubion, trans. Robert Hurley et al., 269–78. Vol. 2 of *The Essential Works of Foucault (1954–84)*. New York: New Press.

———. 2003. *Society Must Be Defended: Lectures at the Collège de France, 1975–1976*. 1975. Trans. David Macey. New York: Picador.

———. 2006. *Psychiatric Power: Lectures at the Collège de France, 1973–74*. 1973–74. Ed. Jacques Lagrange and Arnold I. Davidson. Trans. Graham Burchell. New York: Palgrave Macmillan.

Frazer, Sir James George. 1922. *The Golden Bough: A Study in Magic and Religion*. New York: Macmillan.

Freud, Sigmund. 1955. "Notes Upon a Case of Obsessional Neurosis (The Rat Man)." 1909. *The Standard Edition of the Complete Psychological Works of Sigmund Freud*, vol. 10, ed. and trans. James Strachey, 153–249. London: Hogarth Press.

———. 1963. "Psychoanalytic Notes Upon an Autobiographical Account of a Case of Paranoia (Dementia Paranoides)." 1911. *Three Case Histories*, ed. Philip Rieff, 83–160. New York: Collier Books.

Friedl, Ernestine. 1962. *Vasilika: A Village in Modern Greece*. New York: Holt, Rinehart.

Gaines, Atwood D., ed. 1992. *Ethnopsychiatry: The Cultural Construction of Professional and Folk Psychiatries*. Albany: State University of New York Press.

Gal, Susan. 1991. "Between Speech and Silence: The Problematics of Research on Language and Gender." *Gender at the Crossroads of Knowledge: Feminist Anthropology in the Postmodern Era*, ed. Micaela di Leonardo, 175–203. Berkeley: University of California Press.

Gandolfo, Giancarlo. 1987. *International Economics II: International Monetary Theory and Open-Economy Macroeconomics*. Berlin: Springer-Verlag.

Garcia, Angela. 2008. "The Elegiac Addict: History, Chronicity, and the Melancholic Subject." *Cultural Anthropology* 23 (4): 718–46.

Geertz, Clifford. 1983. *Local Knowledge: Further Essays in Interpretive Anthropology*. New York: Basic Books.

Gilmore, David D. 1987a. "Honor, Honesty, Shame: Male Status in Contemporary Andalusia." *Honor and Shame and the Unity of the Mediterranean*, ed. Gilmore, 90–103. Washington: American Anthropological Association.

———, ed. 1987b. *Honor and Shame and the Unity of the Mediterranean*. Washington: American Anthropological Association.

Giordano, Cristiana. 2008. "Practices of Translation and the Making of Migrant Subjectivities in Contemporary Italy." *American Ethnologist* 35 (4): 588–606.

———. 2011. "Translating Fanon in the Italian Context: Rethinking the Ethics of Treatment in Psychiatry." *Transcultural Psychiatry* 48 (3): 228–56.

Goffman, Erving. 1961a. *Asylums: Essays on the Social Situation of Mental Patients and Other Inmates*. New York: Anchor Books.

———. 1961b. "Fun in Games." *Encounters: Two Studies in the Sociology of Interaction*, 15–81. Indianapolis: Bobbs-Merrill.

Gondles, James A., Jr. 1999. "The Criminal Mind: A Challenge to Corrections." *Corrections Today* 61 (1): 6.

Good, Byron J. 1992. "Culture and Psychopathology: Directions for Psychiatric Anthropology." *New Directions in Psychological Anthropology*, ed. Theodore Schwartz, Geoffrey M. White, and Catherine A. Lutz, 181–205. Cambridge: Cambridge University Press.

———. 1994. *Medicine, Rationality, and Experience: An Anthropological Perspective*. Cambridge: Cambridge University Press.

Gourgouris, Stathis. 1996. *Dream Nation: Enlightenment, Colonization, and the Institution of Modern Greece*. Stanford: Stanford University Press.

Hacking, Ian. 1999. *The Social Construction of What?* Cambridge: Harvard University Press.

Handelman, Don. 1976. "Bureaucratic Transactions: The Development of Official-Client Relationships in Israel." *Transaction and Meaning: Directions in the Anthropology of Exchange and Social Behavior*, ed. Bruce Kapferer, 223–75. Philadelphia: Institute for the Study of Human Issues.

Hart, Laurie Kain. 1999. "Culture, Civilization, and Demarcation at the Northwest Borders of Greece." *American Ethnologist* 26 (1): 196–220.

Healey, David. 1997. *The Antidepressant Era*. Cambridge: Harvard University Press.

———. 2002. *The Creation of Psychopharmacology*. Cambridge: Harvard University Press.

Herzfeld, Michael. 1985. *The Poetics of Manhood: Contest and Identity in a Cretan Mountain Village*. Princeton: Princeton University Press.

———. 1987a. *Anthropology through the Looking-Glass: Critical Ethnography in the Margins of Europe*. Cambridge: Cambridge University Press.

———. 1987b. "'As in Your Own House': Hospitality, Ethnography, and the Stereotype of Mediterranean Society." *Honor and Shame and the Unity of the Mediterranean*, ed. David D. Gilmore, 75–89. Washington: American Anthropological Association.

———. 1991. "Silence, Submission, and Subversion: Toward a Poetics of Womanhood." *Contested Identities: Gender and Kinship in Modern Greece*, ed. Peter Loizos and Evthymios Papataxiarchis, 79–97. Princeton: Princeton University Press.

———. 1992. *The Social Production of Indifference: Exploring the Symbolic Roots of Western Bureaucracy*. Chicago: University of Chicago Press.

———. 2002. "The Absent Presence: Discourses of Crypto-Colonialism." *South Atlantic Quarterly* 101 (4): 899–926.

———. 2005. *Cultural Intimacy: Social Poetics in the Nation-State*. 2nd edn. New York: Routledge.

Hirschon, Renée. 1993. "Open Body/Closed Space: The Transformation of Female Sexuality." *Defining Females: The Nature of Women in Society*, 2nd rev. edn., ed. Shirley Ardener, 51–72. Oxford: Berg.

———, ed. 2003. *Crossing the Aegean: An Appraisal of the 1923 Compulsory Population Exchange between Greece and Turkey*. New York: Berghahn Books.

Holmes, Brooke. 2010. *The Symptom and the Subject: The Emergence of the Physical Body in Ancient Greece*. Princeton: Princeton University Press.

Ierodiakonou, Charalambos. 1983a. "Mobile Units in the Framework of a Rural Community Mental Health Center: Experiences and Results of the First Year." *Ιατρική* 44: 225–32 (in Greek).

———. 1983b. "Primary Care and Mental Health Services in Greece." Publication ICP/MNH 059(1)/9, World Health Organization Regional Office for Europe, Working Group on First Contact Mental Health Care.

———. 1983c. "Psychotherapeutic Possibilities in a Rural Community Mental Health Center in Greece." *American Journal of Psychotherapy* 37 (4): 544–51.

Ierodiakonou, Charalambos, with A. Iakovidis and K. Bikos. 1983. "Mobile Mental Health Units Affiliated with a Provincial General Hospital: Comparison of First and Third Six-Month Periods of Operation." *Materia Medica Greca* 11 (6): 518–22 (in Greek).

Jusdanis, Gregory. 1991. *Belated Modernity and Aesthetic Culture: Inventing National Literature*. Minneapolis: University of Minnesota Press.

Karakasidou, Anastasia. 1997. *Fields of Wheat, Hills of Blood: Passages to Nationhood in Greek Macedonia, 1870–1990*. Chicago: University of Chicago Press.

Karastergiou, A. A., et al. 2005. "The Reform of the Greek Mental Health Services." *Journal of Mental Health* 14 (2): 197–203.

Karpozilos, Apostolos. 1991. "Pontic Culture in the USSR between the Wars." *Journal of Refugee Studies* 4 (4): 364–71.

Kleinman, Arthur. 1988. *Rethinking Psychiatry: From Cultural Category to Personal Experience.* New York: Free Press.

———. 1995. *Writing at the Margin: Discourse Between Anthropology and Medicine.* Berkeley: University of California Press.

———. 1997. "'Everything That Really Matters': Social Suffering, Subjectivity, and the Remaking of Human Experience in a Disordering World." *Harvard Theological Review* 90 (3): 315–35.

Kleinman, Arthur, and Joan Kleinman. 1985. "Somatization: The Interconnections in Chinese Society among Culture, Depressive Experiences, and the Meanings of Pain." *Culture and Depression: Studies in the Anthropology and Cross-cultural Psychiatry of Affect and Disorder,* ed. A. Kleinman and Byron Good, 429–90. Berkeley: University of California Press.

Kokkinos, Dimitris. 1991a. "The Greek State's Overview of the Pontian Issue." *Journal of Refugee Studies* 4 (4): 312–14.

———. 1991b. "The Reception of Pontians from the Soviet Union in Greece." *Journal of Refugee Studies* 4 (4): 395–99.

Konstantopoulos, A. 1995. "The Mental Health Group: Goals, Roles, and Problems." *Psychiatric Reform and the New Frameworks of Psychiatric Care in the National Health System in Greece: Conference Proceedings,* ed. Konstantopoulos, 109–56. "Democritus" National Research Center, Athens, 26–27 November 1993. Athens: Ministry of Health, Welfare, and Social Security. (in Greek).

Lacan, Jacques. 1992. *The Seminar of Jacques Lacan, Book VII: The Ethics of Psychoanalysis, 1959–60.* 1959. Ed. Jacques-Alain Miller. Trans. Dennis Porter. New York: W. W. Norton.

———. 1978. "Of the Subject of Certainty." 1973. *The Seminar of Jacques Lacan, Book XI: The Four Fundamental Concepts of Psycho-Analysis,* ed. Jacques-Alain Miller, trans. Alan Sheridan, 29–41. New York: W. W. Norton.

Lakoff, Andrew. 2005. *Pharmaceutical Reason: Knowledge and Value in Global Psychiatry.* Cambridge: Cambridge University Press.

Lavrendiadis, G., et al. 1987. "The Contribution to Rehabilitation of the 'Returning Patients' Clinic." Paper presented at the Tenth Panhellenic Conference on Psychiatry, Athens, 10–13 September (in Greek).

Legendre, Pierre. 2007. *Dominum Mundi, l'empire du management.* Paris: Mille et une nuits.

Lester, Rebecca J. 2004. "Commentary: Eating Disorders and the Problem of 'Culture' in Acculturation." *Culture, Medicine, and Psychiatry* 28: 607–15.

———. 2009. "Brokering Authenticity: Borderline Personality Disorder and the Ethics of Care in an American Eating Disorder Clinic." *Current Anthropology* 50 (3): 281–302.

Levendusky, P. G., et al. 1983. "Therapeutic Contract Program: Preliminary Report on a Behavioral Alternative to the Token Economy." *Behavioral Research Therapy* 21 (2): 137–42.

Lévi-Strauss, Claude. 1963. "The Sorcerer and His Magic." *Structural Anthropology*, trans. Claire Jacobson and Brooke Grundfest Schoepf, 167–85. New York: HarperCollins.

Lewis, Bradley. 2006. *Moving Beyond Prozac, DSM, and the New Psychiatry: The Birth of Postpsychiatry*. Ann Arbor: University of Michigan Press.

Livaditis, Miltos. 2003. *Culture and Psychiatry: Anthropological and Social Dimensions of Psychopathological Phenomena*. Athens: Papazisi (in Greek).

Livaditis, Miltos, and Theophanis Vorvolakos. N.d. "Gypsies and Prejudice." Unpublished manuscript, Department of Psychiatry, University of Thrace.

Lock, Margaret. 1989. "Commentary—Words of Fear, Words of Power: Nerves and the Awakening of Political Consciousness." *Medical Anthropology* 11 (1): 79–90.

———. 1990. "On Being Ethnic: The Politics of Identity Breaking and Making in Canada; or, *Nevra* on Sunday." *Culture, Medicine, and Psychiatry* 14 (2): 237–54.

———. 1993. "Cultivating the Body: Anthropology and Epistemologies of Bodily Practice and Knowledge." *Annual Review of Anthropology* 22: 133–55.

Luhrmann, Tanya. 2000. *Of Two Minds: The Growing Disorder in American Psychiatry*. New York: Alfred Knopf.

Lupton, Deborah. 1999. *Risk*. London: Routledge.

Madianos, Michalis. 1994. *Psychiatric Reform and Its Development: From Theory to Practice*. Athens: Greek Letters (in Greek).

Madianos, Michalis, and G. Christodoulou. 2007. "Reform of the Mental Healthcare System in Greece, 1984–2006." *International Psychiatry* 4 (1): 16–19.

Mahmood, Saba. 2005. *Politics of Piety: The Islamic Revival and the Feminist Subject*. Princeton: Princeton University Press.

Manos, Nikos. 1997. *Basic Elements of Clinical Psychiatry*. Rev. edn. Thessaloniki: University Studio Press (in Greek).

Manos, Nikos, et al. 1983. "The Value of the Psychosocial Approach in the Treatment of Long-Term Hospitalized Patients." *Hospital and Community Psychiatry* 34 (5): 456–58.

Mastoraki, Jenny. 1998. *Tales of the Deep*. 1983. *The Rehearsal of Misunderstanding: Three Collections by Contemporary Greek Women Poets*, bilingual edn., ed. and trans. Karen Van Dyck, 79–144. Hanover, N.H.: Wesleyan University Press.

Matsa, Katerina. 1989. "The Political Role of the Psychiatrist in Relation to the Legislature." *Proceedings of the Pan-Hellenic Conference on the Synchronization of Greek Legislation on Matters Concerning the Mentally Ill*, ed. Ministry of Health, Welfare, and Social Security (Greece), 65–70. Stavroupolis Psychiatric Hospital of Thessaloniki, 8–9 June 1989 (in Greek).

Maurer, Bill. 2005. *Mutual Life, Limited: Islamic Banking, Alternative Currencies, Lateral Reason*. Princeton: Princeton University Press.

Mavreas, V. G. 1987. "Greece: The Transition to Community Care." *International Journal of Social Psychiatry* 33 (2): 154–64.

McCormick, John. 1999. *Understanding the European Union: A Concise Introduction.* New York: St. Martin's Press.

McKinney, Kelly. 2007. "'Breaking the Conspiracy of Silence': Testimony, Traumatic Memory, and Psychotherapy with Survivors of Political Violence." *Ethos* 35 (3): 265–99.

Mezzich, Juan E., et al., eds. 1996. *Culture and Psychiatric Diagnosis: A DSM-IV Perspective.* Washington: American Psychiatric Press.

Mitrosili, Maria. 1996. "Interview: Psychiatric 'Reform' and Legislation on Mental Health" (in Greek).

Nietzsche, Friedrich. 1967. *On the Genealogy of Morals, and Ecce Homo.* 1887. Ed. and trans. W. Kaufmann. New York: Vintage.

———. 1968. *Twilight of the Idols; The Anti-Christ.* 1888. Ed. and trans. R. J. Hollingdale. Harmondsworth, U.K.: Penguin.

———. 1974. *The Gay Science — with a Prelude in Rhymes and an Appendix of Songs.* 1887. Ed. and trans. W. Kaufmann. New York: Vintage.

———. 1979a. "The Philosopher as Cultural Physician." 1873. *Philosophy and Truth: Selections from Nietzsche's Notebooks of the Early 1870's,* ed. and trans. Daniel Breazeale, 69–76. Atlantic Highlands, N.J.: Humanities Press International.

———. 1979b. "Philosophy in Hard Times." 1873. *Philosophy and Truth: Selections from Nietzsche's Notebooks of the Early 1870's,* ed. and trans. Daniel Breazeale, 101–23. Atlantic Highlands, N.J.: Humanities Press International.

Nuckolls, Charles W. 1992. "Toward a Cultural History of the Personality Disorders." *Social Science and Medicine* 35 (1): 37–47.

Obeyesekere, Gananath. 1990. *The Work of Culture: Symbolic Transformation in Psychoanalysis and Anthropology.* Chicago: University of Chicago Press.

Oran, Baskin. 2003. "The Story of Those Who Stayed: Lessons from Articles 1 and 2 of the 1923 Convention." *Crossing the Aegean: An Appraisal of the 1923 Compulsory Population Exchange between Greece and Turkey,* ed. Renée Hirschon, 97–116. New York: Berghahn Books.

Orphanoudakis, S. 1989. "Involuntary Confinement in the Psychiatric Hospital: Institutional Framework, Constitutional Approaches." *Proceedings of the Pan-Hellenic Conference on the Synchronization of Greek Legislation on Matters Concerning the Mentally Ill,* ed. Ministry of Health, Welfare, and Social Security (Greece), 103–6. Stavroupolis Psychiatric Hospital of Thessaloniki, 8–9 June 1989 (in Greek).

Pandian, Anand. 2008. "Devoted to Development: Moral Progress, Ethical Work, and Divine Favor in South India." *Anthropological Theory* 8 (2): 159–79.

———. 2009. *Crooked Stalks: Cultivating Virtue in South India.* Durham: Duke University Press.

Pandolfo, Stefania. 1997. *Impasse of the Angels: Scenes from a Moroccan Space of Memory.* Chicago: University of Chicago Press.

———. 2006. "'Bghit nghanni hnaya' (Je veux chanter ici): Parole et témoignage en marge d'une rencontre psychiatrique." *Arabica* 53 (2): 232–80.

———. 2007. "The Burning: Finitude and the Politico-Theological Imagination of Illegal Migration." *Anthropological Theory* 7 (3): 329–63.

———. 2008. "The Knot of the Soul: Postcolonial Conundrums, Madness, and the Imagination." *Postcolonial Disorders,* ed. Mary-Jo DelVecchio Good et al., 329–58. Berkeley: University of California Press.

Panourgiá, Neni. 1995. *Fragments of Death, Fables of Identity: An Athenian Anthropography.* Madison: University of Wisconsin Press.

———. 2004. "Colonizing the Ideal: Neoclassical Articulations and European Modernities." *Angelaki* 9 (2): 165–80.

———. 2008. "Fragments of Oedipus: Anthropology at the Edges of History." *Ethnographica Moralia: Experiments in Interpretive Anthropology,* ed. Panourgiá and George E. Marcus, 97–112. New York: Fordham University Press.

———. 2009. *Dangerous Citizens: The Greek Left and the Terror of the State.* New York: Fordham University Press.

Papadimas, L. 1999. "Report to the President of the Commission for the Prevention of Torture and Inhuman or Degrading Treatment or Punishment." Ref. No Γ.Υ./7359 L (25/10/1999), including P. Yiannoulatos, "Response to the Commission's Report," Ref. No. Α3α01κ1750 (22/10/1999). Athens: Ministry of Health and Welfare of the Hellenic Republic.

Papagiorgiou, Dimitris. 1989. "Prosecutorial Jurisdiction in the Involuntary Committal of the 'Dangerous Mentally Ill.'" *Proceedings of the Pan-Hellenic Conference on the Synchronization of Greek Legislation on Matters Concerning the Mentally Ill,* ed. Ministry of Health, Welfare, and Social Security (Greece), 79–90. Stavroupolis Psychiatric Hospital of Thessaloniki, 8–9 June 1989 (in Greek).

Papailias, Penelope. 2005. *Genres of Recollection: Archival Poetics and Modern Greece.* New York: Palgrave Macmillan.

Papasteriou, Dimitris. 1989. "Mental Deficiency in Judicial Practice." *Proceedings of the Pan-Hellenic Conference on the Synchronization of Greek Legislation on Matters Concerning the Mentally Ill,* ed. Ministry of Health, Welfare, and Social Security (Greece), 55–62. Stavroupolis Psychiatric Hospital of Thessaloniki, 8–9 June 1989 (in Greek).

Paraschos, A. I. 1983. "De-Centralized Hospital Care of Chronic Psychotics in Northern Greece: Proposal for Planning in the Framework of the National Health System." *Proceedings of the Tenth Pan-Hellenic Conference of Neurology and Psychiatry, Thessaloniki,* vol. 1, 417–27 (in Greek).

———. 1985. "Present Problems of Continuity of Psychiatric Care in Greece." Internal report, Department of Psychiatry, Aristotle University of Thessaloniki, and B' University Clinic, Stravoupolis Psychiatric Hospital.

———. 1986. "Reactive Psychopathology in the Military Setting." *Hellenic Armed Forces Medical Review* 20 (3–4): 339–52 (in Greek).

Paraschos, A. I., et al. 1980. "Pharmacotherapy of Chronic Schizophrenia: A Fifteen-Year Retrospective Study in a State Mental Hospital." Department of Psychiatry and Neurology, Aristotle University, Thessaloniki (Greece). [Reproduced from source in the archive of the B' University Clinic, Stravoupolis Psychiatric Hospital, 381–88.]

Péristiany, J. G., ed. 1966. *Honour and Shame: The Values of Mediterranean Society*. Chicago: University of Chicago Press.

Perrin, Anna, and Craig Newnes. 2002. "Professional Identity and the Complexity of Therapeutic Relationships." *Clinical Psychology* 15: 18–22.

Petryna, Adriana, Andrew Lakoff, and Arthur Kleinman, eds. 2006. *Global Pharmaceuticals: Ethics, Markets, Practices*. Durham: Duke University Press.

Ploumpidis, Dimitris N. 1995. *History of Psychiatry in Greece: Institutions, Foundations, and Social Context, 1850–1920*. Athens: Exantas (in Greek).

Povinelli, Elizabeth A. 2002. *The Cunning of Recognition: Indigenous Alterities and the Making of Australian Multiculturalism*. Durham: Duke University Press.

Rabinow, Paul. 1983. "Humanism as Nihilism: The Bracketing of Truth and Seriousness in American Cultural Anthropology." *Social Science as Moral Inquiry*, ed. Norma Haan et al., 52–75. New York: Columbia University Press.

———. 1988. "Beyond Ethnography: Anthropology as Nominalism." *Cultural Anthropology* 3 (4): 355–64.

———. 1996. *Essays on the Anthropology of Reason*. Princeton: Princeton University Press.

———. 1997. Introduction to *Ethics, Subjectivity and Truth*, ed. Rabinow, xi–xlv. Vol. 1 of *The Essential Works of Foucault (1954–1984)*. New York: New Press.

———. 2001. "The Problem of Anthropology." David Schneider Lecture presented at the Bi-annual Meeting of the Society for Cultural Anthropology, Montreal, April.

———. 2003. *Anthropos Today: Reflections on Modern Equipment*. Princeton: Princeton University Press.

Rhodes, Lorna A. 2004. *Total Confinement: Madness and Reason in the Maximum Security Prison*. Berkeley: University of California Press.

Rohde, Erwin. 1966. *Psyche: The Cult of Souls and Belief in Immortality among the Greeks*, Vol. 2. Trans. W. B. Hills. New York: Harper and Row.

Rose, Nikolas. 1989. *Governing the Soul: The Shaping of the Private Self*. London: Free Association Books.

———. 1998. *Inventing Our Selves: Psychology, Power, and Personhood*. Cambridge: Cambridge University Press.

———. 1999. *Powers of Freedom: Reframing Political Thought*. Cambridge: Cambridge University Press.

Rutherford, M. J., J. S. Cacciola, and A. I. Alterman. 1999. "Antisocial Personality

Disorder and Psychopathy in Cocaine-Dependent Women." *American Journal of Psychiatry* 156 (6): 849–56.

Sakellaropoulos, Panayiotis, ed. 1995. *Elements of Social Psychiatry and Its Implementation in Greece.* 2 vols. Athens: Papazisi (in Greek).

Santner, Eric L. 1996. *My Own Private Germany: Daniel Paul Schreber's Secret History of Modernity.* Princeton: Princeton University Press.

Sarınay, Yusuf, Hamit Pehlivanlı, and Abdullah Saydam. 2000. *The Pontus Issue and the Policy of Greece: Articles.* Ed. Berna Türkdoğan. Trans. Nihal Cihan and Vildan Şahin. Ankara: Attatürk Research Center.

Saris, A. Jamie. 2008. "Institutional Persons and Personal Institutions: The Asylum and Marginality in Rural Ireland." *Postcolonial Disorders,* ed. Mary-Jo DelVecchio Good et al., 309–28. Berkeley: University of California Press.

Scheper-Hughes, Nancy. 1992. *Death Without Weeping: The Violence of Everyday Life in Brazil.* Berkeley: University of California Press.

———. 2005. "The Last Commodity: Post-Human Ethics and the Global Traffic in 'Fresh' Organs." *Global Assemblages: Technology, Politics, and Ethics as Anthropological Problems,* ed. Aihwa Ong and Stephen J. Collier, 145–67. Malden, Mass.: Blackwell.

Scheper-Hughes, Nancy, and Anne M. Lovell, eds. 1987. *Psychiatry Inside Out: Selected Writings of Franco Basaglia.* Trans. Lovell and Teresa Shtob. New York: Columbia University Press.

Scott, Joan. 2005. "Symptomatic Politics: The Banning of Islamic Head Scarves in French Public Schools." *French Politics, Culture and Society* 23 (3): 106–27.

Sedgwick, Eve Kosofsky. 1992. "Epidemics of the Will." *Incorporations,* ed. Jonathan Crary and Sanford Kwinter, 582–95. New York: Zone.

Seremetakis, C. Nadia. 1991. *The Last Word: Women, Death, and Divination in Inner Mani.* Chicago: University of Chicago Press.

———. 1993. "Durations of Pain: The Antiphony of Death and Women's Power in Southern Greece." *Ritual, Power, and the Body: Historical Perspectives on the Representation of Greek Women,* ed. Seremetakis, 119–49. New York: Pella.

Simon, Bennett. 1980. *Mind and Madness in Ancient Greece: The Classical Roots of Modern Psychiatry.* Ithaca: Cornell University Press.

Sinapi, Michèle. 2008. "Displacements of the 'Shadow Line.'" *Social Science Information* 47 (4): 529–39.

Smay, Diana. 2001. "The Disease of Ritual: Obsessive Compulsive Disorder as an Outgrowth of Normal Behavior." Paper presented at the MARIAL Center Colloquium, Emory University, Atlanta, 7 February.

Spivak, Gayatri Chakravorty. 1994. "Responsibility." *boundary 2* 21 (3): 19–64.

———. 1999. *A Critique of Postcolonial Reason: Toward a History of the Vanishing Present.* Cambridge: Harvard University Press.

Stacey, Jackie. 1997. *Teratologies: A Cultural Study of Cancer.* London: Routledge.

Stefanis, K., and Michalis Madianos. 1980. "Findings and Perspectives on the

Regional Development of Mental Health Services." Ιατρική 38: 241–49. (in Greek).

Stylianidis, Stelios, and V. Papadakos. 2000. "La psychiatrie grecque: Pratiques, expériences et perspectives." L'information psychiatrique 3: 347–55.

Stylianidis, Stelios, and Dimitris Ploumpidis. 1989. "Les reflets de la loi du 30 juin 1838: L'expérience hellénique et l'évolution contemporaine." L'évolution psychiatrique 54 (3): 643–49.

Sullivan, Harry Stack. 1966. Conceptions of Modern Psychiatry. 1947. New York: W. W. Norton.

Szasz, Thomas S. 1974. The Myth of Mental Illness: Foundations of a Theory of Personal Conduct. 1961. Rev edn. New York: Harper and Row.

———. 1979. "The Lying Truths of Psychiatry." Journal of Libertarian Studies 3 (2): 121–39.

Taussig, Michael. 1999. Defacement: Public Secrecy and the Labor of the Negative. Stanford: Stanford University Press.

Ticktin, Miriam. 2005. "Policing and Humanitarianism in France: Immigration and the Turn to Law as State of Exception." Interventions 7 (3): 347–68.

Tountas, Y., P. Karnaki, and E. Pavi. 2002. "Reforming the Reform: The Greek National Health System in Transition." Health Policy 62 (1): 15–29.

Tziaferi, Maria. 1989. "The Institution of Guardianship of the Legally Incapacitated Mentally Ill: Current Legislation, Problems, and Suggested Solutions." Proceedings of the Pan-Hellenic Conference on the Synchronization of Greek Legislation on Matters Concerning the Mentally Ill, ed. Ministry of Health, Welfare, and Social Security (Greece), 62–65. Stavroupolis Psychiatric Hospital of Thessaloniki, 8–9 June 1989 (in Greek).

Valverde, Mariana. 1998. Diseases of the Will: Alcohol and the Dilemmas of Freedom. Cambridge: Cambridge University Press.

Velpry, Livia. 2008. "The Patient's View: Issues of Theory and Practice." Culture, Medicine, and Psychiatry 32 (2): 238–58.

Vergeti, Maria. 1991. "Pontic Greeks from Asia Minor and the Soviet Union: Problems of Integration in Modern Greece." Journal of Refugee Studies 4 (4): 382–94.

Voutira, Eftihia. 1991. "Pontic Greeks Today: Migrants or Refugees?" Journal of Refugee Studies 4 (4): 400–420.

———. 2003. "When Greeks Meet Other Greeks: Settlement Policy Issues in the Contemporary Greek Context." Crossing the Aegean: An Appraisal of the 1923 Compulsory Population Exchange between Greece and Turkey, ed. Renée Hirschon, 145–59. New York: Berghahn Books.

———. 2006. "Post-Soviet Diaspora Politics: The Case of the Soviet Greeks." Journal of Modern Greek Studies 24: 379–414.

———. 2007. "Refugees, Returnees, and Migrants: The Meaning of 'Home' in post-Soviet Russia." *Between Past and Present: Ethnographies of the Post-Soviet World*, ed. Voutira and R. Van Booschoten, 323–43. Athens: Kritiki (in Greek).

Winnicott, D. W. 1971. *Playing and Reality*. London: Tavistock.

———. 1992. *Psycho-Analytic Explorations*. 1989. Ed. Clare Winnicott, Ray Shepherd, and Madeleine Davis. Cambridge: Harvard University Press.

World Health Organization. 2001. "Greece." *Mental Health in Europe: Country Reports from the WHO European Network on Mental Health*, 33–35. Copenhagen: Regional Office for Europe, Health Documentation Services.

Xanthopoulou-Kyriakou, Artemis. 1991. "The Diaspora of the Greeks of the Pontos: Historical Background." *Journal of Refugee Studies* 4 (4): 357–63.

Young, Allan. 1995. *The Harmony of Illusions: Inventing Post-Traumatic Stress Disorder*. Princeton: Princeton University Press.

DOCUMENTS FROM THE EUROPEAN COMMISSION CENTRAL LIBRARY, BRUSSELS

Official Journal of the European Commission

(1) Council Regulation (EEC) No 815/84 on Exceptional Financial Support in Favour of Greece in the Social Field, 26 March 1984. *Official Journal* No L 88/1–3.

(2) Proposal for a Council Regulation (EEC) Amending Regulation (EEC) No 815/84 on Exceptional Financial Support in Favour of Greece in the Social Field, 27 July 1988. *Official Journal* No C 209/6–7.

(3) Economic and Social Committee Opinion on the Proposal for Council Regulation (EEC) No 815/84 on Exceptional Financial Support in Favour of Greece in the Social Field, 23 November 1988. *Official Journal* No C 23/1.

(4) Council Regulation (EEC) No 4130/88 Amending Regulation (EEC) No 815/84 on Exceptional Financial Support in Favour of Greece in the Social Field, 16 December 1988. *Official Journal* No L 362/1–2.

(5) Court of Auditors Special Report No 5/90 on the Implementation of Council Regulation (EEC) 815/84 on Exceptional Financial Support in Favour of Greece in the Social Field, Together with the Replies of the Commission, 31 December 1990. *Official Journal* No C 331/1–13.

(6) Written Question E-981/93 by Alexandros Alvanos (GUE) to the Commission, on the Subject: Delay in Carrying out Measures under Regulation (EEC) No 815/84, 29 April 1993. *Official Journal* No C 332/3–4. Answer Given by Mr. Flynn on Behalf of the Commission, 28 October 1993. *Official Journal* No C 332/3–4.

(1) Proposal for a Council Regulation (EEC), Amending Regulation (EEC) No 815/84 on Exceptional Financial Support in Favour of Greece in the Social Field, 22 July 1988. COM (88) 412 final.

(2) Final Report on the Implementation of Council Regulation (EEC) 815/84 on Exceptional Financial Support in Favour of Greece in the Social Field, 15 December 1995. COM (95) 668 final.

INDEX

✳

addiction: Alexandroupolis substance abuse centers, 287 n. 6; in Gypsy culture, 18, 150–51; to sedatives, 62, 130, 140, 253; as a social and subjective identity, 296 n. 73

Agtzidis, Vlasis, 285 n. 85

alcoholism, 268 n. 29; in antisocial personality types, 151; in Gypsy culture, 145–46

Alexandroupolis: amphitheater, 184–85; child psychiatry institute, 42, 145–46, 221; Community Mental Health Center, 258 n. 7; Gypsy settlements, 144, 147; refugee settlements, 167; substance abuse centers, 287 n. 6

Alexandroupolis General Regional University Hospital: group therapy, 227–29; inpatient psychiatric services, 6, 41–42; new hospital construction, 69, 113–14; outpatient clinic, 127, 150; stigmatization at, 278–79 n. 13; training and seminars, 43–45

Aloperidin (US Haldol), 22, 82, 89, 141, 249

Alterman, A. I., 281 n. 54, 281 n. 57

Anafranil, 141, 189, 286 n. 1, 295 n. 68

anthropology: bracketing truth in, 59, 272 n. 25; and diagnostic techniques, 64–65; of ethics, 12, 261 n. 23; figures of *anthropos*, 11, 259 n. 12; Greek dialogue between psychiatry and, 17, 122, 139; Greek ethnography and, 120–21; linguistic ideology and, 60; medical anthropology, 59, 68, 133–34; Mediterraneanist anthropology, 118–19, 122, 126

antidepressants, 44, 141; treatment in patient case studies, 2, 44, 62, 105, 136, 189

antipsychiatry movement, 30, 60, 272 n. 31

antipsychotics, 141, 249, 286 n. 3; side effects, 82, 115

antisocial personality disorder: among Gypsy outpatients, 18, 117, 151–53, 157–59, 281–82 n. 57; and criminality, 276 n. 80; DSM classification, 86–87, 151, 281 n. 54, 281 n. 57; symptoms or traits of, 18, 151; theories, 152

anxiety disorder: depressive anxiety, 130, 133; "normal" levels of anxiety, 295 n. 69; obsessive-compulsive disorder as a type of, 235, 276 n. 78; outpatient population in Greece with, 189–90; patient case studies, 81, 98, 192, 253; theories, 187–89

child psychiatry, 42, 221; Gypsy children as patients, 145–46

citizenship: "active citizenship" definition, 284 n. 83; Greek citizens and ties to Turkey, 164; of Gypsies in Thrace, 257 n. 3; patient responsibility and, 10, 14, 158; state assistance for, 167

clinical disorders: compared to personality disorders, 88, 157, 276 n. 75, 276 n. 85; DSM classification of, 86; suffering severity of, 90–92

clinical encounters: bipolar case studies, 1, 3, 81–82, 176, 189; borderline personality disorder case study, 217; delusional patient case studies, 46–50, 167–82; depression case studies, 135–37, 191–92; hysteria case study, 128–30; with Muslim psychiatric patients, 123–25, 164; obsessive-compulsive disorder (OCD) case study, 187, 189, 191–92, 232–38, 295 n. 66; personality disorder case study, 221–24; psychotic depression case studies, 62, 99–104, 141–49, 154–55; reactive depression case study, 104–9; schizophrenia case studies, 114–16, 164–65; schizophrenic catatonia case study, 160, 247–50; suicide case studies, 1–2, 80, 153–55, 207, 225; voluntary committal case study, 205–10

clinical knowledge, 13, 40, 59–60, 71

cognitive-behavioral therapy, 7, 43, 188–89, 236

cognitive disorder, 116, 249

cognitive symptoms, 135, 138

Cohen, Lawrence, 68, 219–20, 295 n. 67

Cohen, Stan, 287 n. 14

communication: between patient and therapist, 16–17; dishonest, 73–74, 110, 274–75 n. 64; semantico-referential language and pragmatic, 60–64; significance of meaning in, 67–68; and speech, 65–67

community: Gypsy community, 150–53, 257 n. 3; Muslim population, 5, 123, 161–62, 182, 257 n. 3–4; Pontian community, 165–67, 173–74, 181–82, 284 n. 79; responsibility for psychiatric patients, 14, 17, 24; stigmatization of mental illness in, 5, 17, 123

community-based care: in Brazilian public schools, 282 n. 65; community-based psychiatry, 49, 59, 79; growth in Greece, 35, 39–40; language and diagnosis in, 59, 272 n. 30; patient lying and deception in, 80, 111; patient responsibility in, 12, 14, 19, 121, 137; problem of patient danger and, 200; Sakellaropoulos's textbook on, 26; in Thrace, 126–28, 247

compulsory order, 115, 187, 206, 210, 213

compulsory treatment, 194–95, 202–3, 212

conversion disorder, 134–35, 137–38, 149; symptoms, 130, 132, 138–39

cooperation (συνεργασία), 7, 127, 214, 216, 231–32

cooperatives, agricultural, 35, 42, 44–46, 269 n. 36; patient experiences at, 147, 153, 155, 166, 168

Corin, Ellen, 19, 266 n. 37, 280 n. 44

Crapanzano, Vincent, 65, 67, 271 n. 5, 273 n. 34, 284 n. 81; on linguistic ideology, 60–61; on realism in language in Moroccan culture, 278 n. 5

"crazy" (τρελός/-ή), term usage, 172–73, 237

cross-cultural studies: approaches to eating disorders, 283 n. 70; cultural differences and conflicts, 132–34,

cross-cultural studies (*continued*)
152; therapeutic encounters, 18,
131–32
"cultural pathology," 4, 5, 13, 18, 158;
of Gypsy patients, 122, 139, 152–53,
158
cultural relativism, 120, 146, 152–53,
158, 272 n. 25
culture: "cultural intimacy," 119; "culture of dependency," 287–89 n. 14;
and deception, 120–21; ethnographic studies of, 121–22; Greek
traditional culture, 18, 124, 126,
130, 232; Gypsy, 104, 120–21, 144–
45, 150; Moroccan, 278 n. 5; Muslim, 124–25, 144–45, 280–81 n. 48;
Nietzsche on, 240–41; in postcolonial Australia, 264 n. 33; somatic,
133–34; stereotypes, 119, 159; "subjective culture," 131; traditional culture in Thrace, 137–39, 237
Culture and Psychiatry (Livaditis), 131,
150
culture-bound syndromes, 132–33, 280
n. 30

Danforth, Loring, 280 n. 45
danger: legal concept of, 194–95, 216;
patient "danger to him/herself or
others," 199–205, 210, 234, 287–88
n. 14, 291 n. 31
deception: in clinical encounters,
67, 75–76, 109–10; cultures of, 71,
120–21; objective truth and self-
deception, 55, 274 n. 64; in patient-
therapist relations, 4, 17, 53, 73, 76,
80, 111
deinstitutionalization, 24, 211, 237;
in Brazil, 280 n. 46; in Greece and
Europe, 26, 38
Deleuze, Gilles, 66, 240, 287 n. 14; on
symptomatological method, 241–
42, 298 nn. 13–14
delusion: bizarre and nonbizarre types,

79, 83; categories, 176–77; delusional speech, 79–80, 96, 275 n. 70;
DSM definition, 78–79; patient case
studies, 46–50, 82, 101–4, 167–82
Demetriou, Olga, 278 n. 7
dependency: and patient feelings of
shame and guilt, 192, 236–37; on
state care, 40, 122, 158–59, 287–89
n. 14; therapeutic dynamics of, 5,
127–28
depression, 134–35, 153; DSM classification, 86–87; patient case
studies, 135–37, 191–92; psychotic
depression patient case studies, 62,
99–104, 141–49, 154–55; reactive depression patient case study, 104–9.
See also antidepressants
Derrida, Jacques, 266 n. 38
detention center, for immigrants, 160,
165, 248–50; medical care for inmates, 251–55
d'Halluin, Estelle, 258 n. 5
diagnosis: bipolar disorder, 82; in
compulsory treatment, 194–95, 198,
203; cultural, 131–32, 153, 158; definition of, 53–54; "diagnostic synthesis," 31; discrepancies in treatment, 7; and feigning symptoms
for disability certification, 52–53,
76, 157; gender parameters in, 281
n. 57; as genealogical method,
242–45; as a generative technique,
298 n. 7; interpretation in, 61,
248–49; language and communication importance in, 59–61, 64–68,
272 n. 30; madness and moralism,
240–42, 266 n. 38; metrics, 281
n. 57; personality disorders, 86–87,
91, 276 n. 75, 276 n. 85, 281 n. 54;
practice and moral judgment, 56,
203–4, 273 n. 41; practice and theoretical knowledge division, 68–69;
and problem of patient lying, 17,

72–74, 78–80, 104; psychodynamic procedure and statistical, 75–76; psychopathic terminology, 151–52; somatoform symptoms, 133–34; and suspicions of deception, 110–11; techniques and procedure, 59–60, 79, 97; in transcultural psychiatry, 17–18, 137; as a truth game, 55–59, 74; uncertainty in, 76, 176

Diagnostic and Statistical Manual of Mental Disorders. See DSM

Digenis Akritas, 178

disability certifications: feigning symptoms for, 53–54, 76, 107, 158; issued to Gypsy population, 145, 150, 156; psychiatrists' ambivalence, 157; and subsidies, 16, 22, 25, 45, 167, 209

dispositif (apparatus), 31–33, 268 n. 19

Dreyfus, Hubert, 273 n. 41

DSM (Diagnostic and Statistical Manual of Mental Disorders), 43, 68; bipolar disorder, 82; culture-bound syndromes, 132; delusion, 78–79; division between psychosis and neurosis, 95, 104; factitious disorder, 88; mental illness axes, 86; obsessive-compulsive disorder (OCD), 235; paranoid schizophrenia, 165; personality disorders, 87–88, 90, 281 n. 54, 281 n. 57; psychopathic diagnostic term, 151; statistical diagnosis method, 76

du Boulay, Juliet, 277 n. 4

Dunk, Pamela, 134

Durkheim, Émile, 13

Egypt, piety practices, 259 n. 16, 260 n. 22

ΕΙΥΑΑΠΟΕ (National Institute for the Reception and Resettlement of Repatriated Ancestral Greeks), 167

electroshock treatment, 27, 192, 234

ethics: bioethics, 219–20, 293 n. 53;

bracketing truth in, 59; in contemporary Morocco, 262–64 n. 28; "ethical alibis," 159; ethical concept of subjectivity, 12, 14–15, 20, 259 n. 15; "ethical publicity," 219; ethical reform, 287–89 n. 14; Foucauldian genealogy of, 12; humanitarian ethics, 58, 238; Kantian ethics, 12, 260 n. 22; Lacanian psychoanalytic ethics, 73, 103, 261 n. 26, 274 nn. 61–62; mad ethics, 265 n. 35; meta-ethics, 264 n. 33; moralism and, 16, 229, 231; patient-centered, 293 n. 53; on piety practice in Egypt, 260 n. 22; of responsibility, 13–15, 137–38, 195; on self, 5, 12, 14, 261–62 n. 26

European Currency Unit (ECU), 35–36, 269 n. 36

European Economic Community (EEC), 30, 267 n. 16, 269 n. 36; Greek psychiatric reform projects, 28, 34–36, 42–43

European Union (EU), 4, 30, 37–39, 258 n. 9, 267 n. 16

Ewing, Katherine Pratt, 65

factitious disorder, 88

family, 96, 201, 211, 297 n. 74; hierarchal ties, 132; as an institution in rural Greek society, 127, 237; shame and stigma felt by, 5, 45, 49

Fanon, Frantz, 272 n. 22

Farquhar, Judith, 242 n. 15

Fassin, Didier, 258 n. 5, 282 n. 61

Faubion, James D., 258 n. 10, 260 n. 22

Fotiadis, Haritonas, 198

Foucault, Michel: on antipsychiatry, 272–73 n. 31; on genealogy, 12; on liberalism and power, 193, 212, 273 n. 45; on madness and the modern age, 30, 242–44, 266 n. 38; on moralizing sadism, 192; on "paradox of subjectivation," 260–61 n. 22, 261

Roma, 144, 257 n. 3; suicide rate, 140–41; term usage, 257 n. 3; unemployment, 145, 281 n. 50

hallucinations, 78–79; patient experiences of, 81–82, 115, 143, 176, 208
Handelman, Don, 294 n. 60
Hellenism, 11; neo-Hellenism, 258 n. 10
Herzfeld, Michael, 119, 121–22, 159
Hirschon, Renée, 278 n. 12, 283 n. 76
Holmes, Brooke, 259 n. 15, 260 n. 18
hospitals and health centers: Alexandroupolis Community Mental Health Center, 258 n. 7; Athens psychiatric hospitals and clinics, 27, 35; Komotini General Hospital, 7, 9, 71, 139–40, 252–54; mobile (hospital) units, 6, 41–42, 104, 125, 206; Soufli health center, 22–24; Thessaloniki psychiatric hospital, 35, 42, 45, 189–92, 206, 287 n. 6; Xanthi General Hospital, 251. See also Alexandroupolis General Regional University Hospital; Association for Social Psychiatry and Mental Health
Hughes, Charles C., 280 n. 30
humanitarian psychiatry, 13, 201, 238
human rights, 4, 12, 15, 17, 194; legislation on mental illness, 30, 196–97, 204, 218, 220–21
hypersexuality, 82, 86
hypocrisy: of Greek culture, 118–20, 278 n. 5; in patient-therapist interactions, 3, 22
hysteria: cultural decline in, 134, 280 n. 42; as a form of indirect communication, 64; patient case study, 128–30; and patient dishonesty, 274–75 n. 64; symptoms of, 17, 81, 138, 141, 151, 153

Iakovidis, A., 279 nn. 14–15
Ierodiakonou, Charalambos, 41–42, 126–27, 279 n. 15

ΙΚΑ (Ίδρυμα Κοινωνικών Ασφαλίσεων, Social Insurance Institute), 39, 42, 156, 271 n. 70, 287 n. 6
illusio, 55, 57, 71, 271 n. 12, 274 n. 64
immigrants, 5, 134, 247, 258 n. 5; detention center for illegal, 160, 165, 248–50; Pontian, 150, 161–62, 165–67, 182, 283 n. 77, 284 nn. 78–79
inpatient treatment, 28–29, 35, 41
involuntary committal (ακούσια νοσηλία): cases in Thrace, 128; legislation for, 196–203, 210–13, 290 n. 26, 291 nn. 30–31; and psychiatric reform, 200–202
Islam, 145, 161, 247; ethical practices, 260 n. 22; Islamic financial contracts, 293 n. 59; medieval Islamic scholars, 259 n. 16

Kantian ethics, 12, 260 n. 22
Karpozilos, Apostolos, 283 n. 75
Kleinman, Arthur, 68, 132–33, 280 n. 44
Kokkinos, Dimitris, 285 nn. 85–86
Komotini: community outreach program, 123; General Hospital, 7, 9, 71, 139–40, 252–54; Gypsy neighborhood, 144; mobile (hospital) units, 42, 104; suicide rate, 140

Lacan, Jacques, 73, 103, 261 n. 26, 274 nn. 61–62
Laing, R. D., 58
Lakoff, Andrew, 260 n. 19, 265 n. 34, 271 n. 74
language: barriers with patients, 117, 125, 160, 253–54; and belief, 273 n. 35; diagnosis and significance of, 59–61, 64–68, 272 n. 30; Greek dialects, 161; Nietzsche on illness and, 244; and realism in Moroccan culture, 278 n. 5; semantico-referential language, 60–61, 64

pathology (*continued*)
psychiatry and, 13, 238; of minority patients, 4, 152–53; in personality disorders, 88, 91; psychopathology, 202, 204; sexuality as, 80; shift in clinical profile of, 19
patients: average admission length of treatment, 38, 270 n. 53; counter-moralism practiced by, 16, 66, 138, 231; danger to him/herself or society, 199–205, 210, 234, 287–88 n. 14, 291 n. 31; dehumanization of, 44; dramatization, 150, 152, 154; feigning symptoms of illness, 88, 158; freedom, 18, 27, 194–95, 204, 212, 291 n. 30; Gypsy patients, 139–50, 152–59; integration programs, 42, 167; minority patients, 4, 17–18, 117, 122, 162, 165; nonmedical needs of, 44–45; Pontian patients, 122, 135–38, 160; poverty, 156, 220; residences and group homes, 24, 42, 45, 147, 237, 270 n. 51; rights, 14, 123, 126, 138, 193, 260 n. 22; self-care, 15, 17, 137; unconscious motives, 73–74, 88, 95, 103–4, 109–11
Persians, The (Aeschylus), 183–85
personality disorders: among Gypsy outpatients, 18, 117, 150–59, 281–82 n. 57; compared to clinical disorders, 88, 157, 276 n. 75, 276 n. 85; as a "cultural pathology," 139; difficulty of patients with, 88, 91–92; DSM description, 87–88, 90, 281 n. 54, 281 n. 57; lying as symptomatic of, 86–87, 91; obsessive-compulsive personality disorder, 276 n. 78, 295 n. 69; patient case study, 221–24. *See also* antisocial personality disorder; borderline personality disorder
pharmaceutical treatment, 48, 96, 135, 236, 280 n. 46; humanization of, 13,

44, 271 n. 74; and psychoanalytic practice, 30, 236, 260 n. 19; research, 43, 59, 68
Plato, 11, 259 n. 15, 266 n. 39
Ploumpidis, Dimitris, 201–2, 204
Pomaks: population in Thrace, 5, 161, 257–58 n. 4, 278 n. 7; term usage, 279 n. 24
Pontii (Πόντιοι): community, 5, 173, 178, 181–82; immigrants, 150, 161–62, 165–67, 283 n. 77, 284 nn. 78–79; language, 160–61; Neo Ipsos settlement, 170; psychiatric patients, 122, 135–38
post-traumatic stress disorder (PTSD), 135–36, 247, 249, 292 n. 47
Povinelli, Elizabeth, 264 n. 33
Psychargos, 38, 290 n. 26
psyche (ψυχή): anthropologists of, 259 n. 12; ethical subjectivity of, 12, 65, 137, 287–90 n. 14; Homeric and Platonic usage, 11, 266 n. 39; para-noiacs as theorists of, 181; psychiatric model of human, 11–12; social science of, 15; soul translation, 11, 20, 259 n. 13
psychiatric knowledge, 11, 19, 69, 204; diagnosis as procedure for attaining, 59; psychiatric reform and, 40
psychiatric nosology, 133–34, 198, 211, 265 n. 34
psychiatric reform: compulsory treatment, 193–95; decentralization, 28; deinstitutionalization, 26, 38; EEC memoranda on Greek psychiatry, 34–35; EEC reform projects and reports 35–38; establishment of National Health System, 33–34; events leading up to, 27–30; funding, 35–36, 269 n. 36, 269 n. 40; global transformation, 30–33; humanitarian politics, 4, 12, 15, 17, 19, 43, 194; legislation on men-

ELIZABETH ANNE DAVIS

is an assistant professor in the Department

of Anthropology, in association with

Hellenic Studies, at Princeton University.

This is her first book.

*Library of Congress Cataloging-in-
Publication Data*

Davis, Elizabeth Anne, 1974–
Bad souls : madness and responsibility in
modern Greece / Elizabeth Anne Davis.
p. cm.
Includes bibliographical references
and index.
ISBN 978-0-8223-5093-4 (cloth : alk. paper)
ISBN 978-0-8223-5106-1 (pbk. : alk. paper)
1. Mentally ill—Treatment—Greece—Thrace,
Western. 2. Mental health policy—Greece—
Thrace, Western. 3. Psychiatry—Greece—
Thrace, Western—History. I. Title.
RA790.7.G8D38 2012
362.196′89009381—dc23
2011027453